Biomedicine in the Twentieth Century: Practices, Policies, and Politics

Biomedical and Health Research

Volume 72

Recently published in this series:

Vol. 71. J.-F. Stoltz (Ed.), Cardiovascular Biology: Endothelial Cell in Health and Hypertension – Volume 1

Vol. 70. J. Buckwalter, M. Lotz and J.-F. Stoltz (Eds.), Osteoarthritis, Inflammation and Degradation: A Continuum

Vol. 69. O.K. Baskurt, M.R. Hardeman, M.W. Rampling and H.J. Meiselman (Eds.), Handbook of Hemorheology and Hemodynamics

Vol. 68. J.-F. Stoltz (Ed.), Mechanobiology: Cartilage and Chondrocyte – Volume 4

Vol. 67. R.J. Schwartzman, Differential Diagnosis in Neurology

Vol. 66. H. Strasser (Ed.), Traditional Rating of Noise Versus Physiological Costs of Sound Exposures to the Hearing

Vol. 65. T. Silverstone, Eating Disorders and Obesity: How Drugs Can Help

Vol. 64. S. Eberhardt, C. Stoklossa and J.-M. Graf von der Schulenberg (Eds.), EUROMET 2004: The Influence of Economic Evaluation Studies on Health Care Decision-Making – A European Survey

Vol. 63. M. Parveen and S. Kumar (Eds.), Recent Trends in the Acetylcholinesterase System

Vol. 62. I.G. Farreras, C. Hannaway and V.A. Harden (Eds.), Mind, Brain, Body, and Behavior – Foundations of Neuroscience and Behavioral Research at the National Institutes of Health

Vol. 61. J.-F. Stoltz (Ed.), Mechanobiology: Cartilage and Chondrocyte – Volume 3

Vol. 60. J.-M. Graf von der Schulenburg and M. Blanke (Eds.), Rationing of Medical Services in Europe: An Empirical Study – A European Survey

Vol. 59. M. Wolman and R. Manor, Doctors' Errors and Mistakes of Medicine: Must Health Care Deteriorate?

Vol. 58. S. Holm and M. Jonas (Eds.), Engaging the World: The Use of Empirical Research in Bioethics and the Regulation of Biotechnology

Vol. 57. A. Nosikov and C. Gudex (Eds.), EUROHIS: Developing Common Instruments for Health Surveys

Vol. 56. P. Chauvin and the Europromed Working Group (Eds.), Prevention and Health Promotion for the Excluded and the Destitute in Europe

Vol. 55. J. Matsoukas and T. Mavromoustakos (Eds.), Drug Discovery and Design: Medical Aspects

Vol. 54. I.M. Shapiro, B.D. Boyan and H.C. Anderson (Eds.), The Growth Plate

Vol. 53. C. Huttin (Ed.), Patient Charges and Decision Making Behaviours of Consumers and Physicians

Vol. 52. J.-F. Stoltz (Ed.), Mechanobiology: Cartilage and Chondrocyte, Vol. 2

Vol. 51. G. Lebeer (Ed.), Ethical Function in Hospital Ethics Committees

Vol. 50. R. Busse, M. Wismar and P.C. Berman (Eds.), The European Union and Health Services

Vol. 49. T. Reilly (Ed.), Musculoskeletal Disorders in Health-Related Occupations

Vol. 48. H. ten Have and R. Janssens (Eds.), Palliative Care in Europe – Concepts and Policies

Vol. 47. H. Aldskogius and J. Fraher (Eds.), Glial Interfaces in the Nervous System – Role in Repair and Plasticity

ISSN 0929-6743

Biomedicine in the Twentieth Century: Practices, Policies, and Politics

Caroline Hannaway   EDITOR

2008

IOS
Press
Amsterdam • Berlin • Oxford • Tokyo • Washington, D.C.

ISBN 978-1-58603-832-8
Library of Congress Control Number: 2008920118

Publisher
IOS Press
Nieuwe Hemweg 6B
1013 BG Amsterdam
The Netherlands
fax: +31 20 620 3419
e-mail: order@iospress.nl

Distributor in the UK and Ireland
Gazelle Books Services Ltd.
White Cross Mills
Hightown
Lancaster LA1 4XS
United Kingdom
fax: +44 1524 63232
e-mail: sales@gazellebooks.co.uk

Distributor in the USA and Canada
IOS Press, Inc.
4502 Rachael Manor Drive
Fairfax, VA 22032
USA
fax: +1 703 323 3668
e-mail: iosbooks@iospress.com

LEGAL NOTICE
The publisher is not responsible for the use which might be made of the following information.
PRINTED IN THE NETHERLANDS

In Honor of Victoria A. Harden

Founding Director of the Office of NIH History (1986-2006)

Champion of the History of Twentieth-Century Biomedicine

Contents

Preface.. vii

Inventing the Office of NIH History 1
    Caroline Hannaway

The Socialization of Research and the Transformation
    of the Academy.. 9
    Richard C. Lewontin

Disease Categories and Scientific Disciplines:
    Reorganizing the NIH Intramural Program, 1945-1960 27
    Buhm Soon Park

The National Institute of Mental Health and Mental
    Health Policy, 1949-1965 59
    Gerald N. Grob

Radium and the Origins of the National Cancer Institute 95
    David Cantor

Transplant Nation: The NIH and the Politics of Heart
    Transplantation in the 1960s 147
    Susan E. Lederer

Mobilizing Biomedicine: Virus Research Between Lay Health
    Organizations and the U.S. Federal Government, 1935-1955 171
    Angela N. H. Creager

Genes, Disease, and Patents:
  Cash and Community in Biomedicine 203
    Daniel J. Kevles

The Critical Role of Laboratory Instruments at the Rockefeller:
  Biomedicine as Biotechnology 217
    Darwin H. Stapleton

Clinical Research in Postwar Britain: The Role of the
  Medical Research Council 231
    Carsten Timmermann

Towards a History of "The Vaccine Innovation System,"
  1950-2000 255
    Stuart Blume

Molecularization and Infectious Disease Research:
  The Case of Synthetic Antimalarial Drugs in the
  Twentieth Century 287
    Leo Slater

Scientific Discoveries: An Institutionalist and
  Path-Dependent Perspective 317
    J. Rogers Hollingsworth

Notes on Contributors 355

Index 359

Preface

The editor wishes to acknowledge with gratitude the contributions of the many people and organizations that have made this volume possible. The book is based on a conference that was held at the National Institutes of Health in December 2005 to promote historical research on biomedical science in the twentieth century. The conference was conceived as a way to honor Victoria A. Harden, the founding Director of the Office of NIH History, on her retirement. The conference was sponsored by the Office of Communications and Public Liaison (OCPL) of the Office of the Director, the administrative home at the time of the Office of NIH History. Special thanks to John Burklow, NIH Associate Director for Communications, and Judy Fouche, Administrative Officer, OCPL, for their generous support and encouragement. Financial support for the conference also came from the Foundation for Advanced Education in the Sciences, Inc. The assistance of Henry Metzger, President, Board of Directors, FAES, was much appreciated. The National Library of Medicine provided meeting space and support. The following individuals in the Office of NIH History worked with the editor in important ways too numerous to describe in staging the conference: Victoria A. Harden, Sarah Leavitt, Brooke Fox, Michele Lyons, Leo Slater, Buhm Soon Park, Lisa Walker, and Mary Alvarez. It was a group effort to which all contributed.

Bringing the volume to publication was generously assisted by the support of the Office of Intramural Research (OIR), the administrative location of the Office of NIH History since 2006. The editor thanks Michael M. Gottesman, NIH Deputy Director for Intramural Research, Richard G. Wyatt, Executive Director, OIR, and Alan N. Schechter, Acting Director, Office of NIH History, for their assistance in moving the project forward. She also thanks members of the Advisory Committee to the Office of NIH History, especially its chair Peter Greenwald, for encouragement. Helpful assistance was also provided by the NIH Division of Medical Arts, especially by Bryan Ewsichek, Designer and Project Manager. The editor is very grateful to all the contributors who worked so hard to make their essays lively contributions to the historical analysis of biomedicine in the twentieth century. In addition, thanks are due to Yale Altman, editorial director of IOS Press, for his assistance.

Inventing the Office of NIH History

Caroline Hannaway

It has long been a conundrum in the history of twentieth-century science and medicine why some of the major research institutions and sources of funding for medical research have not received serious and appropriate historical investigation. In the early 1980s, the National Institutes of Health (NIH) was one of these institutions. Neither the contributions of the significant research programs on campus nor the important changes wrought in research programs elsewhere by the infusion of NIH funding had received widespread or systematic recognition in the history of American medicine. One person who has done her level best to change this situation both through her own research and writing and through her directorship of an Office and a Museum dedicated to NIH history over a twenty-year period is Victoria A. Harden. The NIH has been more fortunate than perhaps it knows to have had such a champion, and the history of biomedicine at large has benefited from her encouragement of scholarship in this important research area. This book is an outcome of her enthusiasm.

The volume and its contents are a testimony to the growing interest of scholars in the development of the biomedical sciences in the twentieth century and to the number of historians, social scientists, and health policy analysts now working on the subject. The essays by noted historians and social scientists offer insights on a range of subjects that should be a significant stimulus for further historical investigation. Readers of the book will know more about the NIH's practices, policies, and politics on a variety of fronts, including the development of the intramural program, the National Institute of Mental Heath and mental health policy, the politics and funding of heart transplantation, and the initial focus of the National Cancer Institute. Comparisons can be made with the development of other American and British institutions involved in medical research, such as the Rockefeller Institute and the Medical Research Council. Discussions of the larger scientific and social context of United States federal support for research, the role of lay institutions in federal funding of virus research, the consequences of technology transfer and patenting, the effects of vaccine and drug development, and the environment of research discoveries writ large all offer new insights and suggest questions for further exploration. This collection of essays has much to offer a wide audience.

To appreciate Victoria Harden's contributions to this now thriving research area and to the NIH's understanding of its past, it is necessary to look back at the invention of the Office of NIH History. Harden's interest in the NIH and its history first manifested itself in her Ph.D. dissertation work under the mentorship of Professor James Harvey Young at Emory University and continued during fellowships at the Smithsonian Institution and the Johns Hopkins University. The fruits of her research became public in her book, *Inventing the NIH: Federal Biomedical Research Policy, 1887-1937*, which was published in 1986. This significant volume quickly became a standard reference in tracing the transformation of the one-room Hygienic Laboratory on Staten Island, New York, into a biomedical research institution of national stature and international recognition in Bethesda, Maryland. Harden's next research project began in 1984 when she was invited by the National Institute of Allergy and Infectious Diseases (NIAID) to write a history of Rocky Mountain spotted fever. Richard Krause, the director of the NIAID at the time, believed that such a project would contribute to the understanding of twentieth-century medical research.

Working on this major project might have been enough for many historians, but this was not all that Harden was involved in at that time. In the mid-1980s she got to know DeWitt (Hans) Stetten, Jr., the NIH Deputy Director of Science emeritus, a man whose fierce pride in the NIH made him want to preserve laboratory instruments that were important in biomedical research studies and to make NIH research contributions known to the world. Stetten's vision and ability to maneuver through organizational challenges, difficult in an unwieldy federal agency such as the NIH, and Harden's historical training and energy together came together to begin the creation of an original product.

After months of discussion, on 10 August 1986, Stetten was able to send a memo to members of an Advisory Committee, announcing the good news that the Director of NIH at the time, James Wyngaarden, had approved the Committee's proposal to establish an NIH Museum of Medical Research. The committee decided to put Harden in charge of the new enterprise. This was the formal beginning of what is now the Office of NIH History with its two components, the Historical Research Unit and the Stetten Museum.

Harden was thrown into a challenging situation from the outset of her new responsibilities. The NIH Centennial celebration was coming up in 1987, something in which the new museum should be involved. She was working intensively on her book on Rocky Mountain spotted fever. There was no designated space to display or store historic instruments and no support staff to assist in developing or cataloguing resources. None of these difficulties were to prove easy to resolve through the years, despite Harden's best efforts and those of individual members of the Advisory Committee and NIH administrators. Large amounts of time and energy in the next two decades were to be required to locate spaces to house the office, store historical documents, conserve museum objects, acquire contractors to work on projects, and set up exhibits.

The Museum's opening was set for 21 May 1987, timed to coincide with the opening of the "Windows on the NIH" exhibit, part of the Centennial observances. The five institutes at the NIH established before 1950, the National Cancer Institute, the National Heart, Lung, and Blood Institute, the National Institute of Allergy and Infectious Diseases, the National Institute of Mental Health/ the National Institute of Neurological Disorders and Stroke, and the National Institute of Dental Research (some with different names initially) had all produced individual exhibits on research achievements. By all accounts it was a splendid event, with DeWitt Stetten and his wife Jane doing the ribbon cutting and Surgeon General C. Everett Koop in attendance. Curators of medical collections at the National Museum of American History, Smithsonian Institution, and the National Museum of Health and Medicine came to lend their support to the new endeavor. The exhibit won the 1989 John Wesley Powell prize of the Society for History in the Federal Government, gaining early recognition in the historical community for the fledgling activities of the new enterprise.

Exhibits were important from early on to make the Museum better known to the NIH community and the larger world, and to highlight the achievements of NIH researchers. Marshall Nirenberg's genetic code research and computers in medicine were early subjects. But there soon were others. From the outset, Clinical Center exhibit space was problematic. One of the earliest support staff, and longest serving, that Harden recruited in 1987 was Michele Lyons, who has spent years building up the collection and is now the curator of the Stetten Museum. In 1988 Harden also began seriously to survey the historical resources available on the NIH campus in order to start building the documentation and archival side of the new endeavor.

In 1988 and 1989, Harden began a new initiative that had long-term consequences for the Office, not only in areas of documents collected and oral histories conducted, but also in the holding of conferences to promote important new themes of historical scientific inquiry and in raising the profile of the NIH historical office. In May 1988, Harden had been made co-chair of the AIDS History Group of the American Association for the History of Medicine. Energized by the idea of producing documentary strategies and recommendations for issues relating to AIDS that could benefit from historical inquiry, Harden began an intensive effort to collect documents and records relating to the NIH response to AIDS. Two outcomes of this historical inquiry were significant conferences held on the NIH campus: the first, in March 1989, was a workshop of historians and health policy analysts, which resulted in the publication *AIDS and the Historian*; the second was a broad-ranging conference in1993 with speakers from many diverse fields–scientists and policy makers as well as activists, writers, and historians–which resulted in the much noted volume *AIDS and the Public Debate: Historical and Contemporary Perspectives* (1995). After that research on AIDS history became a major focus of Harden's intellectual inquiry and, in conjunction with the NIAID, she produced an important historical website on NIH contributions to AIDS research for the twentieth anniversary of the first publication on the new syndrome.

The AIDS-related projects led to the recruitment of another support staff person. The editor of this volume began working as historian and editor in the Office in 1992 in conjunction with these projects.

In 1990, the Office of NIH History reached a turning point on several fronts. After time in temporary quarters in three places on campus, Harden's endeavors to have a regular location for the Office were rewarded when it was assigned a suite of rooms on the second floor of Building 31 of the NIH. This was to be its home for many years. Negotiations for additional museum collection space were ongoing. More important, after the death of DeWitt Stetten, the Advisory Committee, under the chairmanship of Alan Schechter, agreed to the establishment of a memorial fellowship in honor of Stetten that would enable scholars to come to the campus and conduct research on projects relating to the history of NIH intramural scientific research. The fellowship was initially funded by the Foundation for Advanced Education in the Sciences, Inc. The first fellow was Caroline Acker, who was interested in the history of the problem of addiction. She was followed by a roster of excellent historians, three of whom, Buhm Soon Park, Leo Slater, and David Cantor, are contributors to this volume. The scholarship of the Stetten fellows and their outreach to the scientific community has given an enormous boost to the range and substance of historical writing about scientific inquiry at the NIH. Harden deserves credit for this, not only for the example of her own research and publishing, but by her determined and sustained advocacy of the need for more research being conducted by others. She has literally put the history of the NIH on the map of historians' consciousness of what happened in American twentieth-century biomedicine.

An important development in the Stetten Fellow program came in 1998, when Advisory Committee member Henry Metzger proposed to the directors of the NIH intramural research programs–known on the campus as "Scientific Directors"–that they fund the Stetten fellowship program directly. This group, under the leadership of NIH Deputy Director of Intramural Research Michael Gottesman, agreed to the proposal, which has allowed for longer-term fellowships and the ability to have more than one fellow at a time, plus the opportunity to have seminars in which fellows and NIH scientists interact. An additional incentive for research on NIH history came in 1997 when Advisory Committee member Henry Fales proposed to members of the family of deceased NIH chemist John J. Pisano that they might support short-term travel grants for scholars to come to use NIH historical collections. The Pisano family was enthusiastic about this project and in 1998 funded the first of more than a dozen grantees whose work has also enriched the historical literature about the NIH. The expectation is that the momentum achieved by these programs will be ongoing in the next chapter of the Office's history.

In the fifteen years after 1990, the Office of NIH History under Harden's direction continued to focus on a broad range of activities. Notable lectures were given by visiting historians, Stetten fellows, and NIH scientists, and new and important exhibits were installed that achieved NIH and public recognition. For example, an exhibit on the revolution in medicine caused by research in genetics was a major enter-prise, as was an exhibit on the Nobel Prize winning work of Martin Rodbell on how cells respond to signals and an exhibit on the notable research of NIH biochemists, Earl and Thressa Stadtman. After 2000, the Office developed in new directions. Despite the ever present issue of storage space, Harden began a serious endeavor to expand the photograph and document collection of the Office of NIH History. This was coupled with an initiative to use new scanning and internet technology to begin placing such materials on the World Wide Web. The rapid expansion of the Office after 2001 and the new level of sophistication in collection activity, web presence, and response to queries were consequent on Harden's ability to hire on contract an associate historian, Sarah Leavitt, and an archivist, Brooke Fox. Group synergy of Office personnel, Stetten fellows, historians, and scientists helped to give the Office of NIH History the profile and level of usefulness on campus and elsewhere that Harden had dreamed of from the beginning in 1986. As all knowledgeable about the NIH appreciate, it is a long way from authorization of an entity to realization. In such an institution, administrative and professional support, designated office, storage, and exhibit space, and an energetic staff are important components of success.

There is still plenty to be done. Documents and instruments continue to arrive at the Office of NIH History in ever increasing numbers.

Oral histories multiply and more are planned. Physical and web exhibits are sought. Potential Stetten Fellows and other scholars are keen to come to the NIH and do research. Conferences are under discussion. It is hoped that this volume of essays honoring Victoria Harden's accomplishments in inventing, and then constructing, the Office of NIH History will be a catalyst for a wide range of substantive research on twentieth-century biomedicine.

The Socialization of Research and the Transformation of the Academy

Richard C. Lewontin

It is a common assumption that the vast increase in public expenditure on health related research in the United States since the Second World War is the direct consequence of the greater demand for scientific medicine in a society of increasing age, increasingly aware of its health. But there is a paradox here. If the state is simply recognizing the demand for a public support of medicine then why has there been no establishment of a socialized system of medical treatment? Why is it politically acceptable to socialize the cost of medical research but not the cost of medical practice? Somehow the socialization of medical practice, "socialized medicine," carries with it the American political taboo of "Socialism," while the socialization of medical research costs is not only an acceptable, but even a demanded, function of the state. The same legislators who adamantly reject a single payer system of medical treatment, vote consistently for an increase in the National Institutes of Health (NIH) budget for research.

The solution to this paradox is to see health-related research as part of a larger problem of the cost of innovation and the cost of technical training in an economic system of private profit maximizing enterprises. In the nineteenth century, technical innovation was largely the product of individual inventors, "garage tinkerers," working at a level that required very low capital inputs and a low level of technical education. Industrial innovations could be made within the manufacturing enterprises themselves without large commitments of large resources. Even medical research, much of which was carried out by professionals like Robert Koch and Louis Pasteur, could be carried out as cottage industries, in small laboratories with perhaps one assistant and a microscope or as extensions of the teaching function in medical schools. To the extent that the investigator needed access to resources like libraries and collections these were within the power of colleges and learned societies to provide.

The immense explosion of technology in the twentieth century made the earlier model for innovation obsolete. No individual enterprise can now provide the resources necessary for progressive technological change. An immense infrastructure in support of innovation is now necessary. No pharmaceutical company, no matter how large or profitable, can afford to carry out the basic research in genetics, cell biology, and biochemistry that underlie the production of new drugs. Nor do they have the freedom to invest in work that may not produce profitable results for ten or twenty years. The typical investment horizon allowable in corporations is three years or less. So a pharmaceutical company may carry out a certain amount of the later stages of drug development and testing in the interest of acquiring a property right in the end product, but it cannot possibly carry out the research that underlies this final product. Nor can any enterprise, no matter how large, create an institution of education needed to produce trained scientists, involving the faculty, laboratories, libraries, and living facilities that characterize universities. The consequence is that modern research and the education needed to produce the research workers must be socialized. In the absence of any other collective institution that can marshal the necessary resources, the state has come to play this role.

Despite what seems to be the obvious need for the state to act as the central provider of the resources for technological change, that need, in itself, has not been sufficient to overcome the hurdle of political consciousness. Individual enterprise is too deeply built into American political ideology. The solution to this contradiction between economic necessity and political ideology has been to invoke the necessities of war as the legitimating special circumstances for the intervention of the state in the organization of research and development. The condition of war solves three problems for the modern capitalist state by providing a legitimation of the state as a provider of subsidies to private enterprise by three routes. First, and most important economically, the state becomes a major purchaser of goods and services. Second, it enables it to provide capital for modernization and of undercapitalized sectors of the economy, as for example, transportation. The third, and the one to which we devote our attention here, is to assume the cost, beyond the resources of even very large enterprises, of creating new technologies that are of immediate military interest but may be of long-term importance to the economy as a whole. Nuclear fission, instrument miniaturization, and machine computation are the obvious recent examples.

The first entry of the federal government into the organization and funding of scientific research was during the Civil War. Lincoln created the National Academy of Sciences, an honorary organization of the American scientific elite, modeled on the British Royal Society, to which the state could turn for advice and expertise on technical questions. The dependence of the state on a small group of older scientists, past their creative prime, was not satisfactory, however, so during the First World War President Woodrow Wilson created the National Research Council (NRC). The Council, which operates under the general direction of the Academy, draws into its activities, on a temporary basis, members of the scientific community as a whole and so can make use of the most productive members of that community on an ad hoc basis. Although the NRC and the Academy are not themselves agencies of the federal government, they are obliged. The NRC is obliged by the terms of its creation to undertake an investigation and evaluation, although not actual laboratory research, on any scientific matter requested and paid for by a government body.

There would appear to be an exception to the rule that state intervention in research and development was from the beginning instituted by war conditions. Agricultural research and education have been a major preoccupation of the federal and state governments since the middle of the nineteenth century. However, there is no exception. The Organic Act which began the Department of Agriculture including its research function and the Morrill Land Grant College Act, which established the State Colleges of Agriculture and Engineering were passed in 1861 and 1862, in the early days of the Civil War. An important task for the new Department of Agriculture was to find ways of replacing Southern agricultural production, especially of cotton, sugar, and silk, which were not only essential for domestic consumption but were also major export commodities.

The case of agriculture also illustrates from its very beginning a feature that became characteristic of federal intervention and which is a central concern of this review. That is the distinction between the source of funds for research and the control of the actual expenditure of those funds. There was a repeated struggle between the federal government and local state institutions over control of funds, a struggle which resulted in the complete victory of the local forces. Over and over, the Congress appropriated funds for agricultural research and turned over those funds to the state agencies for actual implementation. The Hatch Act of 1887 which created the State Agricultural Experiment Stations provided funds to the Experiment Stations to carry out: "researches and experiments bearing directly on the agricultural industry of the United States as may in each case be deemed as having due regard to the various conditions and needs of the various States and territories."[1] That provision reflects the ideology of political institutions which permeates American history, a hostility to central as opposed to local power. This ideology is exemplified in the present in the general relation between the centralized sources of funding for all research and the local power to determine the actual direction of that research.

The occasion of a war as the circumstance that legitimates the socialization of research is not confined to actual military confrontations. The rhetoric of "war" has become the common denominator of all proposals for state intervention beyond its more narrowly circumscribed historical role. In addition to the "Cold War," there has been the "war on drugs," the "war on cancer," and the "war on disease." All of these "wars" have been used to justify an immense expansion in the state support of activities that would normally be thought of as part of civil society.[2]

The State Becomes the Patron of Research

The wartime intervention of the state into the economy during the First World War had only temporary effects on the economy in general and research and development in particular. With the cessation of government procurement programs at the end of the war there was a brief postwar boom of about two years during which the accumulated demand for civilian goods was filled, but this was followed by a long period of stagnation and recession. Until the radical programs of the New Deal there was essentially no input of government funding into the economy. Figure 1 shows the proportion of the Gross National Product (GNP) constituted by governmental functions between 1929 and 1993. At the beginning of the Depression total government expenditures were only about 8 percent of the GNP and, of this, nearly all was spent by local government. The New Deal programs resulted in a rapid rise in federal expenditure, but a concomitant reduction in taxes available to local governments moderated this effect so that by the entry of the United States into the Second World War total public contribution to the GNP was only about 14 percent. As a result of the war this rose rapidly to 45 percent of the GNP, but then dropped back to its prewar level almost immediately after the end of the war.

Figure 1. Proportion of the Gross National Product constituted by all governmental, by local, by federal and by military purchases.

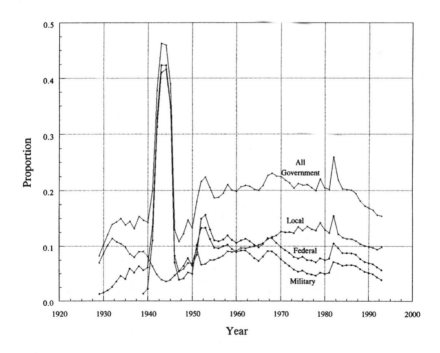

During the war, economists and other government planners recognized that the experience of the period after the First World War would be
repeated after the Second. Paul Samuelson wrote in 1943 of the danger,
after the war, of "the greatest period of unemployment and industrial
dislocation which any economy has ever faced."[3] The solution adopted in
Europe, of a massive state intervention into the peacetime economy, was
clearly politically unacceptable in the United States as a general approach
to a postwar slump. There was, however, one sector that could escape this
constraint and that was scientific research and development. All concerned
parties, including industry, recognized that the socialization of research
and technical education were a structural necessity for long-term prosperity. The Atomic Bomb Project was the most visible example of what
a centralized research effort could produce, but even before its public
recognition it was a model for postwar research.

As early as November 1944, President Franklin D. Roosevelt was
concerned with the role of state-funded research in peacetime. He asked
Vannevar Bush, head of the Office of Scientific Research and Development, to make recommendations for a continuation of the relationship
between the state and scientific research after the war. Bush produced
a manifesto, *Science, The Endless Frontier*, that clearly represented
the interests of the scientific community.[4] The report affirms, first, that
scientific research is the foundation of national prosperity and security.

> New products, new industries and more jobs require
> continuous additions to knowledge of the laws of nature....
> Similarly, our defense against aggression demands new
> knowledge...[which] can be obtained only through basic
> scientific research.[5]

Second, there is no more important task for the state in promoting the economy than its patronage of research and the training of scientific workers:

> The most important ways in which the Government can
> promote industrial research are to increase the flow of new
> scientific knowledge through the support of basic research
> and to aid in the development of scientific talent.[6]

Third, while the state should provide the funds, the control of its disbursement should be vested in the hands of representatives of the same group that is to receive it. Bush proposed a central research funding agency made up of:

> persons of broad interest in and understanding of the peculiarities of scientific research and education.
>
> The agency should promote research through contracts or grants to organizations outside the Federal Government. It should not operate any laboratories of its own.
>
> Support of basic research in public and private colleges and universities and research institutes must leave the internal control of policy, personnel, and the method and scope of the research to the institutions themselves. This is of utmost importance.[7]

We see here an echo of the model of federal support of agricultural research already established in the nineteenth century.

Bush's original vision of a single federal research agency covering all scientific research was not adopted. There was too much opposition from already existing public research entities like the NIH. Indeed, the first attempt to establish a federal agency to fund scientific research without specific subject boundaries, the National Science Foundation (NSF), was at first defeated in Congress in 1946, but was finally established in 1950 during the Korean War. It began with a budget of $100,000, but within ten years this grew by three orders of magnitude, 90 percent of which was disbursed to universities and research institutes under university control.

Total federal funding of research and development was only 74 million dollars on the eve of the American entry into the Second World War and, of that, agricultural research accounted for 40 percent while the rest was largely for military research carried out in government establishments and industrial laboratories. There was no large-scale support of research in universities and in centralized state research institutions. The changes wrought by the development of state support of research can be seen in the postwar history of total government expenditure for goods and

services as contrasted with the postwar support for research. As shown
in Figure 1, with the beginning of Korean War and the Cold War total
government expenditures rose and remained more or less a constant 20
percent of the GNP with an occasional spike until 1986 when it began
its decline to its more recent steady state of about 15 percent. Figure 2
shows the total federal funds for research and development. It might
have been expected that federal research and development expenditures
would have remained in parallel with all federal expenditures but they
have not. The atomic bomb changed all that in ways that would not have
been obvious to its military proponents. Instead, beginning in 1950,
federal research and development funds began an exponential rise reaching a new more or less steady state two orders of magnitude higher than
at the end of the Second World War.

Figure 2. Total federal expenditures on research and development in millions
of constant (1983) dollars.

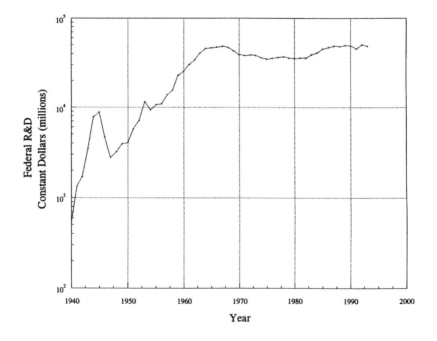

The Relation Between the State and the Academy

Vannevar Bush's model of government funding of research under the effective control of the very community that receives the funds and carries out the research became the rule not only in the National Science Foundation, but in the extramural programs of the National Institutes of Health, the Atomic Energy Commission (AEC, now the Department of Energy, DOE), and even such patently military organizations as the Office of Naval Research and the Defense Advanced Research Projects Agency (DARPA).

Ironically, it was the militarily instigated Manhattan Project that provided a model of work that was very different from the industrial laboratory. The success of a single project of high visibility created a new model for state support of research. The laboratories at Oak Ridge and Los Alamos showed how centrally funded research could accomplish an immensely difficult defined task in a short time, but it also showed that it could be accomplished in a research environment populated by academic scientists who brought to the research institution an academic research culture. The research culture of those institutions was made by professors, many of them European, and their graduate students. While General Leslie Groves was the head of the Los Alamos laboratories, the symbolic image of the atom bomb project became an Italian professor building an atomic pile in the University of Chicago's Stagg Field. After the war, side by side with the essentially military programs of Oak Ridge and, to a smaller extent, Los Alamos National Laboratories there were active biological programs that were only nominally motivated by military concerns about the effect of radioactive fallout. The Biology Division at Oak Ridge, under the leadership of Alexander Hollander, was outside the security screen of the rest of the establishment. On its genetics staff at various times were geneticists who became leaders in the world research community. They began their careers at a time when academic positions and research funds in universities were in low supply and so they could be attracted to the rather isolated situation of a dry county in Tennessee. There they formed a community with an academic culture of lectures, visiting research colleagues, and collaborative research with scientists in universities. With the arrival of Sputnik and the immense increase (using federal funds) of the prosperity of universities, they moved into the external academic world to continue their careers.[8]

The situation in the National Laboratories of the AEC was unusual and temporary. The research activities of the National Institutes of Health illustrate more typically the way in which both intramural and extramural research programs of a state agency are seamlessly joined to the research programs of the academy. The extramural research programs are, of course, carried out physically in academic institutions by research scientists who are academics and these research programs are carried out with funds awarded by a peer review system in which the reviewing peers in Study Sections are drawn from academia. While the final awarding of funds is made by the Councils of the various NIH Institutes, the members of these Councils are for the most part academics and with few exceptions they accept the judgment of the reviewing Study Sections. Thus, it is the community of academic research scientists who usually decide what research is worth doing, who should do it, and how much money should be granted for the work. The result is a self-reinforcing and self-perpetuating consensus on general programs of research in each field. There are exceptions to this scenario, but they do not contradict the influence of the academy. The extramural grant system is administered by full-time NIH program officers. These officers themselves have advanced degrees and have spent some part of their careers carrying out research. They are recognized by the external research scientists as part of the general research community and are part of the social fabric of that community. One of their responsibilities is to know and evaluate the general state of research in particular fields, to organize workshops on questions they regard as important, and, in particular, to recognize gaps in the total program of research and formulate Requests for Research Proposals (RFPs) in an attempt to fill these gaps. They also participate in Council discussions of funding. These program officers, themselves formed in an academic environment, are integrated members of the academic peer system, sharing the assumptions of that community yet standing outside it on a more objective position.

The scientists in the intramural programs of research in the NIH are no less a part of the general academic community. They have had the same formation as those in academia, they participate in and organize the communal professional activities in their field and they share with the rest of the community the same views as to what questions are worth asking. While their research programs are, in principle, more tightly linked to health questions and must be justified as having some relation to issues of health and disease, they nevertheless formulate their own research agendas and in some ways are freer than their external academic colleagues in that they can undertake more long-range projects.

The Transformation of the Academy

A major effect of the increase in research expenditure by the federal government has been a radical transformation in the size, affluence and structure of institutions of higher learning. While the data in Figure 2 show a leveling out of state expenditures on research in the mid-1960s, the proportion of that expenditure awarded to universities rose consistently from 1950 to 1980 then dropped for a short period at the beginning of the 1980s and then resumed its climb (See Figure 3). In 1954

Figure 3. Proportion of federal research and development funds received by colleges and universities including federally funded Research and Development Centers.

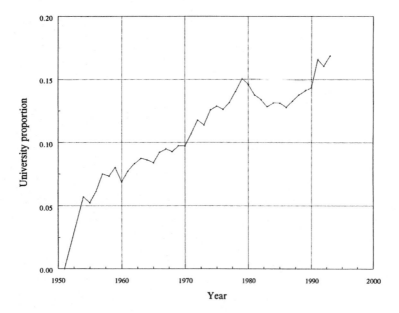

universities received about 5 percent of total federal expenditures for research and development, whereas by the millennium their proportion was about 22 percent. This figure includes not only basic research, which might be thought to be the appropriate function of universities, but also applied research and development. Using the tabulation by the National Science Foundation which is, admittedly, somewhat arbitrary in its distinction between basic and applied research, universities and the research institutes that are associated with them account about for 60 percent of federal expenditures for basic research (their chief competitor being the federal intramural share of 22 percent), 30 percent of applied research and 7 percent of development. The equivalent figures in the 1970s were 50 percent, 23 percent and 4 percent so the university share has grown, but disproportionately for applied research and development.

Clearly a major political concern of the public is with health and it might be expected that universities have benefited from the demand for the solution of persistent problems of health. Indeed, it might be claimed that it is the public preoccupation with health that has been the chief source of the prosperity of academic institutions. As seen by a professor of humanities in a large research university, the Medical School seems to consume a disproportionate share of the university's resources. Certainly professors in the Medical School seem to be extravagantly paid. For example, at the University of Chicago in the middle of the 1960s, the Division of Biological Sciences, which included the Medical School, accounted for half of the entire instructional and research budget. In order to build a new university library the central administration temporarily "borrowed" the Medical School's richest patron from its dean.

A comparison of the growth in government expenditures on research and development in health research with the growth in the total amount assigned to universities shows a remarkable similarity in historical trajectory. The values in Figure 4 compare the total federal expenditure for research and development in universities (Univ), the federal expenditure in universities for health-related research (Univ Health), the federal expenditure in universities for all other research and development (Univ Other) and the total federal budget for health research (Health). Although the curves for health related research are remarkably parallel, even in their year-to-year fluctuations, they do not support the claim that it is health

Figure 4. Total federal expenditures for health-related research and development, total federal expenditures for all research and development in colleges and universities, and federal expenditures in colleges and universities for health- and non-health-related projects.

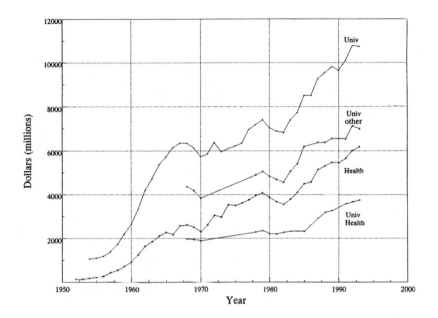

concerns that have driven the pattern because, as Figure 4 shows, health-related research has accounted for only about one-third of federal research and development expenditures in universities, a proportion that has been true over the entire period. That is, the federal support of health-related research in universities is a consequence, not the cause of, the immense general increase in the role of federal grants and contracts in universities that has occurred since the Second World War. That general increase has been driven, rather, by the realization that research and training costs of all kinds must be socialized, the universities being the obvious public service institutions to carry out that function.

We do not need to document in detail the obvious immense change that has occurred in the size of academic institutions since the Second World War. It is sufficient to observe that, in constant dollars, the total budgets of institutions of higher learning in the United States increased by a factor of twenty and the value of their physical plants by a factor of six and the compensation of full-time faculty by two-and-a-half in the 50 years following the war. The annual number of degrees granted increased ninefold. How much of this flows from the socialization of research through government expenditure? Before and immediately after the Second World War, federal expenditures accounted for about 5 percent of university budgets. This rose rapidly, fluctuating between 12 percent and 26 percent but seems to have settled down to about 15 percent of general academic revenues. There is, of course, immense variation among institutions of different sizes and kinds. In general, large and already rich institutions get most of the money disbursed by federal grants and contracts, and the proportion of their total budgets that is received from that source is greater than for smaller colleges and universities. This discrepancy has been constant over the whole period. Over 95 percent of federal expenditures in colleges and universities for research and development are awarded to 10 percent of all such institutions. A mere ten universities accounted for 28 percent of all federal obligations for research and development in 1968 (24 percent in 1990) and fifty universities received 68 percent of the money (64 percent in 1990) the amounts being between 60 million and 500 million dollars annually.

From the standpoint of the operation of large academic institutions, they are heavily dependent on their role as the performers of socialized research. Table 1 shows this dependency as early as 1967, a dependency that shows no signs of having decreased since. It might be claimed that these figures overestimate the need of the institutions since, after all, much of the money is spent on the direct costs of doing the research, and so if there were fewer grants and contracts there would be less need for the funds. Indeed, in the absence of any such grants and contracts the universities could simply return to their original purpose of education. But this claim will not work. Depending upon the year and grant, between 40 percent and 60 percent of the total value of a federal grant for research is in "indirect costs" that go into the general fund of the university for infrastructural support. Obviously, research does incur costs for electricity, heat, and, increasingly, administration and some fraction of those costs would be incurred even in the absence of the research. On the other hand, much of the direct costs, often most, are heavily weighted toward salaries, including graduate student stipends. Faculty salaries are paid from direct

Table 1. Proportion of total institutional income from federal research funds.

Level of Federal Support in 1967	Approximate 1991 Equivalent	Number of Institutions	Ratio of Research Support to Total Budget
$ above 20,000,000	above $140,000,000	14	.355
10,000,000 – 20,000,000	80,000,000 to 140,000,000	15	.303
5,000,000 – 10,000,000	35,000,000 to 80,000,000	31	.241
500,000 – 5,000,000	4,000,000 to 35,000,000	106	.187
100,000 – 500,000	700,000 to 4,000,000	129	.054
1,000 – 100,000	10,000 to 700,000	416	.018

From William V. Consolazio, *The Dynamics of Academic Science*, NSF 67-6 (Washington, D.C.: U.S. Government Printing Office, 1967)

costs either as summer salaries or as some fraction of the full time said to be devoted to the research. The loss of federal grants and contracts for research would mean a major contraction in the educational functions of the institutions.

There is another aspect of the subsidy of the state to academic institutions that is not directly linked to research grants and contracts. Student grant and loan programs, fellowships and work-study, and funds for construction account for 40 percent to 55 percent of federal expenditures in these institutions. In 1990, of the total of 15.21 billion dollars spent by the government in academia, 6.06 billion was for these non-research purposes. The claim that the state spends large sums of money in academic institutions only because they are obvious sites for needed research does not hold up. The major expenditure of funds for educational purposes shows that the state is involved not only in the socialization of research costs, but also in the formation of a managerial and technological cadre without which the operation of the modern economy is impossible. As in the case of research, individual firms, no matter how large, do not have the resources needed. The vastly expanded educated infrastructure needed after the Second World War could only be provided through the socialization of the costs of education.

One result of the large federal expenditure in academic institutions has been a growth in the educational structure and operation of institutions that were once meant to serve a local constituency. North Carolina State College of Agriculture and Engineering became North Carolina

State University as the sources of money changed from state controlled agricultural funds to grants and contracts from the NIH, the NSF, the Department of Energy and the Department of Defense. Many agricultural and technical institutes and teachers' colleges have become state universities with graduate programs and research institutes. Undergraduate institutions like Butler University in Indianapolis, without a graduate program, were enabled to carry out high level research with undergraduates, using federal research funds.

Another result of government funding of research has been a change in the relations of power between faculty members and their employing institutions. An oddity of university employment is that faculty members have the education, social status and specialized craft knowledge typical of self-employed independent professionals like physicians and lawyers, while at the same time they are salaried employees of large institutions that can set the conditions of their work and their compensation. There has been a long struggle in American academic institutions between the faculty and the administration over the degree to which the corporate body can control the conditions of employment and tenure. Before the Second World War, the academics had little power in this struggle. The American Association of University Professors produced a number of manifestos describing what they viewed as the rights of academic freedom and the proper conditions for tenured employment, but it was not until 1958 that any general agreement was reached with administrations. Beginning at the end of the 1950s, the increasing flow of research funds into the universities resulted in a major increase in the size, security and compensation of faculties. Especially in science, because research grants were awarded on the basis of proposals from individual scientists, and because the supply of scientists was smaller than the demand created by the expanding universities, these faculty members acquired a powerful weapon in their struggle for power. If a university administration failed to meet the demands of present or potential faculty members, they would find employment elsewhere. Professors in natural and social sciences could choose between institutions based on how low the teaching load and how large the laboratory would be. In an important sense, these faculty members ceased to be employees and became independent research entrepreneurs free to move and carry with them the entire laboratory enterprise including graduate students and postdoctoral fellows. But the power over the conditions of work did not remain confined to scientists. As salaries rose, tenure became routine and teaching obligations were reduced, the effects spread from scientists to the faculty as a whole. The universities could hardly offer a set of conditions to natural scientists which they refused to professors of Greek.

It is not only in the conditions of work, but in the status of scholarship in general that benefits have accrued from state subsidy of science. The National Endowment for the Humanities has come into existence and although its budget is only 8 percent as large as that of the National Science Foundation and only one sixth of that budget is devoted to research grants, it makes an important contribution to scholarly work. The humanities and the arts have benefited from the aura of legitimation that has arisen from the socialization of research costs. Attacks on subsidized programs in the humanities or the arts must now be made either as part of a general cut back of all federal expenditure on the basis of the quality of a particular program. It cannot be made on the grounds that it is contrary to the nature of the American polity. The socialization of the cost of intellectual work is now a permanent feature of the American economy.

Notes

1. Hatch Act, 1887, Sec 2(6).
2. I am indebted to the late Elinor Barber of Columbia University for the insight that the metaphor of "war" has done such powerful work in public policy issues.
3. Paul Samuelson, "Full Employment After the War," *Postwar Economic Problems*, ed. Seymour E. Harris (New York: McGraw Hill, 1943), pp. 27-53.
4. Vannevar Bush, *Science, The Endless Frontier: A Report to the President* (Washington, D.C.: U.S. Government Printing Office, 1945).
5. Bush, *Science, The Endless Frontier*, p. 5.
6. Ibid., p. 7.
7. Ibid., p. 33.
8. In the mid-1950s, working in the Biology Division at Oak Ridge were, for example, William K. Baker, Daniel Lindsley, Edward Novitski and Larry Sandler, who then dispersed to the Universities of Chicago, Illinois, Oregon and Washington, where they became national and international leaders of genetics.

Disease Categories and Scientific Disciplines: Reorganizing the NIH Intramural Program, 1945-1960

Buhm Soon Park

In the summer of 1986, the United States Congress designated fiscal year 1987 as the "National Institutes of Health Centennial Year" in order to observe the agency's anniversary with appropriate ceremonies and activities. President Ronald Reagan accordingly proclaimed: "The National Institutes of Health, which began as a one-room laboratory at the Marine Hospital on Staten Island in 1887, has become the world's foremost biomedical research center. Its investigators are at the forefront of discoveries that contribute to better health for mankind."[1] In addition to investigations conducted in the National Institutes of Health's (NIH) own "intramural" laboratories, Reagan also noted the importance of the agency's "extramural" program in supporting the activities of non-federal scientists in universities, medical schools, and other research institutions. Indeed, no other federal agency supported more academic research and development (R&D) than the NIH, which had grown since its beginnings into a vast research complex encompassing twelve institutes and several divisions and centers with a hefty budget of $6 billion.[2]

The expansion of the NIH in its first hundred years is most visible in the agency's changing organizational chart. The Hygienic Laboratory, as the one-room laboratory on Staten Island, New York, came to be called, was relocated to the nation's capital in 1891. Subsequently, it moved to a new, separate building in 1904 and had four divisions established along the lines of scientific disciplines (the Divisions of Pathology and Bacteriology, Chemistry, Pharmacology, and Zoology)–the internal structure reflecting the high status of science at the turn of the century within the public health and medical research communities.[3] There was no change to this four-division structure for more than three decades, but it was during this critical period that an expanded role for the federal government in medical research was much considered and debated. As Victoria A. Harden aptly shows, the 1930 renaming of the Hygienic Laboratory as the National Institute of Health was an outcome of the prolonged legislative debates over this issue.[4] By the time the NIH moved from downtown Washington, D.C. to the spacious Bethesda campus in 1939, its position as the research arm of the Public Health Service (PHS) was considerably strengthened with the addition of two new units—the Divisions of Industrial Hygiene and Public Health Methods.[5] A further tweaking during World War II made the NIH an organization of eight components: one institute (the National Cancer Institute, which officially became part of the NIH in 1944); two divisions (Infectious Diseases and Physiology); and five laboratories (Biologics Control, Industrial Hygiene Research, Pathology, Chemistry, and Zoology).[6] The postwar years, however, witnessed the reshuffling of these components and the creation of new institutes along the lines of disease categories, such as heart disease, mental health, arthritis, and allergy. Hence, it has been the National *Institutes* of Health since 1948.

The origins of the "disease category" structure of the NIH and the ramifications of this for the postwar development of the biomedical sciences have not been fully explored in the history of science or the history of medicine.[7] In this paper I focus on the expansion of the NIH intramural program within the categorical framework, as I will be discussing the changing relationship between the NIH and the extra-mural community elsewhere. Each of the seven categorical institutes that constituted the NIH in the 1950s had a different experience in building its intramural program, depending on the existence of previous activities in that particular category within the NIH or the PHS and the level of congressional support for its growth. Unique as individual situations were, I show that there was a common goal among the categorical institutes at the NIH to establish a strong basic research program covering several scientific fields, even if their links to categorical missions might be neither direct nor transparent. It was each institute's Associate Director in charge

Figure 1. Changes in the organization of the NIH. By 1953, seven categorical institutes of the NIH were in operation: the National Cancer Institute, the National Heart Institute, the National Institute of Mental Health, the National Institute of Arthritis and Metabolic Diseases, the National Microbiological Institute (renamed in 1955 as the National Institute of Allergy and Infectious Diseases), the National Institute of Neurological Diseases and Blindness, and the National Institute of Dental Research.

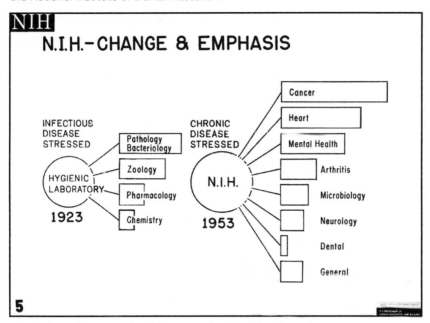

Source: National Institutes of Health, *Data Book 1954*, Office of NIH History.

of research, or "Scientific Director," who exerted a pivotal role in shaping its program. In the 1950s, the Scientific Directors emerged not only as a group that decided a variety of intramural affairs, such as hiring and promotion policies and the resources to share in inter-institute collaborations, but also as the chief interpreters of the relationship between categorical missions and scientific progress.

Shaping the Cancer Program

Not all institutes had to build their intramural programs from scratch in the post-World War II years. A good example is the National Cancer Institute (NCI), which had maintained a remarkable degree of continuity since its establishment in 1937. Carl Voegtlin, the NCI's first director, or

"Chief" as he was called at that time, was a pharmacologist-turned-cancer-researcher with a broad knowledge in the field. Voegtlin was in complete charge of the research activities of his intramural scientists, who were all assembled in one building after 1940, and yet he had no firm organizational pattern in mind. Instead, he preferred to see a series of multidisciplinary groups formed to tackle specific problems, with his senior scientists acting as temporary chairmen of the groups. Voegtlin placed great emphasis upon this flexible, team-oriented approach to cancer research where no predominant theories existed, but at the same time he had a subtle influence upon the direction of research by giving suggestions, not direct orders, backed up with the funds he could allocate.

Several research lines to which Voegtlin gave high priority included the biochemical characterization of tumor tissue, carcinogenesis in tissue culture, nutritional factors in tumor origin and growth, and studies of gastric cancer. He also chaired scientific conferences, held once a month or at his request, at which new findings and research plans were discussed. Occasionally, prominent speakers were invited to give a talk at these events. In addition, Voegtlin made it a rule that the intramural staff send their papers to the *Journal of the National Cancer Institute*, a new publication managed by the NCI and edited by himself.[8]

Upon his retirement in 1943, Voegtlin was succeeded by Roscoe R. Spencer, who had built strong credentials as a microbe hunter, especially for his heroic contribution to the development of a successful vaccine against Rocky Mountain spotted fever.[9] But Spencer possessed a short résumé as a cancer researcher. As one of his colleagues observed, "His interests in cancer were primarily at a philosophical level, with cancer as an example of species adaptation in a multicellular organism."[10] Devoid of towering authority in cancer research, Spencer was not an effective administrator, either. Under his editorship, for example, the institute's journal began to atrophy from a diminishing number of contributions, partly because of the war, and partly because of Spencer's failure to force his staff to follow the publication rules set by his predecessor. Nor did he display political acumen. Spencer's 1946 testimony before the House Appropriations Subcommittee, which was mistakenly construed as the NCI's hesitancy in taking up an immensely expanded budget, did not earn him much trust from the Public Health Service's senior officers or from powerful cancer research advocates. The next year Spencer was replaced by Leonard A. Scheele.

Scheele was a veteran PHS officer who had had experiences of serving as a quarantine officer, a state health officer, a special cancer fellow at the Memorial Hospital in New York, an officer-in-charge of the National Cancer Control Program, a chief of the Medical Division of Civilian Defense, and an assistant chief of the NCI before becoming its director in 1947. Scheele's interests were not so much in cancer research per se as in cancer prevention and control. With his expertise more in administration than in bench work, Scheele made an important contribution by formalizing the internal structure of the NCI into three branches: the research branch, with six sections of biology, biochemistry, biophysics, chemotherapy, endocrinology, and pathology at Bethesda, and a seventh section of a combined laboratory-clinic unit in San Francisco; the research grants branch; and the cancer control branch. The research grants branch was de facto an administrative arm of the National Advisory Cancer Council, which dealt with NCI's extramural programs and traditionally did not meddle with intramural affairs. The cancer control branch had a multifaceted mission of administering cancer grants to state health agencies, loaning radium to hospitals, and promoting cancer teaching programs in medical schools.[11] These activities appeared foreign and suspect to most intramural scientists. They wondered: "Should public health activities be at the NIH, or at administrative bureaus related to state functions? Is the close proximity of such activities to research desirable, wishfully thus being able to translate the findings of research to practical application with least delay? What are the differences and similarities between research grants and control grants?"[12] Indeed, the dilemma of locating the cancer control program and the intramural program side-by-side manifested itself later: the cancer control branch was abolished in 1957, and then made a comeback after the 1971 National Cancer Act.

Scheele appointed Harry Eagle, a noted microbiologist with a strong academic and public health background, as chief of the research branch. Eagle had been director of the Venereal Disease Research Laboratory and Laboratory of Experimental Therapeutics at the Johns Hopkins University for twenty years before entering the PHS during World

War II. At the NCI, Eagle's influence was most noticeable in the development of a simplified, commercially applicable technique for preparing tissue cultures by modifying the complex *in vitro* procedures previously devised by NCI's Wilton R. Earle and Johns Hopkins's George Gey. Eagle was, however, too much of a bench scientist to stay in an administrative position, and too much of an outsider to deal with individualistic intramural scientists. After two years he decided to leave the NCI and continue to pursue his research interests at another institute of the NIH, the Microbiological Institute, where he later became chief of the Laboratory of Cell Biology.[13]

It was widely believed that Jesse P. Greenstein, a biochemist who joined the NCI in 1937, had drawn up the blueprint for the seven scientific laboratories during Scheele's reorganization. An author of the two-volume classic, *Biochemistry of Cancer*, with volumes published separately in 1948 and 1954, Greenstein led the field with great authority. "Greenstein may have become the director of the Institute, but preferred to retain his hands on his retorts rather than to get involved in the paper problems of others. Had he accepted [the position], the intramural program may have emerged much more structurally centralized and directed than it became under the benevolent laissez-faire of J. R. Heller,"[14] recalled one of his colleagues.

In 1948 John R. Heller was selected as director of the NCI by Scheele, who had just been appointed the Surgeon General of the Public Health Service. Like his predecessor, Heller was a veteran commissioned officer having spent most of his career in the PHS's Venereal Disease Division, of which he served as chief. Heller was known as a skilled administrator, but had little experience in cancer research. During his twelve-year tenure as the NCI director, Heller seldom made important decisions or presented controversial opinions on scientific subjects by himself, always following the advice of his trusted intramural staff. In 1952, he successfully lured away G. Burroughs Mider from the University of Rochester to fill the position of chief of the research branch. This position had been newly upgraded, and its occupant was renamed the NCI's Associate Director in charge of research. By that time, the term "Scientific Director" had been used NIH-wide for a person in that capacity.

Mider was no stranger to the NCI. He first came in 1939 as a research fellow and stayed for two years before taking a faculty position at Cornell Medical College. He also spent a year at the University of Virginia, and from there he moved to the University of Rochester as professor of cancer research and research associate in surgery. While maintaining the overall internal structure of the NCI, Mider modified the laboratory research part to strengthen clinical research and provide patient care before the opening of the Clinical Center in 1953. He created two new branches: the research medicine branch composed of sections of endocrinology, environmental cancer, and nutrition and metabolism; and the clinical medicine and surgery branch, which had sections of surgery, medicine, and clinical chemotherapy. His approach to cancer research was well expressed in the 1952 NCI annual report: "The research program of the National Cancer Institute must continue to be comprehensive. It must take advantage of each advance in science and technology. It must be integrated with the total effort in cancer research throughout the world but retain sufficient flexibility to make possible the shift in emphasis from one area to another as the need arises."[15] Mider constantly pursued a balanced expansion of both scientific and clinical cancer programs in the 1950s.

Old Programs in a New Organization

To some old-timers at the NIH, it was perplexing that diseases as amorphous as arthritis and metabolic disorders could be packaged together and assigned to an institute that had a tradition of conducting a broad array of basic research. To others, it was ironical that the microbiology program with a long history of studying and combating infectious diseases became the last, among the seven institutes of the NIH in the 1950s, to adopt a title bearing the names of diseases. The National Institute of Arthritis and Metabolic Diseases (NIAMD) and the National Institute of Allergy and Infectious Diseases (NIAID)–the direct descendants of research programs from the time of the Hygienic Laboratory–did not have to build whole new sets of intramural research programs. The main problem for the two institutes was rather of an administrative nature: how to reinterpret the mission of each individual laboratory in the light of new categorical mandates, and how to foster the unity between old, laboratory-oriented programs and new, clinically oriented ones.

The decision to create the National Institute of Arthritis and Metabolic Diseases was part of a compromise made in the postwar years between voluntary health organizations lobbying for the creation of separate institutes in major disease categories and the Public Health Service opposing the proliferation of an unmanageable number of categorical institutes on campus. The deal, mediated by legislators in Congress, was written in August 1950 as the Omnibus Medical Research Act. It granted the Surgeon General discretion to create new institutes. Though born with a disease-oriented mission, the NIAMD embarked upon its intramural program with four science-oriented laboratories (the Laboratories of Chemistry, Biochemistry and Nutrition, Physical Biology, and Pathology). These laboratories had been constituents of the Experimental Biology and Medicine Institute (EBMI), a short-lived institute that might have been called "the Institute of Basic Medical Sciences" at the time of its inception in 1947.[16]

The man who presided over the transition from the EBMI to the NIAMD was William Henry Sebrell, Jr. An expert in nutritional studies of diseases at the NIH for decades, Sebrell demonstrated a skill for research administration and a sense of research politics. He served as director of the EBMI for three years, became the NIAMD's first director, and, subsequently, took over directorship of the entire NIH in October 1950. Sebrell's successor at the NIAMD was Russell M. Wilder, an internationally renowned nutritional researcher from the Mayo Clinic and Foundation. Wilder took the lead in creating a clinical research program oriented toward specific disease problems, ranging from arthritis and rheumatism to diabetes, endocrine disorders, and other metabolic diseases. Because of ill health, Wilder resigned in June 1953 and was succeeded by Floyd S. Daft, an organic chemist-turned-biochemist who had served as the NIAMD's assistant director of basic research.[17]

The reorientation of the basic research program proceeded at a gradual pace, but not without anxieties. Claude Hudson, the face of the NIH's chemistry program for more than two decades, announced his retirement in 1951, and Paul A. Neal, chief of the Laboratory of Physical Biology, followed suit. There were also several major losses among young scientists, including Arthur Kornberg, who left to become head of the Department of Microbiology at Washington University School of Medicine in St. Louis.[18] To a certain degree, turnover of scientific staff was simply a part of the natural process of senior members retiring and junior ones leaving for better jobs, but there was also a considerable amount of apprehension over the changes underway in the NIAMD. Kornberg, for instance, could not help having the impression that "the advent of the Clinical Center and the disease-oriented institutes would stifle basic research at NIH."[19]

For this reason, it was crucial for Daft to recruit someone as scientific director of the institute who could provide strong intellectual leadership for both scientists and clinicians and foster a sense of togetherness among the intramural staff members. In 1954, after about a year of searching, Daft finally appointed DeWitt Stetten, Jr., as the NIAMD's Scientific Director. Having an M.D. and a Ph.D. from Columbia University, Stetten had built a distinguished career as a biochemist, especially in the study of gout, and he was also a medical educator who had written a textbook in biochemistry and taught the subject at Columbia and Harvard. Stetten appreciated the value of a multidisciplinary approach to the problems of diseases, but put strong emphasis upon a researcher's freedom to choose his or her own topic. "A continuing problem with the scientific direction of an institute such as NIAMD," he wrote in the 1956 annual report, "is the degree to which it is profitable to try to influence the choice of problems by our scientists." He then argued:

> Certainly the direction of the program can be influenced in the selection of new staff members to fill vacancies created either by new positions or by the departure of present staff. Also it is possible, by the distribution of support among the several laboratories, to enhance the production in an area where this seems desirable. It appears highly probable, however, that per research dollar spent, the greatest return will be secured if the mature scientist is allowed and encouraged to select the problems on which he will work. It is our belief that the meritorious and experienced investigator will in

general be the wisest judge of his field of endeavor. The most important function of the Scientific Directors therefore, is in the selection of senior scientists, in their encouragement, and in the attempt to procure for them those facilities which they may require for the fulfillment of their mission.[20]

Articulate and persuasive, Stetten emerged as the champion of elitism and minimalism in research administration within the circle of the Scientific Directors at the NIH.

In the meantime, another set of old programs–the Division of Infectious Diseases, the Division of Tropical Diseases, the Biologics Control Laboratory, and the Rocky Mountain Laboratory–were joined together in 1948 in the newly created Microbiological Institute. This institute was renamed four years later as the National Microbiological Institute (NMI), which then became the National Institute of Allergy and Infectious Diseases in 1955.[21] The NIAID had some difficulties from the beginning, because the advances in prevention and treatment of infectious diseases, marked by the development of antibiotics during World War II, precipitated a decline in public concern about such diseases and a change in funding patterns for research. Between 1948 and 1954, in fact, the study of infectious diseases had dropped from first to eighth place in terms of federal and private funding for medical research.[22] A chart was also circulated at that time among policy makers and health reformers in order to illustrate dramatic changes in the death rates for various diseases in the past decades. "I recall becoming terribly annoyed at a chart," said a former director of the NIAID, "that was proposed for showing to some influential group–I don't know whether it was Congress or another group–which showed the death rates for cancer and heart disease going up steeply and the death rate for infectious disease going down sharply. I think I got it stopped all right, but . . . it took quite an effort to get people to think of infectious diseases as still a serious health problem."[23]

In this context, the title change in 1955 was a significant event for the NIAID. It meant an end to several years of frustration with congressional indifference and the lack of direction for future developments. For instance, the Microbiological Institute had an extramural program

Figure 2. Mortality of major diseases between 1900 and 1950.

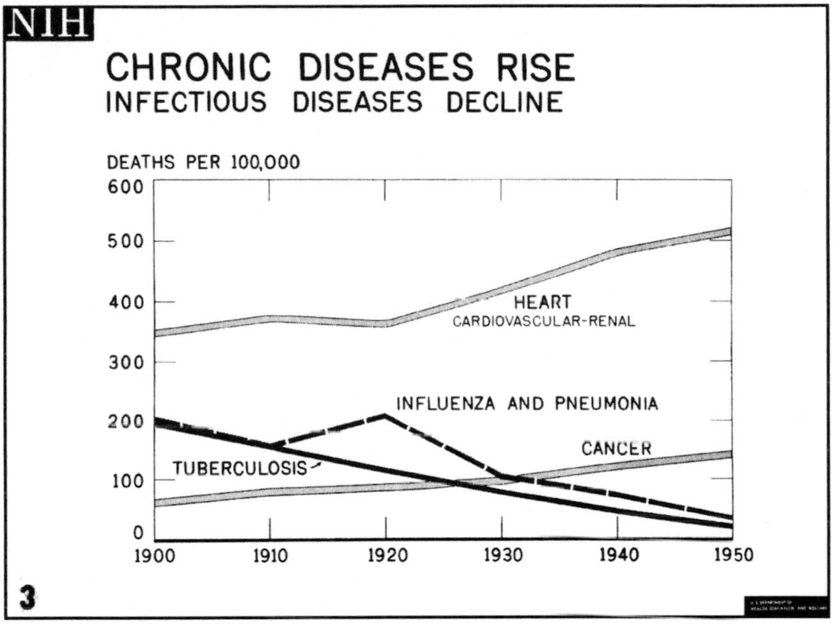
NIH
CHRONIC DISEASES RISE
INFECTIOUS DISEASES DECLINE
DEATHS PER 100,000
600
500
400
300
200
100
0
HEART
CARDIOVASCULAR-RENAL
INFLUENZA AND PNEUMONIA
CANCER
TUBERCULOSIS
1900
1910
1920
1930
1940
1950
3

Source: National Institutes of Health, *Data Book 1954*, Office of NIH History.

in 1951 to administer two million dollars in research grants and fellowships, but no advisory council of its own was assembled to review grant applications and set institutional policies. The Surgeon General's National Health Advisory Council assumed this role until 1956, and this arrangement opened the door for the NIH Director and other senior officers of the PHS to influence the process of research planning from the start. The National Microbiological Institute's director, Victor H. Haas, did not exert much influence upon the intramural program, either, as the institute's four constituent research units had been pursuing well-defined research missions of their own for decades. Having previously served as a medical officer in charge of the PHS's malaria investigations, Haas conformed to the existing structure and authority, rather than shaking things up. He also had to fight an uphill battle in Congress. Between 1952 and 1955, the level of extramural funding for the NMI was almost flat (around $2 million), and there was no substantial budget increase for the intramural program ($3-4 million), except the portion for the creation of a new clinical program under the Laboratory of Clinical Investigation. In other areas, the expansion of promising programs or the initiation of new activities took place only by curtailment or abandonment of less promising or unproductive projects.[24]

Although not as imposing a director as he might have been, Haas quietly pursued some changes within the boundaries of financial and administrative constraints. He understood that the greatest strength of the institute was its ability to redirect research in response to new problems or new research opportunities, and a record of successful instances of this flexibility is well documented. For example, Q fever investigations were replaced by studies on the Coxsackie viruses, which in turn were changed to a respiratory virus project. Also, a pertussis study became modified to include Q fever epidemiology, the epidemiology of minor illness, and influenza vaccine evaluation.[25] Haas and his research staff identified several new areas of investigation, such as allergic disorders, which afflicted a large number of the population. Haas reported in 1955: "Using presently available personnel and physical resources of the intramural operation, it would be practicable to reorient certain current projects so that there would be a more definite relationship to immunology and particularly allergy than is presently provided for. Some reorientation of this nature could be done in each of the Institute's major Laboratories, including the clinical operation."[26]

It is difficult to determine how much the decision to strengthen allergy research was affected either by pressure groups and concerned legislators, or by the Surgeon General and his advisors, or by Haas and his NMI researchers. But the consequences were clear. In June 1955, the Laboratory of Biologics Control was taken out of the NMI and elevated to the status of the Division of Biologics Standards, and the NMI was renamed as the NIAID in December. The next year, the National Advisory Allergy and Infectious Diseases Council was formed. Dorland J. Davis, formerly chief of the Laboratory of Infectious Diseases, was appointed to be Scientific Director of the institute, and Congress nearly doubled NIAID appropriations for fiscal 1957 to $13.3 million. Davis was excited as he described the upcoming changes in the 1956 annual report: "The increasing interest and responsibility for advancing knowledge in basic immunology, hypersensitivity phenomenon, and allergy, as reflected in the recent change of Institute name, were implemented by plans to coordinate existing intramural investigations in these fields and to supplement them with new studies." "The beginning of this permanent program," he also said optimistically, "is being made by concentration on the laboratory and basic aspects of immunology with the intention to expand into clinical investigation as promising leads develop, investigators conceive original projects, and facilities become available."[27] A few more laboratories, including the Laboratory of Immunology, were established in the late 1950s, and, by then, the NIAID had caught up with other categorical institutes in terms of connecting itself with the general public while conducting and supporting a broad spectrum of basic and clinical research.

James A. Shannon's Wartime Experience

The National Heart Institute (NHI), established in 1948, was faced with a different set of problems in forming its intramural program. In the first place, the NHI inherited only a small group of research programs scattered around the Public Health Service. One of the NHI's programs was a research unit on cardiovascular diseases, which had been in operation since 1931 and became part of the NIH's Division of Infectious Diseases in 1937. This unit conducted clinical and laboratory studies on the origins of rheumatic fever at hospitals in Washington, D.C., and also carried out epidemiological studies on heart-disease mortality around the country, but its activities were severely curtailed during World War II.[28] Another research unit in operation was a gerontology clinic located at the Baltimore City Hospitals, the institution that became part of the NIH's Division of Physiology during the war.[29] A third research unit was the Heart Disease Epidemiology Study at Framingham, Massachusetts. It had been established in 1948 as a field station of the Bureau of State Services of the PHS. In 1948-1949, these research units were transferred to the NHI, but there was still the daunting task of building laboratory-based research programs. Cassius J. Van Slyke, the appointee as director of the NHI, did not seem the ideal person for this job. He was a career PHS officer who had worked on the experimental study of venereal diseases and subsequently made a key contribution to the administration of research grants as chief of the

Division of Research Grants. A large portion of Van Slyke's time was also spent in drawing up general policies for the NHI's grant and fellowship program with the members of the National Advisory Heart Council. It took a combined effort of the NIH's Director and Associate Director, i.e., Rolla E. Dyer and Norman Topping, to find a man to construct the intramural program of the Heart Institute from planning to staffing. They were finally able to persuade James A. Shannon, then director of the research institute of the pharmaceutical company, E. R. Squibb & Sons, in New Jersey, to take the position of the NHI's Scientific Director in 1949.[30]

Shannon was not a specialist in heart diseases. He was an authority in renal physiology, best known for the development of accurate methods for measuring the glomerular filtration rate in the kidneys.[31] For such a scientifically ill-defined field as the study of heart disease, however, his broad knowledge and administrative experience were deemed to matter the most. Shannon had received his M.D. and Ph.D. from New York University and served on the faculty of its department of physiology and medicine. In 1941, he assumed the responsibility of directing the NYU Research Service at Goldwater Memorial Hospital, where he formed a team of researchers in renal physiology to work back and forth between their laboratories and the patient beds.[32] But then Shannon's group turned its focus to the development of antimalarial drugs as part of the military-civilian coordination of malaria research, and also because Shannon chaired the National Research Council's panel for clinical trials of new drugs.[33]

The wartime experience at Goldwater significantly changed Shannon's perception of the federal role in medical research. First and foremost, Shannon realized that he had the possibility of being able to lead organized research with almost unlimited resources while not having to restrict too much the spirit of freedom in the research of the scientists. He had no reservations about working for the NIH. As he later recalled: "It was new. No one had been there before, and I inherited no sins."[34] After a few months in office, Shannon developed a three-layered structure for the NHI's intramural program–laboratories for basic science, clinics for patient care, and combined laboratory and clinical sections[35]–drawing on the wartime malaria project that had coordinated a variety of research done by organic chemists, pharmacologists, physiologists, and clinicians.[36]

Table 1. Intramural Staff of the National Heart Institute, 1952.

Conceptual Categories	Titles of Labs or Clinics	Chiefs and Their Previous Positions
Laboratory	Cellular Physiology	Christian Anfinsen (Harvard)
	Chemical Pharmacology	Bernard Brodie (NYU)
	Chemistry of Natural Products	Evan Horning (U. Pennsylvania)
Clinics	Surgery	Not yet filled
	Gerontology	Nathan Shock (Baltimore City Hospitals)
	General Medicine and Experimental Therapeutics	Luther Terry (Johns Hopkins)
Laboratory and Clinical*	Kidney and Electrolytes Metabolism	Robert Berliner (NYU)
	Metabolism	Christian Anfinsen (Harvard), temporary
	Cardiovascular Hemodynamics	Not filled
	Technical Development	Bert Boone (Temple)
	Physiology and Pharmacology of the Autonomic Nervous System	Not yet filled

*Titles of research units in this category start with "The Laboratory of."

Yet to persuade top-quality scientists to forsake their academic careers and join government laboratories was no simple matter. First, Shannon began to contact his former colleagues at Goldwater, who universally admired his leadership.[37] "All he had to do was whistle, and people came running," one of his Goldwater associates recalled[38] but, in reality, Shannon had to convince these colleagues that they would be able to cut through government red tape. Robert Berliner, Bernard B. "Steve" Brodie, Robert Bowman, and Sidney Udenfriend, all of whom had set their career paths in academia, eventually became his staff again. Shannon also searched for scientific talent through the so-called "old boys' network" of department chairmen and deans of medical schools. One of his greatest catches was Christian B. Anfinsen, assistant professor of biological chemistry at Harvard Medical School, who had also been involved in the wartime malaria project. Shannon's recruits also included Evan C. Horning, an organic chemist at the University of Pennsylvania; Bert R. Boone, a developer of the electrocardiograph at Temple University Medical School; and Luther L. Terry, assistant professor at the Johns Hopkins University School of Medicine. Shannon penciled in Stanley J. Sarnoff, associate professor of physiology at Harvard, and Eugene Braunwald, a recently minted M.D. from NYU, as his main targets for the Laboratory of Cardiovascular Hemodynamics. He also persuaded Andrew G. Morrow, a young faculty member at Johns Hopkins, to take up the cardiovascular surgery clinic. By the time Shannon decided to move to the Office of the Director of the NIH in 1952 as Associate Director for Intramural Research, the intramural program of the National Heart Institute had been placed on a solid basis.[39]

The Joint Intramural Program

The formation of the intramural programs of two other institutes–the National Institute of Mental Health (NIMH) and the National Institute of Neurological Diseases and Blindness (NINDB)–bore a striking resemblance to that of the National Heart Institute's, although the two institutes were confronted with extraordinary circumstances.[40] The NIMH had to endure a three-year ordeal of being authorized but not officially established until 1949 because of the lack of appropriations. In addition, the institute's visibly community-oriented function of providing social services and training mental health workers gave ample reason for critics to doubt whether or not the NIH would be a better home for it than any of the other bureaus of the Public Health Service. Most important, there was a great deal of skepticism about the scientific nature of mental health research that would include behavioral and social sciences. Robert H. Felix, who had led the way to the creation of the institute and served as its first director, recalled: "This wasn't the most friendly climate. . . . I got nothing but misunderstanding. . . . We weren't respectable. Clinical research in psychiatry wasn't even research. There wasn't any basic research going on. We weren't doing any physiology, or chemistry and so forth."[41] The NINDB encountered a similar situation. Though established in 1950, the NINDB received no direct appropriations earmarked for its extramural and intramural programs for three years. Nor did it have a director until October 1951 when Pearce Bailey was recruited from the neurology program of the Veterans Administration. Bailey managed to initiate programs, one by one, with a budget given as part of the NIH Director's operating expenses. Characterized as "the first cause of permanent crippling and the third cause of death," neurological diseases and sensory disorders drew much attention from concerned citizens and health organizations, but there were only a handful of schools that offered specialized training in this field.[42]

After spending a few years searching for someone to build the NIMH intramural program, Felix finally could make an offer to Seymour S. Kety, professor of clinical physiology at the University of Pennsylvania. A rising star in the physiological study of blood flow and energy metabolism in the human brain, Kety was understandably uncertain about whether physiologists, not psychiatrists, could thrive in a government institute specifically targeted towards mental illness. Felix then made a strong sales pitch to him: "I am a psychiatrist, not a scientist. You are the scientist. You will have free range to hire staff, an unrestricted budget, and beds in the new Clinical Center, scheduled to open in 1953."[43] The unique opportunity to direct the research program of what Felix believed would be "the greatest institution for the study of the brain and behavior that the world has ever seen,"[44] the deep pockets of the federal government, and the strong assurance of research freedom to conduct multidisciplinary studies were prospects too enticing to pass up. Kety accepted the offer in May 1951 and became the NIMH's Scientific Director. Not long after that, the range of Kety's authority was further expanded to the NINDB, as the two directors, Felix and Bailey, made a tactical decision to pool their resources to develop a joint basic research program. Aside from providing a practical benefit for the slow-starting NINDB, the two men purported to see synergistic effects that could come from combining basic research in neurological and mental diseases.

Kety was truly the James Shannon of the NIMH and the NINDB. He spent several months drawing up a blueprint for this joint venture, mostly along the lines of scientific disciplines, not specific diseases, and then embarked upon an intensive recruiting campaign, heavily tilted toward scientists in the universities but also open to researchers in the military services and the PHS. The nine-laboratory structure Kety proposed in late 1952 clearly revealed his vision of a balanced, multi-disciplinary approach, covering the broad areas of biological, behavioral, and clinical exploration: biophysics, biochemistry, neurophysiology, pharmacology, anatomical sciences, experimental neuropathology, experimental psychology, epidemiology, and socio-environmental studies. The laboratories would be comprised of two to four sections, which represented further specialized fields (endocrinology, cellular pharma-cology, etc.), specific body parts or functions (spinal cord, vision and special senses, etc.), and other categories (community studies, animal behavior, etc.).

The laboratories that had their roots in the PHS's Division of Mental Hygiene or the NIH's other institutes, such as the Laboratory of Neuro-physiology and the Laboratory of Socio-Environmental Studies, were established immediately, but the others had to go through the arduous process of staffing, especially that of recruiting laboratory chiefs among top-class scientists. Like Shannon, Kety was confronted with academic prejudice against the federal research establishment, and again like Shannon, he could only offer exceptionally high salaries for a limited number of scientists, a promise of research freedom, and the excitement of working in a brand-new institute without having to worry about writing grant proposals. By the time Kety stepped down in 1956 to return to his bench work, the joint NIMH-NINDB intramural basic research program had taken the form of eight laboratories and one field station (the Addiction Research Center), a slight alteration from his original plan. This joint program continued for four more years before eventually being split into two in 1960.[45]

In parallel to the laboratory-oriented basic research program jointly developed by the NIMH and the NINDB, the two institutes' patient-oriented clinical research programs began to take shape. Felix asked Robert A. Cohen, the clinical director of Chestnut Lodge, a small psychoanalytic hospital in Maryland, to join the NIMH to take charge of its clinical research program. A holder of the dual degrees of M.D. and Ph.D. (in neurophysiology), Cohen had previously had a long career of working for the federal government as a medical officer of the U.S. Naval Reserve during World War II. He was a consultant in psychiatry to the National Naval Medical Center, and a member of the Panel on Human Relations and Morale of the Department of Defense, but none-theless he had reservations about accepting Felix's offer. Like Kety, however, Cohen was sold on the unprecedented opportunity he would have to craft a clinical research program from the beginning. By 1958, under his guidance, the NIMH program had grown to have three clinical branches, three laboratories that were integrated with Kety's joint pro-gram, five wards in the Clinical Center, a children's residential treatment center, and a center at St. Elizabeths Hospital.[46] In the meantime, Bailey tapped alumni of the Montreal Neurological Institute, one of the well-known training grounds for neurologists, to fill the key positions in the NINDB's clinical research program, including G. Milton Shy, who was appointed as the clinical director and at the same time as chief of one of the program's four branches. Eventually, Shy became the Scientific Director of the NINDB after its joint basic research program with the NIMH was dissolved.[47]

Space, Money, and Image: Conundrums of Dental Research

As has been described, each institute had to cope with the opportunities and challenges presented in various contexts during its formative years. But none had experienced the kind of problems that the National Institute of Dental Research (NIDR) encountered. For about ten years after its establishment in 1948, the NIDR struggled not only to find the space to house its researchers, but also to secure the funds for both its intramural and extramural programs and to overcome prejudices against dental research among many medical researchers. This decade was a crucial period in which the NIDR had to survive and became recognized as a legitimate member of the NIH community.

Almost from the start, the NIDR's position in leading the nation's dental health research effort was precarious, because there were two other competing divisions within the Public Health Service: the Division of Dental Public Health (in the Bureau of State Services) and the Division of Dental Resources (in the Bureau of Medical Services). These divisions were primarily charged with traditional public health duties, such as providing education on dental health, training health workers, and treating patients in federal or local facilities. However, they were also involved in research projects like the study of the effects of fluoride on the development of dental caries, and their relation to the NIDR was further complicated because of ambiguity in the 1948 National Dental Research Act as to whether dental research appropriations should be used exclusively for the NIDR or for all the dental health programs of the PHS. NIH director Rolla E. Dyer wanted to separate the NIDR's research activities from the PHS's control and treatment programs as much as possible, but he thought that, given the overlapping functions of the new institute and the two divisions, it would be more practical to receive appropriations for all the dental programs and then allocate specific funds to the NIDR. Surgeon General Scheele accepted Dyer's recommendations. It was thus the PHS chief dental officer, not the NIDR director, who had the responsibility for reporting the nation's dental health activities to Congress and discussing the proposed budget with legislators. This situation continued until 1960 when the House Appropriations Committee allowed the NIDR to submit a separate budget.[48]

The extramural program of the NIDR was set in motion in 1949 immediately with the formation of the National Advisory Dental Research Council, which was composed of dental experts and lay advocates. For its intramural program, there was already a core research group of less than a dozen investigators at the NIH, mostly in the section on dental research in the Laboratory of Physiology of the Experimental Biology and Medicine Institute. The chief of the group was H. Trendley Dean, a commissioned officer who had led dental research at the NIH since 1931 and had been one of the prime movers for the creation of the NIDR. It was thus no surprise that Dean was appointed as the NIDR's first director. Dean was actively engaged in recruiting additional staff members and tweaking the overall structure of the program along the lines of laboratory research and clinical research, a pattern commonly adopted at the NIH. On the side of laboratory research, he established sections on oral biochemistry, oral bacteriology, functional morphology, and epidemiology; and on the clinical side, he planned to create sections for dental and periodontal diseases, dental equipment and materials, and growth and development.[49]

But the thorny question was the location of these programs. Dyer insisted that the NIDR should be located on the grounds of the Bethesda campus as an integral part of the NIH. One option was to house the NIDR research staff either in the future Clinical Center or in a space vacated by other institutes. This idea was rejected by Dean and other senior staff of the NIDR who favored the other option of constructing a separate new building for dental research, as authorized by the 1948 National Dental Research Act. It took ten years to get the construction bill signed into law, however, and the ordeal finally ended with the opening of a new building for dental research in 1961. Until that time, the NIDR's intra-mural program was dispersed in various places: some of the research work stayed in Bethesda, but other sections had to be carried out at field stations, including one at the PHS Hospital on Staten Island, New York, and another at the Eastman Dental Dispensary of Rochester, New York. The NIDR also maintained an office at Grand Rapids, Michigan, in connection with the water fluoridation studies. A 1955 report clearly indicated the acute space problem:

> By being an integral part of the National Institutes of Health, this Institute has access to exceptional research facilities and consultive services which could not be provided otherwise. The scope of the research program of the Institute allows the widest range of scientific freedom to its staff. The only detrimental aspect of the environment is the lack of ade-quate laboratory space which handicaps activities in several important research areas.[50]

The inadequate laboratory space was not the only major problem. The level of funding for the NIDR, always the lowest within the NIH, reflected both the lack of congressional support and the shortage of dental researchers.[51] The NIDR's funding situation was much relieved when it received $6 million in appropriations for fiscal year 1957, includ-ing $3.7 million for grants and fellowships. This was a quantum leap from the half million dollars appropriated in the previous year for these budget items. It was the first time that the amount of extramural funding exceeded that of intramural funding for the NIDR.[52]

The NIDR's third major problem was staffing. Recruiting top-class senior scientists or young talent required special efforts by all institutes, but the NIDR was faced with a unique situation. First, few graduates from dental schools elected research or teaching careers. Very little basic research was taught and conducted in dental schools, and fellowships and scholarships to support graduate education for research careers were generally few. The recruitment of non-dental scientific personnel was not easy, either. "Too few persons who prepare for research careers in the basic sciences ever consider dental research," the NIDR recognized in a 1955 report. "This may be attributed to many factors, such as the feeble emotional appeal of dental diseases, the usual lack of on-the-campus communication between graduate schools and dental schools, the general knowledge that funds for the support of dental research are hard to get and that research-teaching positions on dental school staffs are very limited."[53] Although the situation was gradually improving in the fellowship area, thanks to the NIDR's extramural program, finding investigators competent in fields of clinical research (namely, those who had graduate training in basic sciences and had received specialty training after graduation) was further complicated by the enormous salary disparity between dental researchers and practitioners.

Under these circumstances, the appointment of Seymour J. Kreshover as the Scientific Director of the NIDR in 1956 was especially noteworthy. A holder of three doctoral degrees–a D.D.S. from the University of Pennsylvania School of Dentistry, a Ph.D. in clinical medicine and pathology from Yale University, and an M.D. from New York University School of Medicine–Kreshover had impressive research credentials in the fields of oral pathology and embryology and congenital malformations.[54] Not only was he able to reinvigorate the intramural program with his enthusiasm, but he also helped to upgrade the general image of dental research within the NIH community. "In the relatively brief span of 12 years since the establishment of the National Institute of Dental Research, the unfolding pattern of program activities has been characterized, perhaps most significantly, by a redefinition of dentistry's scope of research," he said in the 1960 annual review of the program. To Kreshover, the intellectual hierarchy or barrier between dental research and other scientific and medical research should be abolished. He argued:

> With early emphasis directed toward the development, on a foundation of existing scientific knowledge, of a rational basis for understanding the natural history of the teeth and their supporting structures in health and disease, there rapidly evolved an era of unprecedented productivity. Today's assets may be measured, in part, by the removal of much of the artificial but traditionally structured separation of dental research from the total body of the biological and medical sciences. With this accomplishment has come new breadth,

new responsibility, and new meaning to dental research. How better to herald this new era of understanding than not, without a raising of eyebrows, the essentially unchanged direction and significance of a scientist's research program as he moves organizationally to or from one of the other categorical Institutes of the NIH.[55]

Kreshover's remarks reflected the new opportunities that had opened for dental research. Like medical research on other body parts or physiological functions, dental research became perceived as firmly grounded on scientific reasoning and methodology. There was no longer the need to attach "oral" to the titles of laboratories and branches, as is revealed in the 1960 organizational chart of the NIDR intramural program. They were now the Laboratory of Biochemistry, the Laboratory of Microbiology, the Laboratory of Histology and Pathology, the Epidemiology and Biometry Branch, and the Clinical Investigations Branch. One has to look at the titles of sections to find such terms as "dental caries" and "calcification." Otherwise, it is almost impossible to tell whether these laboratories and branches belonged to the NIDR or to other categorical institutes.

The Dual Structure of the NIH Intramural Program

Kreshover's observation on the personnel movement across categorical institutes, i.e., along disciplinary lines, indicated the existence of the disciplinary structure in operation within the categorical one. This dual structure—formally categorical but informally disciplinary—was developed as a distinct feature of the NIH intramural program. The idea of creating a new institute devoted to a specific discipline, such as an Institute of Biochemistry, was still floating but not warmly received. Sebrell, the NIH Director from 1950 to 1955, recalled discussions on how to structure research on the Bethesda campus. "One approach envisioned a large autonomous organization in biochemistry, housed in one building, that would serve all the Institutes," he said. "And there was a great deal of argument for this—greater interchange of information, closer association, and so on. What we finally adopted was the opposite: every Institute having its own laboratory of biochemistry. I never felt any unhappiness with this."[56]

A similar proposal was submitted in the late 1950s to create an Institute of Physical Biology, one that would house state-of-the-art physical instruments in one building and provide services for other institutes. Stetten, the NIAMD's Scientific Director, was the man behind this idea, which did not materialize because of the lack of appropriations for the construction of such a building.[57] It was a hard sell in Congress. On the contrary, the benefits of housing different disciplines in one categorical institute were obvious in terms of funding expediencies. But there were other reasons, as Sebrell pointed out:

> I think it would have been a mistake had we created disciplinary institutes, and I was very happy to see the categorical programs go ahead on their own with independent biochemical research units in several institutes. I think this was the way to do it: scientists working in the same general field, but with different ideas, different labs, a certain amount of independence and competition. If a biochemical Institute had been created, I think we would have had real troubles.[58]

In a sense, the NIH intramural program was a microcosm of the whole biomedical enterprise that grew by leaps and bounds in the postwar context. The dual review system of the extramural program—one tier of review by study sections composed of specialists in research fields, and the other by advisory councils composed of specialists and laymen— was gradually put in place to deal with concerns about the potential conflict between the disciplinary organization of science and the categorical funding. The scientists were assured that their proposals would be reviewed by their peers, but at the same time they had to accept the new rules of the game by which societal needs would be seriously considered in research funding. At stake was the research freedom of individual investigators in the new era of federal funding for biomedical research. Where to draw the line between research freedom and research planning? How to steer the nation's fast-growing biomedical research enterprise without encroaching upon the autonomy of universities and medical schools? Indeed, the extramural community faced the same kind of conundrum as its intramural counterpart did in understanding and handling the tension between the categorical mission and the scientific aims of research.

Notes

I am deeply grateful to Victoria A. Harden for my intellectual and professional growth at the NIH. Alan N. Schechter has been a source of insightful perspectives on the NIH and NIH people, past and present. I also wish to express my thanks to Philip Chen, P. Boon Chuck, Caroline Hannaway, and Henry Metzger for their invaluable comments on earlier versions of this article.

1. Ronald Reagan, "National Institutes of Health Centennial Year: A Proclamation," 15 Oct. 1986; Senate Joint Resolution 395, "To designate the period October 1, 1986, through September 30, 1987, as 'National Institutes of Health Centennial Year,'" 13 August 1986, 99th Congress, 2nd Session. Both documents, along with a number of news clippings, are collected in Judi Abramson, "Centennial Highlights," Office of NIH History, NIH, Bethesda, Maryland.

2. The 1987 NIH obligation for academic R&D was $3.9 billion, more than a half of the total, $7.3 billion, for all federal agencies. In contrast, the National Science Foundation's contribution was $1 billion. Daniel S. Greenberg, *Science, Money, and Politics: Political Triumph and Ethical Erosion* (Chicago: University of Chicago Press, 2001), Appendix, Table 4. For the study of the NIH around 1987, see Institute of Medicine, *A Healthy Intramural Program: Structural Changes or Administrative Remedies?* (Washington D.C.: National Academies Press, 1988).

3. John Harley Warner, "Ideals of Science and Their Discontents in Late-Nineteenth-Century American Medicine," *Isis*, 1991, *82*: 454-78; Elizabeth Fee, *Disease and Discovery: A History of the Johns Hopkins School of Hygiene and Public Health* (Baltimore, Maryland: Johns Hopkins University Press, 1987), chap. 1; Nancy Tomes, *The Gospel of Germs* (Cambridge, Massachusetts: Harvard University Press, 1998).

4. Victoria A. Harden, *Inventing the NIH: Federal Biomedical Research Policy, 1887-1937* (Baltimore, Maryland: Johns Hopkins University Press, 1986).

5. Public Health Service, *Annual Report of the Surgeon General of the Public Health Service of the United States for the Fiscal Year 1939* (Washington, D.C.: U.S. Government Printing Office, 1939). Among the four existing divisions, the larger Division of Pathology and Bacteriology was broken up into three smaller Divisions of Infectious Diseases, of Pathology, and of Biologics Control. The NIH was also responsible for administering the newly established National Cancer Institute.

6. Public Health Service, *Annual Report of the United States Public Health Service for the Fiscal Year 1944* (Washington, D.C.: U.S. Government Printing Office, 1944).

7. This can be contrasted with the vast body of literature on the history of the physical sciences during the Cold War. For a general overview of the NIH's transformation after World War II, see Harden, *Inventing the NIH*, epilogue; Daniel M. Fox, "The Politics of the NIH Extramural Program, 1937-1950,"

Journal of the History of Medicine and Allied Sciences, 1987, *42*: 447-66; Stephen P. Strickland, *Politics, Science, and Dread Disease: A Short History of United States Medical Research Policy* (Cambridge, Massachusetts: Harvard University Press, 1972); Donald C. Swain, "The Rise of a Research Empire: NIH, 1930 to 1950," *Science*, 1962, *138*: 1233-38; G. Burroughs Mider, "The Federal Impact on Biomedical Research," in *Advances in American Medicine: Essays at the Bicentennial*, ed. John Z. Bowers and Elizabeth F. Purcell, 2 vols. (New York: Josiah Macy, Jr., Foundation and the National Library of Medicine, 1976), 2: 806-71. On the role of voluntary health organizations in emphasizing the categorical approach to medical research, see Angela N. H. Creager, *The Life of a Virus: Tobacco Mosaic Virus as an Experimental Model, 1930-1965* (Chicago: University of Chicago Press, 2002), and her article in this volume. On some of the social factors that attracted academic researchers to the NIH intramural program, see Buhm Soon Park, "The Development of the Intramural Research Program at the National Institutes of Health after World War II," *Perspectives in Biology and Medicine,* 2003, *46*: 383-402.

8. On Voegtlin's style of research administration, see Michael B. Shimkin, "As Memory Serves–An Informal History of the National Cancer Institute, 1937-57," *Journal of the National Cancer Institute*, 1977, *59*: 559-600. For the history of NCI in general, see William A. Yaremchuk, "The Origins of the National Cancer Institute," *Journal of the National Cancer Institute*, 1977, *59*: 551-58; Richard A. Rettig, *Cancer Crusade: The Story of the National Cancer Act of 1971* (Princeton, New Jersey: Princeton University Press, 1977); James T. Patterson, *The Dread Disease: Cancer and Modern American Culture* (Cambridge, Massachusetts: Harvard University Press, 1987); Nancy Carol Erdey, "Armor of Patience: The National Cancer Institute and the Development of Medical Research Policy in the United States, 1937-1971" (Ph.D. thesis, Case Western Reserve University, 1995).

9. Victoria A. Harden, *Rocky Mountain Spotted Fever: History of a Twentieth-Century Disease* (Baltimore, Maryland: Johns Hopkins University Press, 1990).

10. Shimkin, "As Memory Serves," p. 573.

11. See David Cantor's article in this volume.

12. Shimkin, "As Memory Serves," pp. 589-90.

13. For the NCI's contributions to the development of tissue culture technique, see Virginia J. Evans and Katherine K. Sanford, "The Tissue Culture Section, NCI," in *NIH: An Account of Research in Its Laboratories and Clinics*, ed. DeWitt Stetten, Jr., and W. T. Carrigan (New York: Academic Press, 1984), pp. 88-98. On Harry Eagle, see A. Gilman, "Presentation of the Academy Medal to Harry Eagle, M. D.," *Bulletin of the New York Academy of Medicine,* 1970, *46*: 666-69.

14. Shimkin, "As Memory Serves," p. 575.

15. Public Health Service, *National Institutes of Health, Report for the Period July 1, 1951 to December 31, 1952* (NIH internal document), p. 4, NIH Library, Bethesda, Maryland. There is no specific indication as to who wrote this

introductory statement for the part on laboratory research, although it was most likely written by G. Burroughs Mider. In later annual reports, however, the names of Scientific Directors appeared on such introductions.

16. Public Health Service, General Circular No. 12, "Establishment of the Experimental Biology and Medicine Institute in the National Institute of Health," (11 December 1947), (Revised 8 October 1948), Record Group (RG) 443, Entry, Box 70, National Archives, College Park, Maryland. The Laboratory of Physical Biology was added in 1948 to the EBMI, which had originally been comprised of three units: the Division of Physiology, the Chemistry Laboratory, and the Pathology Laboratory. They were respectively renamed as the Laboratory of Biochemistry and Nutrition, the Laboratory of Chemistry and Chemotherapy, and the Laboratory of Pathology and Pharmacology. For the ideal of basic science at the time of the creation of the EBMI, see R. D. Lillie to Rolla E. Dyer (14 November 1947), RG 443, Entry, Box 70, National Archives.

17. For biographical information on Wilder and Daft, see National Institutes of Health, *NIH Almanac 1969*, pp. 41-42, Office of NIH History. On the role of Sebrell in recruiting Wilder, see William Henry Sebrell, "Oral History Interview," by Albert Siepert, William T. Carrigan, and John E. Fletcher, 8-9 December 1970, p. 174, National Library of Medicine (NLM), Bethesda, Maryland.

18. Among others who left the NIH before 1955 were J. L. Strominger who took a Markle Scholarship (administered by Washington University School of Medicine in St. Louis); Elijah Adams who accepted an offer of an associate professorship at New York University School of Medicine; E. A. Hawk who left to direct clinical nutrition investigations for the Upjohn Company; George E. Daniel who accepted "a much more responsible and remunerative research position" with the Armed Forces; and James Peers who became head of the Department of Pathology at Loyola University, Chicago. See National Institutes of Health, "The Program of the National Institute of Arthritis and Metabolic Diseases," Part V, a report submitted to the National Science Foundation Special Committee on Medical Research in 1955, MSC 419, Box 2, Folder 12, NLM.

19. Arthur Kornberg, *For the Love of Enzymes: The Odyssey of a Biochemist* (Cambridge, Massachusetts: Harvard University Press, 1989), p. 129. According to a survey conducted in the early 1950s, there were "substantial minorities," who did "feel that the proposed benefits [of establishing the Clinical Center] are not likely to be realized." University of Michigan Survey Research Center, *Human Relations in a Research Organization: A Study of the National Institutes of Health* (NIH Internal Report, 1953), General Summary, pp. 12-46, Office of NIH History.

20. National Institute of Arthritis and Metabolic Diseases, *Report of Program Activities, 1956* (NIH internal document), p. 22, NIH Library.

21. Public Health Service, General Circular No. 55, "Establishment of the Microbiological Institute in the National Institutes of Health" (8 October 1948), RG 443, Entry, Box 70, National Archives. The three research units were renamed respectively as the Laboratory of Infectious Diseases, the Laboratory of Tropical Diseases and the Laboratory of Biologics Control. There was no name change for the Rocky Mountain Laboratory.

22. Charles V. Kidd, "American Universities and Federal Research Funds" (Ph.D. dissertation, Harvard University, 1957), pp. 41, 283-84.

23. Dorland J. Davis, "Oral History Interview," by Victoria A. Harden, 27 February 1985, Office of NIH History. Also quoted in Harden, *Rocky Mountain Spotted Fever*, p. 225. Harden gives a detailed account of how this changed perception about infectious diseases affected the research program tackling Rocky Mountain spotted fever.

24. The Microbiological Institute was established by PHS Organization Order No. 20 of General Circular No. 55, effective 1 November 1948. This title was officially changed to the "National Microbiological Institute" on 30 March 1951, by Organization Order No. 29 of General Circular No. 51, Supplement 7, which was issued to restate the institutional mission encompassing the extramural as well as intramural programs. On the general overview of research activities and the budget situation of this institute up to 1955, see National Institutes of Health, "The Program of the National Microbiological Institute," a report submitted to the National Science Foundation Special Committee on Medical Research, MSC 419, Box 3, Folder 10, NLM. On the years between 1950 and 1953, see Public Health Service, *National Institutes of Health, Report for the Fiscal Year July 1, 1950 to June 30, 1951*, pp. 109-46; Public Health Service, *National Institutes of Health, Report for the Period July 1, 1951 to December 31, 1952*, pp. 99-124.

25. National Institutes of Health, "The Program of the National Microbiological Institute," Part III, p. 2.

26. Ibid., pp. 2-3. For the reasons why "allergy" was adopted instead of "immunology," see Sheldon G. Cohen and William R. Duncan, "Immunology and NIAID, 1887-1970," in *National Institute of Allergy and Infectious Diseases*, ed. Harriet R. Greenwald and Victoria A. Harden (Bethesda, Maryland: National Institutes of Health, 1987), pp. 82-84. Based on their personal communications with Hass, Cohen and Duncan wrote: "Instead, in the choice of *allergy* for the Institute's new name, consideration was given to the scientific acceptability of this term within a global interpretation that would include the study of immune functions and disorders. At the same time, it would satisfy those who believed that NIH had lacked involvement with and concern for that large segment of the public afflicted by allergic disorders."

27. National Institute of Allergy and Infectious Diseases, *Annual Report of Program Activities 1956* (NIH internal document), p. 1, NIH Library.

28. See, for example, Public Health Service, *Annual Report of the Surgeon General of the Public Health Service of the United States for the Fiscal Year 1940* (Washington, D.C.: U.S. Government Printing Office, 1941), pp. 66-68.

29. Public Health Service, *Annual Report of the United States Public Health Service for the Fiscal Year 1944* (Washington, D.C.: U.S. Government Printing Office, 1944), p. 31.

30. For Van Slyke's biographical information, see National Institutes of Health, *NIH Almanac 1969*, p. 30. It was also Dyer and Topping who persuaded Van Slyke to take the directorship of the NHI. Topping recalled, "The first thing Van Slyke said was that the institute needed a Scientific Director." Topping also said that he had known Shannon during the war for Shannon's important role in malaria research, and that he began to court Shannon when they met at a scientific meeting in early 1949. Norman Topping, *Recollections* (Los Angeles: University of Southern California Press, 1990), pp. 104-5. For a sketchy, personal account of the history of the institute, see Ernestine Taylor Lanahan, *A Salute to the Past: A History of the National Heart, Lung, and Blood Institute Based on Personal Recollections* (Bethesda, Maryland: National Institutes of Health, 1987).

31. On Shannon, see Thomas J. Kennedy, Jr., "James Augustine Shannon," *Biographical Memoirs of the National Academy of Sciences*, 1998, *75*: 357-78.

32. As the science writer Robert Kanigel has observed, "Goldwater was a preview of what he would do, on a larger scale, at the National Institutes of Health." Robert Kanigel, *Apprentice to Genius: The Making of a Scientific Dynasty* (Baltimore, Maryland: Johns Hopkins University Press, 1993), p. 18.

33. Irvin Stewart, *Organizing Scientific Research for War: The Administrative History of the Office of Scientific Research and Development* (Boston: Little, Brown and Company, 1948), pp. 114-15; Margaret Humphreys, *Malaria: Poverty, Race, and Public Health in the United States* (Baltimore, Maryland: Johns Hopkins University Press, 2001), pp. 140-54.

34. Barbara J. Culliton, "NIH Policymaker: A Fundamentalist Takes the Number Two Spot at NIH," *Science News*, 15 March 1969, *95*: 263-64.

35. On the three-layered structure of the intramural program of the NHI, see Public Health Service, *National Institutes of Health Report 1950-51*, pp. 45-100; Public Health Service, *National Institutes of Health Report 1951-52*, pp. 41-85. See also Margaret W. Rossiter, "IOM Case Study of the National Heart, Lung, and Blood Institute," a draft in January 1984 for the Panel on Historical Issues of the Committee for the study of the Organizational Structure of the National Institutes of Health, Office of NIH History.

36. On the wartime malarial program as a model for research coordination at NIH, see Leo B. Slater, "Malaria Chemotherapy and the 'Kaleidoscopic' Organisation of Biomedical Research During World War II," *Ambix*, 2004, *51*: 107-34; Marcel H. Bickel, "Das amerikanische Malaria-Programm (1941-1946) und seine Folgen für die biomedizinische Forschung nach dem Zweiten Weltkrieg," *Gesnerus*, 1999, *56*: 107-19.

37. Kanigel, *Apprentice to Genius*, pp. 20–30.

38. Kanigel, *Apprentice to Genius*, pp. 66-89, quote on p. 69. See also Kennedy, "Laboratory of Kidney and Electrolyte Metabolism," pp. 328-29.

39. For more information on how Shannon staffed the intramural program of the National Heart Institute, see Park, "Development of the Intramural Research Program." pp. 391-94.

40. On the early history of the NIMH and the NINDB, see Ingrid G. Farreras, Caroline Hannaway, and Victoria A. Harden, eds., *Mind, Brain, Body, and Behavior: Foundations of Neuroscience and Behavioral Research at the National Institutes of Health* (Amsterdam: IOS Press, 2004); and Lewis P. Rowland, *NINDS at 50: An Incomplete History Celebrating the Fiftieth Anniversary of the National Institute of Neurological Disorders and Stroke* (New York: Demos Medical Publishing, 2003). See also Gerald N. Grob, *From Asylum to Community: Mental Health Policy in Modern America* (Princeton, New Jersey: Princeton University Press, 1991), chap. 3.

41. Robert Felix, "Oral History Interview," by George Rosen, 8 February 1963, MSC 203, Box 1, Folder Felix, NLM, quoted in Farreras, et al., eds., *Mind, Brain, Body, and Behavior*, p. 10. See also Sebrell, "Oral History Interview," pp. 145-46. Sebrell said: "Then, as the treatment of mental disease with drugs came along, Felix began to change. But the type of mental research they were doing for awhile in the Clinical Center did not appeal to me. Being the kind of research man I was, I didn't call it research. They had a man who played a guitar for the little murderous children as a research project."

42. On the history of neurology in the United States, see Russell N. DeJong, *A History of American Neurology* (New York: Raven Press, 1982); Lawrence C. McHenry, "The Founding of the American Neurological Association and the Origin of American Neurology," *Annals of Neurology*, 1983, *14*: 153-54; William F. Windle, ed., "The Beginning of Experimental Neurology," *Experimental Neurology*, 1976, *51*: 277-80. For Bailey's view, see Pearce Bailey, "National Institute of Neurological Diseases and Blindness: Origins, Founding, and Early Years (1950 to 1959)," in *The Nervous System: A Three-Volume Work Commemorating the 25th Anniversary of the National Institute of Neurological and Communicative Disorders and Stroke, Vol. 1: The Basic Neurosciences*, ed. Donald B. Tower and Roscoe O. Brady (New York: Raven Press, 1975), pp. xxi-xxxii; idem, "American's First National Neurologic Institute," *Neurology (Minneap.)*, 1953, *3*: 321. See also Pearce Bailey, "Oral History Interview," by Wyndham D. Miles, 7 October 1964, OH 149, Box 1, NLM. Quote is from the interview, which is cited in Farreras, et al., eds., *Mind, Brain, Body, and Behavior*, p. 21.

43. Seymour S. Kety, "Oral History Interview," by Lewis P. Rowland, 2 Apr. 2000, quoted in Rowland, *NINDS at 50*, p. 24.

44. Seymour S. Kety, "Mental Illness and the Sciences of Brain and Behavior," *Nature Medicine*, 1999, *5*: 1114. For Kety's biographical information, see Philip S. Holzman, "Seymour S. Kety," *Nature Medicine*, 2000, *6*: 727.

45. On the formation of this joint program, see Farreras, et al., eds., *Mind, Brain, Body, and Behavior*, pp. 33-56.

46. Ibid., pp. 57-63. On Cohen's recollections, see ibid., pp. 183-200; and on his clinical research of schizophrenia, see Robert A. Cohen, "Studies on the Etiology of Schizophrenia," in *NIH: An Account of Research in Its Laboratories and Clinics*, ed. Stetten, Jr., and Carrigan, pp. 12-34.

47. The Montreal Neurological Institute, founded in 1934 at McGill University by the Rockefeller Foundation, the neurology program of the Veterans Administration, and the NINDB, filled the academic training gap during the early years of neurological studies, according to Donald B. Tower who was a section chief in Shy's Medical Neurology Branch and would eventually become the institute director. See Donald B. Tower, "The 1950s Clinical Program at the NINDB," in Farreras, et al., eds., *Mind, Brain, Body, and Behavior*, pp. 295-300; Tower, "Neurosciences–Basic and Clinical," pp. 46-70.

48. The Public Health Service's dental health organizations evolved over time. The 1944 PHS Reorganization Act consolidated the position of chief dental officer at the level of an assistant surgeon general in the PHS, and a section on dental health was established in the Bureau of State Services. In 1949 the function of this section was enlarged and divided into the Division of Dental Public Health and the Division of Dental Resources. In 1960, these two merged to form the Division of Dental Public Health and Resources. On the legislation of the National Dental Research Act, Dyer's effort to make the new institute an integral part of the NIH, and the rivalry over dental research in the PHS, see Ruth Roy Harris, *Dental Science in a New Age: A History of the National Institute of Dental Research* (Rockville, Maryland: Montrose Press, 1989), chaps. 4 and 6.

49. For the laboratory research programs of the NIDR in the early 1950s, see Public Health Service, *National Institutes of Health, Report for the Period July 1, 1951 to December 31, 1952*, pp. 103-6. No clinical program was yet established.

50. National Institutes of Health, "The Program of the National Institute of Dental Research," Part V, a report submitted to the National Science Foundation Special Committee on Medical Research, MSC 419, Box 3, Folder 1, NLM.

51. In 1955, the NCI would get $25 million; NHI $19 million; NIMH $18 million; NIAMD $11 million; NINDB $10 million; NMI (i.e., NIAID) $8 million; and NIDR $2 million. There was also $6 million appropriated for non-categorical general research and service activities. Dean, who retired in 1953 from the NIDR directorship, complained strongly to the National Science Foundation special committee investigating the administration of the NIH: "This disparaging amount, $2,136,000, does not even represent the amount expended by the National Institute of Dental Research for research. Included in this sum are the amounts spent by the Services' dental

public health activities in the Bureau of State Services, and the amount spent by the Division of Dental Resources in the Bureau of Medical Services." H. Trendley Dean to Joseph W. Pisani, 9 September 1955, MSC 419, Box 1, Folder 14, NLM. The NSF special committee recommended no major expansion of the NIH intramural program and no increase in the number of categorical institutes but agreed that, "in general, the present level of support of the intramural programs of all Institutes except those of Microbiology and of Dental Research is adequate." Special Committee on Medical Research, "Medical Research Activities of the Department of Health, Education and Welfare," December 1955, pp. 22-23, MSC 419, Box 1, Folder 1, NLM.

52. National Institutes of Health, *NIH Almanac 1969*, p. 49, Office of NIH History.

53. National Institutes of Health, "The Program of the National Institute of Dental Research," pp. 1-3.

54. National Institutes of Health, *NIH Almanac 1969*, p. 49. In 1966, Kreshover was appointed director of the NIDR, succeeding Francis A. Arnold, Jr., who became the PHS's chief dental officer.

55. National Institute of Health, *Review of Intramural Research 1960* (NIH internal document), p. 343, Office of NIH History.

56. Sebrell, "Oral History Interview," p. 141.

57. "Physical Biology Building," minutes of the Scientific Directors' meeting, 21 December 1959, Office of NIH History. See also minutes of 20 January 1960, 3 February 1960, and 16 March 1960.

58. Sebrell, "Oral History Interview," p. 141.

The National Institute of Mental Health and Mental Health Policy, 1949-1965

Gerald N. Grob

"For too many Americans with mental illnesses, the mental health services and supports they need remain fragmented, disconnected and often inadequate, frustrating the opportunity for recovery. Today's mental health care system is a patchwork relic–the result of disjointed reforms and policies. Instead of ready access to quality care, the system presents barriers that all too often add to the burden of mental illnesses for individuals, their families, and our communities." These were the words of Chairman Michael F. Hogan in transmitting the final report of George W. Bush's President's New Freedom Commission on Mental Health in 2003.[1]

That the mental health system would be so troubled at the beginning of the twenty-first century would have come as a shock to the advocates of change who had labored long and hard after World War II to abolish traditional mental hospitals and create a new system that would provide care and treatment of persons with serious mental disorders in the community. Indeed, they believed that a new era had been inaugurated with the passage of the Community Mental Health Centers Act of 1963. In their eyes a novel institution would replace obsolete and ineffective institutions and thus transform mental health policy in fundamental ways.

What were the origins of a new policy that eventually came to be known as deinstitutionalization, and why did it fail to live up to its promise? What role did the federal government in general and the National Institute for Mental Health (NIMH) in particular play in hastening policy changes? Why did novel policies fail to achieve goals that, at least in theory, held out the promise of a better life for persons with severe and persistent mental illnesses?

The answers to these intriguing questions are anything but simple. A variety of factors played a role in creating alternatives to institutional care of persons with mental disorders: humanistic and egalitarian ideologies that were so common after 1945 (in part a response to the perceived threat of totalitarian regimes); the emphasis on environmental etiologies in the social and behavioral sciences; the emergence of a literature that was critical of mental hospitals (as well as other institutions) and their dehumanizing impact upon individuals; the spiraling costs associated with hospital care; the introduction of new biological and psychosocial therapies; and radical critiques of capitalist societies. Equally important was the entrance of the federal government into a policy arena traditionally reserved for states. Moreover, the unique structure of American politics gave rise to a process of change that transformed policies and led to outcomes that were neither anticipated nor desired.

******

At the time of their creation in the early nineteenth century asylums were widely regarded as the symbol of an enlightened and progressive nation that no longer ignored or mistreated its insane citizens. The justification for such institutions appeared self-evident: they benefited the community, family, and individual by offering effective treatment for acute cases and humane custodial care for long-duration cases. In providing such services, states met their ethical responsibilities and contributed to the general welfare by limiting, if not eliminating, the spread of disease and dependency. By 1945 state hospitals had a daily resident population of about 430,000; approximately 88,000 were first-time admissions.

Yet, within a short time, mental hospitals slowly began to lose their social and medical legitimacy as the prevailing consensus on mental health policy dissolved. The experiences of the military during World War II in successfully treating soldiers manifesting psychiatric symptoms and returning them to their units led to a faith that outpatient treatment in the community was more effective than confinement in remote institutions that shattered established social relationships. The war also hastened the emergence of psychodynamic and psychoanalytic psychiatry with its emphasis on the importance of life experiences and socioenvironmental factors. Taken together, these changes contributed to the belief that early intervention in the community would be effective in preventing subsequent hospitalization and thus avoiding chronicity. Finally, the introduction of psychological and somatic therapies (including, but not limited to, psychotropic drugs) held out the promise of a more normal existence for persons with mental illnesses outside of institutions.[2]

By themselves these developments might not have resulted in major policy changes. What was required was a catalyst capable of transforming policy by shifting authority from forty-eight state governments to a central agency having a vision of a national policy. The role of catalyst was taken by the federal government, whose functions had increased dramatically as a result of the Great Depression of the 1930s and World War II. After 1945 it assumed a leadership role in the formulation of social welfare and health policies.

Traditionally, mental health had been a state responsibility. Prior to World War II the federal government played virtually no role. A Division of Mental Hygiene had been created within the Public Health Service (PHS) in 1930, but it dealt largely with narcotic addiction. In the late 1930s, Dr. Lawrence Kolb, its head, led an effort to create a National Neuropsychiatric Institute modeled in part after the National Cancer Institute (established in 1937). The initiative, however, failed as war-related concerns overwhelmed domestic issues.[3]

By 1945 conditions appeared propitious for change. Under Surgeon General Thomas Parran, the PHS had begun to lay the foundation for a major extramural research program within the National Institute of Health. The enactment of the Hill-Burton Act the following year, which provided generous subsidies for hospital construction, was another symbol of an expanding federal role. At the same time an emerging health lobby began to promote massive federal funding for biomedical research. Nowhere was the growing support for medical science better reflected than in President Harry S. Truman's Scientific Research Board, which not only expressed faith in medical progress but insisted on the necessity of a "national policy."[4]

These initiatives, however, excluded mental disorders despite the fact that hundreds of thousands of patients resided in the nation's state hospitals.

Psychiatry, once an elite specialty, had become a stepchild within medicine and lacked the prestige of other specialties. The task of integrating mental health within the burgeoning federal biomedical policy role was undertaken by Dr. Robert H. Felix, who had succeeded Kolb as head of the Division of Mental Hygiene.

Born in Kansas in 1904, Felix received both his undergraduate and medical degrees from the University of Colorado in 1926 and 1930, respectively. He interned at Colorado General Hospital, and subsequently was awarded a Commonwealth Fund Fellowship in psychiatry. He spent the next two years as a resident working under Franklin G. Ebaugh at Colorado Psychopathic Hospital in Denver. Ebaugh was an early proponent of what subsequently became known as community psychiatry, and in 1940 published an important work emphasizing the need to treat patients with mental disorders in general hospitals and thus avoid lengthy confinement in state institutions.[5] Felix's experiences and training under Ebaugh created an incipient hostility toward institutional care.

Because the Great Depression had made it difficult to succeed in private practice, Felix joined the PHS in 1933 and spent the next eight years at several federal institutions. In 1941 he was assigned to the Johns Hopkins University for training in public health, and received an M.P.H. degree. This experience had a profound impact on his understanding of psychiatry. Taking a public health approach, he became convinced that knowledge of the epidemiology of mental diseases was crucial and that the social and behavioral sciences had much to contribute to an understanding of mental pathology. After a brief stay at the U.S. Coast Guard Academy in Connecticut, he returned to the Mental Hygiene Division and shortly thereafter replaced Kolb as its chief in late 1944.[6]

Parran, undoubtedly one of the most influential figures ever to occupy the office of Surgeon General, was especially supportive of younger career officers and he urged Felix to think about new responsibilities for the Division of Mental Hygiene. Felix in turn resurrected Kolb's proposal for an institute, but in sharply expanded form. Kolb had been primarily concerned with research. Felix was by no means opposed to research. His agenda, however, was to expand substantially the role of the federal government and to use its authority to move away from an institutional toward a community-based policy. In late 1944 he prepared a memorandum sketching out his views. Parran was enthusiastic and promptly put Felix in touch with several key officials at the Federal Security Agency (predecessor of the Department of Health, Education, and Welfare), including Mary Switzer, an individual who played an influential role in federal health and rehabilitation policy in the postwar decades. Together they drafted legislation creating a National Psychiatric Institute whose functions included but transcended research. The draft gave the proposed institute a role in the education and training of professional personnel and in providing psychiatric services. Although denying that he was engaged in lobbying (and perhaps violating the provisions of the Hatch Act), Felix was clearly using his position to influence the legislative process in subtle but significant ways despite the fact that (with the exception of Parran) he had little support within the PHS.[7]

Felix's charisma, his mastery of bureaucratic and organizational politics, and his vision of a sharply expanded role for psychiatry were traits that enabled him to negotiate the treacherous terrain of the Washington scene. He also cultivated close relationships with members of Congress, relationships that were strengthened by his willingness to provide them with assistance in coping with family members and relatives who had psychiatric problems. Felix's draft of the legislation was characteristic. Its broad–even vague–provisions gave him freedom to move in the direction he thought appropriate.[8] Equally important, he believed that basic policy changes were a necessity, but rarely concerned himself with details. For the next twenty years, he and the NIMH were to play crucial roles in the shift from an institutional to a community policy.

The context of American politics only enhanced Felix's importance. From the 1940s to the 1960s, strategically placed individuals and small groups had the ability to play major roles in policy formulation. Federal bureaucrats such as Felix and Mary Switzer, laypersons such as Mary Lasker, and a congressional health lobby that included Senator Lister Hill and Representative John Fogarty, could influence health policies in fundamental ways. After 1970, by contrast, interest groups representing constituencies based on gender, race, class, and ethnicity assumed greater importance. The proliferation of interest groups introduced a new element and gave policymaking a quite different character, thus diminishing the role of individuals.

With a draft in hand and with the support of a small coterie of individuals that included Mary Lasker (who was then beginning her influential career as an advocate for federal funding of biomedical research), Felix sought a cooperative member of Congress to introduce the legislation. Through Switzer, he met J. Percy Priest, a sympathetic Tennessee congressman with an interest in psychiatry and persons with mental illnesses. Acting in a precipitous manner, Priest introduced the bill into the House of Representatives in March 1945. A few months later Claude Pepper, a New Deal Democrat from Florida, sponsored similar legislation in the Senate. After extended hearings in both houses of Congress and assiduous lobbying by Felix and other psychiatric leaders, the bill passed and was signed into law by President Truman on 3 July 1946.[9]

The passage of the National Mental Health Act and formal creation of the NIMH in 1949 thrust the federal government directly into mental health, an arena historically reserved for state governments. The legislation had three basic goals: support of research into the causes, diagnosis, and treatment of psychiatric disorders; training of mental health personnel by providing individual fellowships and institutional grants; awarding grants to states to establish clinics and treatment centers and to fund demonstration studies dealing with the prevention, diagnosis, and treatment of neuropsychiatric disorders. The act provided for a six-member National Advisory Mental Health Council to provide advice and to recommend grants as well as for the creation of the NIMH and an intramural research program. The law authorized $30 million per annum for state programs and research and $7.5 million for a home for the NIMH.[10]

******

The significance of the National Mental Health Act lay not in its specific provisions, but rather in its general goals and, more important, the manner in which it was interpreted and implemented. Indeed, federal policy in succeeding decades would ultimately be shaped less by congressional mandates and appropriations than by the outlook of officials such as Felix charged with the responsibility for administering programs and distributing funds.

By the time he had become NIMH director, Felix's views about the proper shape of mental health policy had matured. Although he remained friendly with both psychodynamic and somatic psychiatrists, he was never identified with either group. Felix's approach reflected the absence of clinical experience in dealing with persons with severe and persistent mental illnesses. Hence he favored a broad public health approach. His underlying belief was that mental disorders represented "a true public health problem," the resolution of which required knowledge about the etiology and nature of mental illnesses, more effective methods of prevention and treatment, and better-trained personnel. Felix shared many of the views of Paul V. Lemkau of Johns Hopkins, an able and influential proponent of a public health approach and author of an important text on the subject. Public health, according to Felix, was concerned with the "collective health" of the community. Unlike clinicians who dealt with individuals, public health workers emphasized "the application and development of methods of mass approach to health problems," including mental illnesses. The NIMH mental health program was designed "to help the individual by helping the community; to make mental health a part of the community's total health program, to the end that all individuals will have greater assurance of an emotionally and physically healthy and satisfying life for themselves and their families."[11]

Felix's agenda required radical changes in the prevailing institutional policy. In a suggestive article in 1948 he and R.V. Bowers insisted that mental hygiene had to be concerned "with more than the psychoses and with more than hospitalized mental illness." Personality, after all, was shaped by socioenvironmental influences. Psychiatry, in collaboration with the social sciences, had to emphasize the problems of the "ambulatory ill and the preambulatory ill (those whose probability of breakdown is high)." The community, not the hospital, was psychiatry's natural habitat, and practitioners had to play a vital role in creating a healthier social order. Only the "reintegration of community life" offered the possibility of reducing mental disorders.[12] Indeed, three years earlier Felix argued that psychiatry had an obligation to "go out and find the people who need help–and that means, in their local communities." Hostile to mental hospitals, he emphasized that the greatest need was for large numbers of outpatient community clinics. Such institutions would avoid the stigmatization associated with mental hospitals and point the way to effective preventive programs.[13] Indeed, the "guiding philosophy" of the NIMH, he told his American Psychiatric Association (APA) colleagues in 1949, "is that the prevention of mental illness, and the production of positive mental health, is an attainable goal."[14]

Cognizant that his policy goals were not achievable in the immediate future, Felix worked to make the NIMH a force in the mental health arena. A shrewd bureaucrat, he persuaded the Surgeon General to place the NIMH within the National Institutes of Health (NIH) rather than the Bureau of State Services, thus linking his organization with other research-oriented entities such as the National Cancer Institute. That the NIMH was indirectly involved in funding services as well as research and training was largely ignored. Indeed, demonstration clinics were placed under the rubric of research. In so doing, Felix was able to exploit the identification of mental health with biomedical science during the 1950s.[15]

The internal organization of the NIMH reflected its broad goals. The Professional Services Branch dealt with long-term planning. Biometrics assumed responsibility for data gathering and analysis. Under the direction of Morton Kramer, this branch worked to develop standardized classifications for data collection that would in turn create the foundation of psychiatric epidemiological analysis. Publication and Reports was charged with the dissemination of information about mental disorders and their prevention. Three extramural branches—Research, Community Services, and Training—were responsible for implementing the grants program (which ultimately accounted for more than three-quarters of the total annual appropriation).[16]

The NIMH also developed a small but significant intramural research program. In 1951 Felix recruited Seymour S. Kety as scientific director, who was given great latitude in developing the program. During the 1950s the intramural program emphasized three kinds of activities: biological research, including neurochemistry, biochemistry, neurophysiology, neurobiology, and neuropharmacology; behavioral research in psychology and such subspecialties as sociology and social anthropology; and clinical investigations in psychiatry and medicine. Nevertheless, Felix was preoccupied with fostering community services, alternatives to hospitalization, and prevention of mental disorders, and hence was never closely involved with the intramural program. Indeed, he saw it largely as a means of gaining congressional support.[17]

******

That Felix's goal was a radical policy transformation was evident in the manner in which he interpreted the National Mental Health Act. In testimony before a congressional subcommittee in 1948, he maintained that the act precluded the use of federal funds for the support of hospitalization in state institutions. Such funds were rather to be used by states to create clinics and other alternatives to institutionalization. The ideal was to have one outpatient mental health clinic for each 100,000 of population; rural areas would be served by traveling clinics. Moreover, it was evident that Felix's vision went far beyond individuals with mental illnesses. He told the subcommittee that if the "mentally ill" included the "emotionally disturbed" as well as those requiring "counseling or guidance or advice," the total would be around eight to ten million persons.[18]

From the very beginning, Felix and the NIMH undertook a variety of innovative activities designed to demonstrate that there were more effective ways of fostering mental health and diminishing the incidence of mental disorders. They included assistance to states, the inclusion of the behavioral sciences and non-medical personnel in mental health activities, and the awarding of research grants. The NIMH provided grants-in-aid to states to assist them in establishing and improving their mental health services. By 1947 every state and territory had designated an agency to prepare plans detailing the use of federal funds and maintaining liaison with the NIMH. Although funds could be used for a variety of purposes, federal officials encouraged states to develop additions, if not alternatives, to traditional mental hospitals. Slowly but surely the NIMH began to create a national constituency favorably disposed to new policy initiatives.[19]

At the outset, congressional funding for the NIMH was modest. Yet Felix was able to deploy small resources in a way that furthered his goal of broadening and moving mental health activities into the community. The state grant-in-aid program, for example, rose from $2 million to $4 million between 1948 and 1958. Yet its impact was by no means of minor significance. By 1951 the NIMH had assisted 342 clinics that served almost 110,000 individuals. Moreover, state matching funds exceeded federal grants. When the NIMH conducted its first survey of outpatient clinics in the mid-1950s, it found nearly 1,300 in existence. In efforts to further its goals, the NIMH also created several demonstration clinics. The first was in Prince Georges County in Maryland, which served both as a showplace for members of Congress and a facility to train NIMH personnel. The most significant impact of the state assistance program, however, was the relationships that developed between the NIMH and health professionals employed in community institutions. The result was the creation of a new professional constituency that grew with leaps and bounds during the second half of the twentieth century. Its members would contribute to the effort to shift mental health services from state hospitals to community institutions, thus creating a potential conflict with their hospital brethren.[20]

That the NIMH—as well as state officials and organizations such as the Milbank Memorial Fund—waxed enthusiastic about community programs was obvious. Nevertheless, little attention was devoted to program evaluation. Claims of accomplishment and effectiveness rested on ideology and faith, and were rarely, if ever, accompanied by empirical data. As early as 1950, a committee of the NIMH National Advisory Mental Health Council recommended that funds be allocated to develop methods "for determining the effectiveness of community mental health programs."[21] Five years later council members expressed concern over "the vagueness surrounding the whole problem of community mental health."[22] After surveying the literature, a subcommittee conceded that there was a "thinness of the efforts of evaluation" as well as "a confusion of levels of conceptualization."[23]

To be sure, the NIMH was not alone in heralding the importance of community mental health clinics and programs. During the 1950s, as well as in later decades, rhetoric rather than data often shaped policy discussions. The belief that many individuals—including those with severe and persistent mental illnesses—could be treated in outpatient clinics was an article of faith even though there was virtually no supporting data. Indeed, data that contradicted prevailing beliefs were all but ignored. A study of the effectiveness of hospital and clinic treatment in comparable psychiatric cases in California resulted in disquieting results. From a sample of state hospital admissions, investigators screened 504 patients in the hope of referring half to clinics. Only 57 were identified as candidates for clinic referral; 20 of the 57 were referred; and 6 were accepted, of whom only 2 kept appointments and demonstrated improvement. The investigators concluded that there were "marked discontinuities in functions" of hospitals and clinics. Individuals requiring a social support network were unsuitable for clinic treatment. The study did not challenge the viability of clinics. But the evidence suggested that the manner in which clinics were conceptualized required modification, and that far greater attention had to be paid to the development of linkages between hospitals and clinics.[24]

Ironically, some of the data calling into doubt many of the generalizations about mental hospitals and the viability of community mental health clinics in treating individuals with severe and persistent mental disorders were generated by Morton Kramer, who served as the chief of the Biometrics Branch from 1949 to 1975.[25] In a pioneering study of more than 15,000 patient cohorts admitted to Warren State Hospital in Pennsylvania between 1916 and 1950, he and his colleagues found that the probability of release of first admissions within twelve months increased from 42 to 62 percent between 1919/1925 and 1946/1950. That many state hospitals had deteriorated dramatically because of the decline in funding during the Depression of the 1930s and the loss of personnel during World War II was true. Yet Kramer's data as well as other studies suggested that popular perceptions of mental hospitals as warehouses and "snakepits" were not entirely accurate. To put it another way, a high proportion of chronic and aged patients in public mental hospitals led many to overlook the reality that substantial numbers of individuals were admitted, treated, and discharged in less than a year. Subsequent studies revealed that the experiences of Warren State Hospital were by no means atypical, suggesting that some patients benefited from hospitalization.[26]

Other data raised even more serious issues. A community policy was based on the expectation that individuals with serious and persistent mental disorders could be treated in non-institutional settings. Underlying this belief were several assumptions: that such individuals had a home; that they had a sympathetic family or other person willing and able to assume responsibility for their care; that the organization of the household would not impede rehabilitation; and that the patient's presence would not cause undue hardships for other family members. In 1960, however, 48 percent of all institutionalized individuals were unmarried, 12 percent were widowed, and 13 percent were divorced or separated. A large proportion of patients, in other words, may have had no families to provide care. The assumption that patients could reside in the community with their families while undergoing rehabilitation was hardly consistent with such data. Indeed, a community-based policy required a range of supportive services that included, but was not limited to, housing. Obviously known to Felix and many of his staff who set the agenda that eventually led to the passage of the Community Mental Health Centers Act in 1963, such data were rarely considered. Moreover, in 1958 nearly a third of all hospitalized patients were sixty-five or older and were incapable of surviving on their own in a community setting. If not provided with care in institutions, what would happen to this group?[27]

Nor were the difficulties of evaluating community-based policies unique. At the same time that Felix was emphasizing a public health agenda, a quite different approach to the treatment of mental disorders was emerging. During the 1950s the introduction of such major tranquilizing drugs as chlorpromazine and reserpine (marketed as Thorazine and Serpasil) as well as antidepressants (iproniazid and impramine) appeared to inaugurate a new era in psychiatry. Although the APA expressed concern about aggressive marketing practices and the indiscriminate use of drugs, there was little doubt that the reception of the new pharmacological agents was favorable and enthusiastic. Their introduction, however, raised once again the thorny problem of evaluation.

At the NIMH, Kramer had become increasingly preoccupied with problems associated with efficacy studies. In 1956 he turned his attention to the new tranquilizing drugs. He first noted that little was known about their safety, their short- and long-term effects, or appropriate dosage levels for different patients and diagnoses. Second, hospital admissions and retention rates were governed by multiple factors, and to attribute the recent decline in hospital populations to drugs was an error. Kramer therefore called for well-designed studies to evaluate therapies. Such studies, he wrote, had to include "carefully defined diagnostic groups of patients, comparable control groups, carefully specified therapeutic plans and staffing patterns, and specific objective criteria for evaluating results of treatment and for determining condition at time of release."[28]

Kramer's cautious approach was shared by Felix as well as staff members from the social and behavioral sciences. By that time many mental health researchers had been chastened by previous unsatisfactory efforts to determine the efficacy of shock therapy and lobotomy, and they were determined to avoid if possible the rapid deployment of therapies of questionable utility. In 1955 Felix appointed an ad hoc committee to study the drug issue. The following year members attending a joint conference sponsored by the NIMH and the National Research Council agreed that the problem of evaluation could not be solved by the kinds of crude clinical trials employed in the past.[29]

External pressures quickly embroiled the NIMH in public controversy for the first time since its creation. The successes of new antibiotic drugs, the activities of pharmaceutical firms, and publicity in the mass media created an almost mystical faith in the redemptive powers of medications. The introduction of such major tranquilizing drugs as chlorpromazine and reserpine was equated to the discovery of antibiotics and the polio vaccine. Mike Gorman, the indefatigable and influential lobbyist who was Mary Lasker's spokesperson, emerged as the champion of the new drugs. He was especially critical of those psychiatrists who were raising troublesome questions and preventing their deployment. In testifying before Congress in 1956 he accused Felix of "dodging this problem of drug evaluation."[30] A few months later he publicly excoriated Felix and referred to Kramer's monograph on evaluation as "drivel."[31]

Felix was distressed by the controversy, but insisted that the NIMH had an obligation to determine efficacy and risks. Any evaluation had to ascertain whether drugs prepared patients for earlier release from the hospital than would otherwise be the case. There was also a need to understand what "drugs do for and to patients, the kinds of changes they induce that are truly psychiatric in nature as distinguished from physiological only, the differential effects by diagnostic categories, age, sex, etc." Gorman's proposal for large-scale studies might serve a public-relations function, but would not meet the needs of clinicians.[32] With some reluctance, Felix bowed to congressional pressure and agreed to establish the

Psychopharmacology Service Center within the NIMH. Evaluation studies proved so problematic that the unit did not begin a collaborative research project involving nine institutions until 1961. Completed in 1964, the study proved a minor landmark because of its relatively sophisticated methodology. The results seemed to demonstrate that phenothiazine therapy for acute cases of schizophrenia was superior to placebos.[33]

******

The pace of change in the years following the end of World War II, however rapid, did not satisfy psychiatric activists. In 1953 Kenneth E. Appel, then APA president and professor of psychiatry at the University of Pennsylvania, called for a study to deal with the "breakdown crisis in the administration of state hospital functions." His model was the famous report by Abraham Flexner on medical education in 1910, a report that hastened the process of change. The eventual result was the creation of the Joint Commission on Mental Illness and Health (JCMIH) in 1955. There was unanimous agreement that the commission would be more effective if it were sponsored by professional organizations rather than the federal government. The lead was taken by the APA and American Medical Association (AMA). In mid-1955 Congress passed the Mental Health Study Act. Under its provisions the federal government endorsed the creation of the JCMIH (which remained a nongovernmental body) and provided a modest level of funding to facilitate its work. During its six-year existence, the commission sponsored a series of studies that culminated with the publication of its famous *Action for Mental Health: Final Report of the Joint Commission on Mental Illness and Health 1961.*[34]

Action for Mental Health provided a compelling case for change. The problem was "the unmet need—those who are untreated and inadequately cared for." Founded to provide therapy and care, state mental hospitals had become dumping grounds for individuals outside the pale of normal society. The report called for much larger investments in research; a national recruitment and training program to alleviate staff shortages and minimize jurisdictional conflicts within the mental health professions; and the creation of community clinics and general hospital psychiatric units. It recommended that no state mental hospital with more than 1,000 beds be constructed, and that institutions with more than 1,000 beds "be gradually and progressively converted into centers for the long-term and combined care of chronic diseases, including mental illness." To achieve such goals, the members of the JCMIH called for a doubling of expenditures for public mental patient services in five years and a tripling in ten. They also asked for a major increase in the federal share; at the end of ten years the national government would pay for 58 percent of all mental health expenditures; the state and local share would be 33 and 8 percent, respectively.[35]

Action for Mental Health was more of a smorgasbord than a precise blueprint that could easily become law; at most it suggested a general direction. What was required was the translation of its broad goals and numerous recommendations into a specific legislative agenda, and then to persuade the executive and legislative branches of the federal government of the necessity to act. Such a task was by no means simple. The JCMIH, after all, represented a relatively narrow constituency. In the larger world of American politics mental health advocates had to compete with a variety of other interest groups, all seeking to advance their own agenda.

The reception of *Action for Mental Health*, although generally favorable, was by no means uncritical or one-sided. Many members of the APA felt that the emphasis on psychotherapy and lay practitioners, as well the failure to give credit to the new psychopharmacology, were misplaced. The American Psychological Association, on the other hand, was critical of the "medical model of mental health and illness."[36]

The sharpest criticism came from state officials. State commissioners of mental health were ambivalent; they questioned whether a national program could take local differences into account. Individuals long identified with traditional state hospitals believed that many of the data and recommendations in the report represented personal opinions and ideology and ignored reality. Newton Bigelow, editor of *Psychiatric Quarterly* and a major figure in the New York state hospital system, insisted that public institutions played a vital role in caring for and treating individuals with severe mental illnesses, a group all too often ignored by psychiatrists in private practice. He also noted the omission of any "humane planning" in *Action for Mental Health* for the large numbers of aged persons in mental hospitals. His most damning criticism was reserved for the recommendation to create institutions for persons with chronic illnesses. "Who will say that there is no hope for this person as opposed to that one in this day of remission of chronic illness?" If anything, there was a pressing need to raise hospital standards rather than to eliminate them. Bigelow's criticisms were echoed by many other state officials.[37]

That the JCMIH had recommended a much greater role for the federal government in mental health was hardly surprising. The experiences of the New Deal and expansion of federal social programs had persuaded many that the national government was better qualified than its state counterparts to deal with pressing social problems. Indeed, the prevailing consensus was that most states had failed to meet their social welfare responsibilities. The tendency to denigrate state governments was also accompanied by an idealization of local communities and local control. This perception, which played an increasingly important role in the 1960s, tended to promote a vision of a federal-local government partnership that bypassed state authority not only in mental health, but in other domestic welfare programs as well as civil rights legislation. Felix and his associates shared these beliefs. In their eyes, states lacked both the knowledge and capacity to undertake meaningful changes; they remained wedded to obsolete mental hospitals. NIMH officials, therefore, were supportive of community alternatives. Committed to a public health approach, they desired to create a system capable of providing therapeutic and preventive services within defined geographical areas.

The internal reaction of NIMH officials to an early draft of the JCMIH final report was revealing. Philip Sapir, chief of the Research Grants and Fellowships Branch, believed that many parts were "pedestrian, platitudinous, rehashes of previous statements, half-truths, or untruths." The draft was "so incredibly bad that there seems almost no point in making specific criticisms."[38] Richard H. Williams of the Professional Services Branch was more polite, but noted that the document failed "to bring much wisdom to the material available."[39] Felix thought that the Commission had placed too much emphasis on "hospital care of patients" and ignored more effective community-based alternatives. The proposal to create hospitals for chronically ill patients was "obsolete."[40]

Despite hostility toward the recommendations of the JCMIH, NIMH officials lacked a specific legislative agenda of their own before 1961. This was not true of state officials and hospital psychiatrists, most of whom resented the attacks on their institutions. Nor were they necessarily opposed to the creation of community-based facilities that had links to hospitals. They persuaded the Surgeon-General to create an Ad Hoc Committee on Planning for Mental Health Facilities. At the beginning of 1961 its members offered a series of recommendations that sharply differed from the JCMIH program. They recommended a plan that provided for partial state support for the replacement of institutional care by the kinds of community mental health services adopted in the mid-1950s by New York and California.[41]

The inauguration of President John F. Kennedy and his call for a New Frontier augured well for those pushing for basic changes in mental health policy. The Democratic Party platform had pledged federal support for research, training, and community mental health programs. Kennedy's staff was equally supportive. Yet the administration was by no means unified. The President and his sister Eunice Shriver were primarily concerned with retardation. Moreover, Shriver was hostile toward psychiatrists because of their seeming preoccupation with persons with psychological problems and mental disorders and neglect of the retarded. Nine months after taking office, Kennedy created the President's Panel on Mental Retardation. At the same time he was facing pressure from others in his administration as well as Congress to take corresponding action in the mental health field.[42]

Caught between conflicting forces, Kennedy followed the advice of Myer Feldman (a key staff advisor) and created an Interagency Task Force on Mental Health at the end of 1961 to consider the recommendations of the JCMIH. Chaired nominally by Abraham Ribicoff, Secretary of the Department of Health, Education and Welfare (DHEW) and his successor Anthony Celebrezze, the group included such figures as Daniel Patrick Moynihan from the Department of Labor, Robert Atwell from the Bureau of the Budget, Felix and his deputy Stanley Yolles, as well as several others.[43]

Several months earlier the NIMH, at the urging of Atwell (who favored non-institutional services), had begun work on a position paper that would provide an alternative to the JCMIH recommendations. Completed in November 1961, the document reflected the unique character of the

NIMH. Most NIH institutes were preoccupied with basic biomedical research. The NIMH, by contrast, was interested primarily in service delivery systems. Its service orientation reflected the public health background of many of its staff and their aversion to traditional mental hospital care.

The NIMH's position paper began with a complimentary allusion to the work of JCMIH, but then went on to express disagreements with many of its recommendations. It specifically rejected the Commission's underlying presumption that the core problem was the care and treatment of persons with mental disorders. The focus rather should have been on "the prevention of mental illness and . . . maintenance of mental health." The document was particularly critical of the recommendation that large state hospitals be converted into centers for the care of persons with chronic illnesses. It recommended a larger federal role and subsidies to encourage states and communities to upgrade their activities in the prevention and treatment of mental disorders.[44]

Two other task forces created by Felix completed their work in the spring of 1962. The first dealt with the status of state mental hospitals. "Despite improvements," the group reported, "the traditional large State mental hospital continues to be the focal point of negative attitudes toward psychiatric treatment." These institutions fostered dependency and were governed by an archaic administrative structure. The task force urged the development of new approaches and the use of federal funds to assist states in formulating new policies.[45]

The second task force offered a comprehensive proposal that mirrored the NIMH preference for a community-oriented public health approach. Its members began with the claim that progress in preventing mental illnesses and the growing commitment to community responsibility for the care, treatment, and rehabilitation for persons with mental illnesses led to an inescapable conclusion, namely, that comprehensive community mental health programs would make it possible "*for the mental hospital as it is now known to disappear from the scene within the next twenty-five years.*" The report supported the creation of a radically new institution—a community center, as compared with a more traditional clinic. Centers would offer a broad spectrum of services and programs: diagnosis and evaluation; inpatient care; day and night care programs;

twenty-four-hour emergency services; rehabilitation; consultative services to community agencies; public information and education; and supervision of foster care. Ultimately, all services within communities and regions–preventive, therapeutic, educational–would be absorbed by comprehensive centers serving designated populations within specific geographical areas. Careful state planning and a dramatic increase in federal funding for planning, training, research, and construction would foster the development of such centers. The role of the NIMH would undergo a corresponding increase; an expanded staff would provide advice and oversee the creation of these new agencies. Oddly enough, the report left a continuing albeit modest role for traditional mental hospitals.[46]

The slowness of the administration to develop a specific legislative agenda came under criticism from both figures such as Gorman as well as key congressional figures.[47] The House Committee on Appropriations, noted Representative John E. Fogarty in March 1962, "was disappointed that the budget did not include any plans for implementing the [JCMIH] Report. . . . The committee feels that the Executive Branch had been remiss in its duties in not having a plan for implementation before Congress."[48]

The following month Kennedy's interagency task force began its work in earnest. Influenced by Felix, its members were enthusiastic about the NIMH proposal to create centers. They accepted without question the claim that new knowledge about diagnosis, treatment, and prevention offered the potential for an exciting new policy departure that could really make a difference and that the population of state hospitals could be halved within a decade. To be sure, there were differences within the task force. Some members felt that states were obsolete and that an effective policy required not only federal funding, but a measure of federal control. Others did not want to bypass states and hoped that persuasion and education might achieve the goal of reshaping mental health policy. Several issues remained unresolved, including funding mechanisms and regulations. Nor did the group address the problem of staffing the projected two thousand centers or their impact upon federal-state-local relationships. In the end, members agreed that the NIMH proposal to create community mental health centers (CMHCs) and to eliminate the state mental institution as it now stood represented the best policy choice.

The goal was to have five hundred centers in operation by 1970 and an additional fifteen hundred a decade later. They recommended federal grants for construction and a decreasing subsidy for operating costs.[49]

That the interagency task force had partly ignored–if not rejected–the recommendations of the JCMIH was obvious. Equally significant, in the absence of any empirical data, it had recommended the creation of an entirely new institution that would presumably replace traditional mental hospitals. Indeed, the new policy was based on an ideological foundation that reflected the rhetoric of community superiority that was so popular during the 1960s. The paradoxes and contradictions of this policy were profound and its consequences would only become apparent in succeeding years. The presumption was that federal beneficence and wisdom, on the one hand, and community involvement on the other, would lead to the creation of a new institution that would overcome the myopic inability of states to provide for the welfare of persons with severe mental disorders. In effect, the task force had recommended centralized direction and local autonomy while implicitly weakening the role of states.

Celebrezze, although initially opposed to the use of federal subsidies for operating funds, reversed himself and supported the recommendations of the task force. Public policy had to incorporate two overriding objectives: first, the promotion of mental health and the prevention of mental illness; and second, an emphasis on cure rather than incarceration. He therefore endorsed the creation of a comprehensive CMHC, which would be "the foci of future mental health activities." In effect, he had rejected the recommendations of the JCMIH in favor of those of Felix and his colleagues at the NIMH.[50]

In the autumn of 1962 the stage was set for some form of presidential decision. When Kennedy was shown a draft of the message to Congress, he simply accepted in a somewhat uncharacteristic manner the recommendations of his advisors. In early 1963 he forwarded a message to Congress urging the passage of a law to make the CMHC the centerpiece of mental health policy. What was required was a "bold new approach" that would make it possible "for most of the mentally ill to be successfully and quickly treated in their own communities and returned to a useful place in society." The federal government would provide construction grants and short-term subsidies for staffing.[51]

In the Senate the President's message met with a favorable reception. The supportive testimony before Lister Hill's subcommittee was orchestrated by organizations and individuals long active in the mental health field. Felix echoed their claims. "I am as certain as I am that I am sitting here," he told the committee in impassioned rhetoric,

> that within a decade or two we will see the size of these mental hospitals, the population of these mental hospitals, cut in half. I wish to God I could live and be active for 25 more years, because I believe if I could, I would see the day when the State mental hospitals as we know them today would no longer exist, but would be a different kind of institution for a selected few patients who needed specialized types of care and treatment.[52]

Supporters of the bill faced a slightly different situation in the House. Oren Harris, chair of the Committee on Interstate and Foreign Commerce, had few links to the mental health lobby. Nor did the public hearings before a House subcommittee go as well as those in the Senate. Celebrezze's presentation was so ineffectual that part of it was excised from the printed record. Several committee members also raised serious concerns. Paul Rogers–who was by no means unsympathetic–expressed doubts about the feasibility of staffing the projected centers with qualified personnel, a point that had been raised earlier by Michael March of the Bureau of the Budget. In reviewing the Interagency Task Force-DHEW plan, March had concluded that it was not feasible because of the shortage of qualified personnel to staff the projected two thousand CMHCs. The schools of social work or nursing lacked the capacity to meet projected needs. Equally significant, the goal of dramatically increasing the number of psychiatrists might have the inadvertent effect of reducing the supply of general practitioners as well as specialists, thus exacerbating other health problems. There was also considerable concern over whether temporary financial support for staffing could actually be phased out.[53]

Despite some concerns, the hearings in both chambers were largely celebratory. Boisfeuillet Jones–who had played a key role in the Interagency Task Force–told the House committee that the CMHC "will make possible caring for the emotionally disturbed, the mentally ill, and

. . . assist in preventing mental illness through training of ministers, of social workers, of teachers, of police officers, of juvenile court representatives in the community in order that mental health will be promoted."[54] The proceedings were dominated by a partnership of professional authority and political deference. There was no inclination to evaluate the claim that CMHCs would be capable of dealing with persons with severe and persistent mental disorders who required a broad range of services that included such basic necessities as housing. Although there was agreement about the need for continuity of care and integration of services, the administrative and organizational problems involved in implementing a community-oriented policy were never addressed. Faith that a new institution would resolve existing problems created a euphoric atmosphere that facilitated favorable congressional action.

Despite broad support, the legislation faced several obstacles. In the House the opposition of the American Medical Association to the provision providing federal subsidies for staffing led to partisan bickering. Moreover, there was potential for conflict between the advocates of mental retardation and mental health. Anticipating problems, Senator Lister Hill persuaded the administration to support the merger of mental health and mental retardation into a single bill. In an omnibus bill, the staffing provision might recede in significance, given the popularity and noncontroversial nature of the more popular mental retardation bill. The bill passed the Senate with only one dissenting vote. Those opposed to the staffing provision in the House were unyielding, and ultimately the bill passed both houses without its inclusion. The bill was signed into law by President Kennedy on 31 October 1963.[55]

The mental health provisions of the Mental Retardation and Community Mental Health Centers Construction Act of 1963 were relatively simple. The legislation provided a three-year authorization for grants totaling $150 million for fiscal years 1965 through 1967 for construction; the federal share ranged between one- and two-thirds. To be eligible, states had to submit a comprehensive plan; designate an agency to administer the plan as well as an advisory council with broad representation; and establish a construction program based on a statewide inventory of existing facilities and needs. The designated state agency would then forward individual construction applications to Washington for final approval.[56]

For Felix and the NIMH the passage of the CMHC legislation represented both a personal and organizational triumph. In their eyes the foundation had been laid for a fundamental change in the manner in which American society dealt with mental illnesses and other emotional disorders. The legislation, proclaimed Felix,

> reflects the concept that many forms and degrees of mental illness can be prevented or ameliorated more effectively through community oriented preventive, diagnostic, treatment, and rehabilitation services than through care in the traditional–and traditionally isolated–state mental hospital. The act is designed to stimulate state, local, and private action. It is based on the belief that it will be possible to reduce substantially, within a decade or two, the numbers of patients who receive only custodial care–or no care at all–when they could be helped by the application of one or more of the modern methods of dealing with emotional disturbances and the mental illnesses.[57]

******

The passage of the CMHC legislation was but a beginning. The provisions of the act were vague. The essential services that CMHCs were required to provide were not defined, but left to DHEW. The meaning and actual operation of the legislation, therefore, would reflect the views of DHEW officials responsible for writing the regulations and defining standards.

At the very outset, an internal bureaucratic struggle took place within the PHS. The staff of the Bureau of State Services, which had responsibility for overseeing hospital construction under the Hill-Burton Act of 1946, wanted jurisdiction. Felix and his colleagues at the NIMH, by contrast, interpreted the act as mandating a service system and not as one limited to construction of centers. They believed that the act of 1963 was the logical culmination of a process begun by the passage of the National Mental Health Act of 1946, which had authorized the creation of the NIMH and given it responsibility for research, training, and service. In a bureaucratic struggle, Felix easily prevailed; responsibility for writing the regulations and administering the program remained within the NIMH.[58]

The writing of the regulations was completed by the spring of 1964. Promulgated by a small group that included Felix, Bertram Brown, and four other individuals, they defined five essential services that each CMHC was required to provide: inpatient services, outpatient services, partial hospitalization (including day care); twenty-four-hour emergency services; and consultation and educational services for community agencies and professional personnel. The regulations also encouraged, but did not mandate, states to provide other diagnostic, rehabilitative, precare and aftercare services, training, research, and evaluation.[59]

On several major issues the regulations were silent. They did not stipulate which professional group would have primary responsibility for administering centers, although psychiatrists were to control the clinical program. Nor did the regulations (or, for that matter, the legislation) define the meaning of community. Since Felix and his colleagues found that political, geographical, ethnic, or socioeconomic boundaries did not work, they fell back on numbers. They defined what a community was by stipulating a population range of 75,000 to 200,000.[60]

In most respects the regulations embodied the visions of both NIMH officials and advocates of community care and treatment. They were issued without asking for comments or criticisms. Even state officials who supervised a large mental health system were ignored. To be sure, these officials were required to develop comprehensive plans, to divide their jurisdiction into geographical areas, and to rank and approve locally developed proposals for funding. In practice, however, the regulations diminished state authority by creating a decentralized system that shifted authority to local communities.

Perhaps the most curious aspect of the regulations was the omission of any mention of state hospitals. In one sense this was understandable, given the faith that they would be replaced by CMHCs. Nevertheless, the absence of linkages with a system that still cared for nearly half a million persons and admitted about 300,000 each year was striking. If centers were designed to provide comprehensive services and continuity of care, how could they function without linkages to state hospitals? Indeed, the absence of specific linkages facilitated the development of an independent system of centers that ultimately catered to a quite different clientele.

The final element in the new community-oriented system–legislation providing for federal support for staffing CMHCs–was in place within fifteen months after the promulgation of the new regulations. A series of fortuitous events had created a very different political climate. The accession of Lyndon Johnson to the presidency in late 1963 and his overwhelming victory in the election of 1964 brought to the White House a shrewd, forceful, and determined individual. Johnson used his talents to push through Congress his Great Society program. Committed to civil rights and to measures designed to alleviate the burdens of poverty and extend access to health care, he oversaw passage of legislation that had a profound impact upon the lives of millions of Americans.

In the autumn of 1964, Felix retired to become dean of St. Louis University School of Medicine. The staff that he had put together during his nearly two decades as the director of the NIMH, however, ensured that there would be no policy shifts. With the support of the administration, Stanley Yolles (who succeeded Felix) developed a plan that went even further than the staffing provision that had been deleted from the act of 1963. Aware that budgetary pressures precluded any substantial infusion of state funds for the support of centers, Yolles proposed federal funding not merely to staff centers, but for additional mental health services in local communities. Less sensitive than his predecessor to state authorities, he urged that funds go directly to communities.[61]

Although state officials were critical, they were in no position to prevail. Moreover, the AMA, which had played an important role in defeating the staffing provision in 1963, was now preoccupied with the impending Medicare and Medicaid legislation. By this time the House was more sympathetic. In testimony before Oren Harris's committee, Yolles insisted that the legislation was designed to assist community mental health services and thus to hasten the disappearance of mental institutions. "There is no direct link between the community program and the State hospital program," he added in revealing words.[62]

That those committed to new policies turned to the federal government was understandable. By this time there was a pervasive belief–not necessarily shared by all–that the national government was better qualified than its state counterparts to deal with pressing social problems. Indeed, the prevailing consensus was that most states had failed to meet their social welfare responsibilities. The tendency to denigrate state governments was also accompanied by an idealization of local communities and local control. This perception, which played an increasingly important role in the 1960s, tended to promote a vision of a federal-local government partnership that bypassed state authority not only in mental health, but in other domestic welfare programs as well as civil rights legislation.

In early August, Johnson signed the legislation into law. The act gave DHEW the authority to provide grants for staffing new centers and new services. Awards were to be based on relative needs of states for services, their financial situation, and their population. This was a departure from a formula-based system (such as Hill-Burton), and gave NIMH officials considerable decision-making authority while bypassing state authorities. The bill authorized an expenditure of $73.5 million for three years. Congress also mandated a declining level of support beginning at 75 percent and falling to 30 percent. The final regulations followed those of 1963. Centers were given responsibility for the "mental health of the community, . . .the prevention of mental illness and the more rapid and complete recovery of persons affected with mental illness in the community, . . . [and] the development of improved methods of treating and rehabilitating the mentally ill."[63]

******

By 1965 the final elements of a national program were in place. Although Felix had retired the year before, he and his colleagues at the NIMH had played major roles in creating a new institution that would supposedly replace an archaic institutional system that had been in place for well over a century. Yet, within a decade, it had become clear that the CMHC program had done little to improve the lives of persons with severe and persistent mental illnesses. Why had such a promising policy that was designed to shift care and treatment from institutions to the community failed to achieve its objectives?

That the federal government reneged on its promise to create 2,000 centers by 1980 is obvious. By the late 1960s the war in Vietnam had taken center stage. Domestic issues tended to lose their priority, and funding for construction and staffing declined dramatically. Between 1966 and 1970, 274 centers were funded; in the succeeding decade an additional 480 were the beneficiaries of federal subsidies. By 1980 only 754 centers had been funded. Senator Daniel Patrick Moynihan, who had served on Kennedy's Interagency Task Force, charged that the failure to construct and staff the projected 2,000 centers and the concomitant discharge of patients from mental hospitals was responsible for the creation of a large population of "homeless, deranged people."[64]

Moynihan's observations, however poignant, are hardly sustained by a careful analysis of the activities of those centers that were created. The fact of the matter is that the euphoria and rhetoric surrounding the acts of 1963 and 1965 concealed an inner ambiguity about the precise nature and functions of centers. Indeed, from their very beginnings, most CMHCs served largely a new set of clients who better fit the orientations of mental health managers and professionals trained in a psychodynamic tradition and a faith in the efficacy of prevention. The treatment of choice at most centers was individual psychotherapy, an intervention especially adapted to a middle-class educated clientele who did not have severe disorders and which was congenial as well to the professional staffs composed largely of social workers and clinical psychologists. CMHC personnel rarely gave persons with severe and persistent mental disorders a high priority. Such individuals, after all, presented daunting problems. They were not always easy to manage; they often required comprehensive care, and many were poor candidates for psychotherapies. Needs that in mental hospitals were minimally satisfied were not easily met in community settings. Who would ensure that persons with severe mental disorders would have access to housing, food, support systems, and jobs? To provide for such persons in the community, in other words, was arduous and time-consuming. Under such circumstances centers tended to respond to local pressures for services to non-mentally ill constituencies. Most CMHCs, charged APA President Donald G. Langsley in 1980, were offering "preventive services that have not yet been proven successful" and "counseling and crisis intervention for predictable problems in living." "A critical consequence of these events," he added, "has been the wholesale neglect of the mentally ill, especially the chronic patient and the deinstitutionalized."[65]

Within a decade after the passage of the acts of 1963 and 1965 it was clear that CMHCs had neither replaced mental hospitals nor provided services for persons with severe mental disorders. Moreover, those who had warned of the problem of providing psychiatric personnel to staff centers proved prescient. Between 1970 and 1977 the number of full-time psychiatrists per center fell from 6.8 to 4.2. In 1973, 56 percent of CMHC directors were psychiatrists; by 1977, the comparable figure was 22 percent. Centers were now staffed by clinical psychologists, social workers, or nonprofessional staff–groups that had neither interest in nor experience with persons with severe disorders.[66]

Nor did centers play a significant role in the decline of the mental hospital population after 1965. The first wave of deinstitutionalization actually followed the enactment of Medicare and Medicaid in 1965, which encouraged the construction of nursing home beds. The Medicaid program also provided a payment source for patients trans-ferred from state mental hospitals to nursing homes and general hospitals. States could thus direct patients to other facilities and have the federal government assume half to three-quarters of the costs. This incen-tive encouraged a mass transinstitutionalization of long-term patients, primarily elderly patients with dementia who were housed in mental hospitals for lack of other institutional alternatives. The second wave of deinstitutionalization occurred during and after the 1970s. By then, the existence of such federal entitlement programs as Social Security Disability Insurance (SSDI) and Supplementary Security Income for the Aged, the Disabled, and the Blind (SSI) encouraged states to discharge patients from mental hospitals, since federal payments would presumably enable them to live in the community. These individuals were also eligible for medical coverage under Medicaid, food stamps, and public housing.[67]

The availability of federal entitlements by the early 1970s provided resources that enabled persons with serious mental disorders to reside in the community. Hospital populations declined rapidly. But the states' policy decisions to reduce public hospital populations and to make admission to these institutions more difficult, along with other changes in public attitudes, treatment ideologies, and social and economic factors, supported a confusing array of organized and unorganized settings for treating persons with mental disorders. Treatment in the community for clients with multiple needs, after all, posed severe challenges as compared with mental hospital care. In the community (and particularly in large urban areas) clients were widely dispersed, and their successful management depended on bringing together needed services administered by a variety of bureaucracies, each with their own culture, priorities, and preferred client populations. Although there were sporadic (and occasionally successful) efforts to integrate these services (psychiatric care and treatment, social services, housing, social support) in meaningful ways, the results in most areas were at best dismal. The institutional disarray and absence of service integration forced many patients with serious mental illnesses to survive in homeless shelters, on the streets, and even in jails and almshouses.[68]

If CMHCs played little or no role in the hastening the decline of long-term institutionalization, they did help to shift the focus away from persons with serious and persistent mental disorders. Indeed, their greatest impact was to provide services for those seeking assistance to deal with problems of living. Their growth paralleled the expansion of psychiatric diagnostic categories in the latter half of the twentieth century, a development perhaps best mirrored in the publication of DSM-III in 1980 and subsequent editions.[69]

The history of the role of the NIMH in mental health policy in the two decades following the end of World War II offers a sobering lesson. It suggests that there is a price to be paid for implementing ideology ungrounded in empirical reality, and for making exaggerated claims. The ideology of community mental health and the facile assumption that treatment and residence in the community of persons with severe and persistent mental disorders would promote adjustment and integration did not take into account the subsequent social isolation, exposure to victimization, inducement to substance abuse, and homelessness. The assumption that CMHCs would assume responsibility for the aftercare and rehabilitation of persons discharged from mental hospitals proved erroneous. The absence of mechanisms of control and accountability permitted CMHCs to focus on new populations of more amenable and attractive clients with less severe problems.

The same was true of provisions in the acts of 1963 and 1965 relating to the prevention of mental illnesses and the promotion of mental health.

To be sure, their popularity reflected the postwar faith in human agency, that disease was not inevitable and could be avoided by conscious and purposive actions. In fact, the prevention of mental illness and the promotion of mental health were little more than attractive slogans. Given that neither the etiology nor the pathology of mental illnesses was understood, how could strategies be developed that would prevent such disorders and promote mental health?

That the outcome of policy decisions in the postwar decades was far removed from original intentions is obvious. This is not in any way to suggest that Felix and his staff should have known better. Human beings have great faith in their ability to shape and mold the world in ways they think desirable. They rarely recognize that such faith is partly misplaced, if only because reality is far more complex than is generally recognized. Nor are they cognizant of the fact that the adoption of new policies leads to behavioral change on the part of others, thus giving rise to unanticipated consequences. Nowhere are these generalizations better illustrated than in the development of mental health policy from the 1940s to the 1960s.

Notes

1. New Freedom Commission on Mental Health, *Achieving the Promise: Transforming Mental Health Care in America, Final Report* (DHHS Pub. no. SMA-03-3832: Rockville, Maryland: 2003), p. 1.
2. Gerald N. Grob, *From Asylum to Community: Mental Health Policy in Modern America* (Princeton, New Jersey: Princeton University Press, 1991), chaps. 1 and 2.
3. Gerald N. Grob, *Mental Illness and American Society, 1875-1940* (Princeton, New Jersey: Princeton University Press, 1983), pp. 308-15.
4. President's Scientific Research Board, *Science and Public Policy*, 5 vols.(Washington, D.C.: Government Printing Office, 1947), 1: 3, 113-18; Daniel M. Fox, *Health Policies, Health Politics: The British and American Experience, 1911-1963* (Princeton, New Jersey: Princeton University Press, 1986), pp. 158-60; Stephen P. Strickland, *Politics, Science, and Dread Disease: A Short History of United States Medical Research Policy* (Cambridge, Massachusetts: Harvard University Press, 1972), chaps. 2-3.
5. Franklin G. Ebaugh, *The Care of the Psychiatric Patient in General Hospitals* (Chicago: American Hospital Association, 1940).
6. Biographical material culled from Felix interview by Dr. Jeanne Brand, 2 April 1964, W. D. Miles Oral History Collection, History of Medicine

Division, National Library of Medicine (hereinafter cited as NLM), Bethesda, Maryland; Felix interview by Daniel Blain, Blain Papers, Box 24, Folder 7, Archives of the American Psychiatric Association (hereafter AAPA), Washington, D.C.; Felix interview by Milton J. E. Senn, 8 March 1979, Senn Collection, OH76, NLM.

7. Felix interview by Brand, NLM; Alanson W. Willcox to Felix, 20 February 1945 (with draft bill), Mary E. Switzer Papers, Schlesinger Library, Radcliffe College, Cambridge, Massachusetts; Mary Switzer interview, 1966, OH 161, APAA.

8. Felix interview by Brand, NLM.

9. Grob, *From Asylum to Community*, pp. 50-53; Felix interview by Brand, NLM; Mary E. Switzer to Karl A. Menninger, 14 March 1945, Switzer File, Menninger Foundation Papers, Kansas Historical Society, Topeka, Kansas; 79-1 Congress, *National Neuropsychiatric Institute Act: Hearing before a Subcommittee of the Committee on Interstate and Foreign Commerce, House of Representatives. . .1945* (Washington, D.C.: U.S. Government Printing Office, 1945); 79-2 Congress, *National Neuropsychiatric Institute Act: Hearings before a Subcommittee of the Committee on Education and Labor, United States Senate. . .1946* (Washington, D.C.: U.S. Government Printing Office, 1946).

10. Chap. 538, *U.S. Statutes at Large*, 60 (1946): 421-26.

11. Robert Felix, "Mental Disorders as a Public Health Problem," *American Journal of Psychiatry*, 1949, *106*: 401-6. See Paul V. Lemkau, *Mental Hygiene in Public Health* (New York: McGraw-Hill, 1949).

12. Robert Felix and R.V. Bowers, "Mental Hygiene and Socio-Environmental Factors," *Milbank Memorial Fund Quarterly*, 1948, *26*:125-47.

13. Felix, "Mental Public Health: A Blueprint," presentation at St. Elizabeths Hospital, 21 April 1945, Felix Papers, NLM.

14. Felix, "Mental Disorders," pp. 401-6.

15. Felix interview by Brand, NLM.

16. Ibid.; Robert Felix, *Mental Illness: Progress and Prospects* (New York: Columbia University Press, 1967), pp. 49-50.

17. Seymour S. Kety interview by Daniel Blain, 14 May 1973, Blain Papers, APAA; John Clausen interview by Milton J. E. Senn, 30 March 1973, Senn Collection, OH20, NLM; Jeanne L. Brand and Philip Sapir, eds., "An Historical Perspective on the National Institute of Mental Health," February 1964, mimeograph document prepared as sec. 1 of the NIMH Report to Dean E. Woolridge, chairperson, NIH Study Committee, pp. 69-79; Ingrid G. Farreras, Caroline Hannaway, and Victoria A. Harden, eds., *Mind, Brain, Body, and Behavior: Foundations of Neuroscience and Behavioral Research at the National Institutes of Health* (Amsterdam: IOS Press, 2004), p. 196 et passim.

18. 80-2 Congress, *Hearings before the Subcommittee of the Committee on Appropriations House of Representatives . . . on the Department of Labor-Federal Security Agency Appropriation Bill for 1949* (Washington, D.C.: U.S. Government Printing Office, 1948), Part 2, pp. 271-87.

19. PHS Mental Hygiene Division, "Annual Report for Fiscal Year 1947," pp. 5-6, typed copy in NIMH Records, Subject Files, 1940-51, Box 82, National Archives (NA), Washington, D.C.; Robert Felix, "The Relation of the National Mental Health Act to State Health Authorities," *Public Health Reports*, 1947, *62*: 46-47; Robert Felix, "The National Mental Health Program—A Progress Report," ibid., 1948, *63*: 837-39. I examined the NIMH records when they were still at the Washington National Record Center, Suitland, Maryland.

20. PHS Mental Hygiene Division, "Annual Report, Fiscal 1948," pp. 4, 8-9, NIMH, "Annual Report, Fiscal 1949," pp. 9, 12, and table 5, typed copies in NIMH Records, Subject Files 1940–51, Box 82, NA; Jerry W. Carter, "The Community Services Program of the National Institute of Mental Health, U.S. Public Health Service," *Journal of Clinical Psychology*, 1950, *6*: 113-14; Anita K. Bahn, V. B. Norman, *Outpatient Psychiatric Clinics in the United States, 1954-55, PHS Public Health Monograph No. 49* (1957): 40; National Advisory Mental Health Council, Minutes of Meeting, 8-9 November 1954, p. 8, RG 90, NA.

21. National Advisory Mental Health Council, Minutes of Meeting, 11-12 December 1950, pp. 11-14, RG 90, NA.

22. Ibid., 9-11 March 1955, pp. 5-7.

23. NIMH, *Evaluation in Mental Health. . .Report of the Subcommittee on Evaluation of Mental Health Activities, Community Services Committee, National Advisory Mental Health Council, PHS Publication 413* (1955), pp. 1, 3, 57.

24. Harold Sampson, D. Ross, B. Engle, and F. Livson, *A Study of Suitability for Outpatient Clinic Treatment of State Mental Hospital Admissions*, California Department of Mental Hygiene, Research Report No. 1 (1957). A briefer version appeared under the title "Feasibility of Community Clinic Treatment for State Mental Hospital Patients," *Archives of Neurology and Psychiatry*, 1958, *80*: 71-77.

25. See Jonas H. Ellenberg, "A Conversation with Morton Kramer," *Statistical Science*, 1997, *12*: 103-7.

26. Morton Kramer, H. Goldstein, R. H. Israel, and N. A. Johnson, *A Historical Study of the Disposition of First Admissions to a State Mental Hospital: Experience of the Warren State Hospital during the Period 1916-50*, PHS *Publication 445* (1955), and the same authors' "Application of Life Table Methodology to the Study of Mental Hospital Populations," in American Psychiatric Association, *Psychiatric Research Reports*, 1956, *5*: 49-87.

27. Morton Kramer, "Epidemiology, Biostatistics, and Mental Health Planning," in American Psychiatric Association, *Psychiatric Research Reports*, 1967, *22*: 27; idem, *Some Implications of Trends in the Usage of Psychiatric Facilities for Community Mental Health Programs and Related Research*, PHS *Publication 1434* (1967); American Psychiatric Association, *Report on Patients Over 65 in Public Mental Hospitals* (Washington, D.C.: American Psychiatric Association, 1960).

28. Morton Kramer, *Facts Needed to Assess Public Health and Social Problems in the Widespread Use of the Tranquilizing Drugs*, PHS *Publication 486* (1956).

29. Jonathan O. Cole and R.W. Gerard, eds., *Psychopharmacology: Problems in Evaluation* (Washington, D.C.: National Academy of Sciences, National Research Council, 1959). This volume printed the proceedings of the Conference on the Evaluation of Pharmacotherapy in Mental Illness.

30. 84-2 Congress, *Labor-Health, Education, and Welfare Appropriations for 1957: Hearings before the Subcommittee on Appropriations. . .Senate* (Washington, D.C.: U.S. Government Printing Office, 1956), pp. 1298-1300, 1308ff.

31. Gorman speech, Trenton, N.J., 4 February 1957, Gorman Papers, NLM.

32. 85-1 Congress, *Departments of Labor, Health, Education, and Welfare Appropriations for 1958: Hearings before the Subcommittee of the Committee on Appropriations House of Representatives* (Washington, D.C.: U.S. Government Printing Office, 1957), pp. 851-78; Felix to William C. Menninger, 5 March 1957, Menninger to Felix, 11 March 1957, Felix Memo to Surgeon General, PHS, Re: Public Attack by Mr. Mike Gorman, 13 February 1957, William C. Menninger Papers, Kansas Historical Society, Topeka, Kansas.

33. NIMH Psychopharmacology Service Center Collaborative Study Group, "Phenothiazine Treatment in Acute Schizophrenia," *Archives of General Psychiatry*, 1964, *10*: 246-61.

34. The history of the JCMIH is covered in Grob, *From Asylum to Community*, pp. 180-238.

35. *Action for Mental Health: Final Report of the Joint Commission on Mental Illness and Health* (New York: Basic Books, 1961), pp. xxv, 8, 22-23, 26-85, 93, 213-95.

36. Grob, *From Asylum to Community*, pp. 210-16.

37. Newton Bigelow's criticisms appeared in the *Psychiatric Quarterly*, 1959, *33*: 148-65; 1961, *35*: 576-85 (quotations from pp. 581-82), 777-84; 1962, *36*: 151-64, 754-67; 1963, *37*: 153-65; 1965, *39*: 347-54; 1966, *40*: 357-66; 1969, *43*: 568-73.

38. Philip Sapir to Felix, 23 October 1959, NIMH Records, Mental Health Subject Files 1957-60, Box 7, NA.

39. Richard H. Williams to Felix, 22 October 1959, *ibid*.

40. Felix to John R. Seeley, 25 February 1959; Felix interview by Brand, NLM; Felix interview by Blain, Blain Papers, AAPA; Felix, "Implications and Implementation of the Joint Commission Report at the National Level," speech at the Governors' Conference, November 1961, Felix Papers, NLM; Felix to Special Assistant to Secretary, Health and Medical Affairs, DHEW, 27 September 1961, Bertram S. Brown Papers, NLM.

41. *Planning for Facilities for Mental Health Services: Report of the Surgeon General's Ad Hoc Committee on Planning for Mental Health Facilities*, PHS *Publication 808* (1961), pp. ii-v, 2-5, 25-34.

42. Grob, *From Asylum to Community*, pp. 219-20; Edward D. Berkowitz, "The Politics of Mental Retardation during the Kennedy Administration," *Social Sciences Quarterly*, 1980, *61*: 128-41. The Myer Feldman (Kennedy's special assistant) interview is especially revealing: see vol. 7, pp. 304-7, vol. 14, pp. 1-30, John F. Kennedy Library, Boston, Massachusetts.

43. John F. Kennedy to Abraham Ribicoff, 1 December 1961, White House Central Files, Box 338, Folder HE 1-1, Kennedy Library; Henry A. Foley, *Community Mental Health Legislation: The Formative Process* (Lexington, Massachusetts.: Lexington Books, 1975), pp. 33-37.

44. "National Institute of Mental Health Position Paper on the Report of the Joint Commission on Mental Illness and Health," November 1961 (quotation from p. 8), NIMH Records, Miscellaneous Records 1956-67, Box 1, NA.

45. "Report of [NIMH] Task Force on the Status of State Mental Hospitals in the United States," 30 March 1962, Brown Papers, NLM.

46. "Preliminary Draft Report of NIMH Task Force on Implementation of Recommendations of the Report of the Joint Commission on Mental Illness and Health," 5 January 1962, and "A Proposal for a Comprehensive Mental Health Program to Implement the Findings of the Joint Commission on Mental Illness and Health," April 1962, pp. 10 (quote), 12, 34-35, et passim, NIMH Records, Miscellaneous Records, 1956-67, Box 1, NA.

47. Mike Gorman to Myer Feldman, 19 February 1962, White House Central Files, Box 338, Folder HE 1-1, Kennedy Library; Mike Gorman interview by Daniel Blain, 7 October 1972, pp. 27-29, Blain Papers, AAPA; John E. Fogarty speech, "The Responsibility of the Federal Government in the Fight Against Mental Illness," 6 March 1962, copy in William C. Menninger Papers, Kansas Historical Society;

48. 87-2 Congress, *House Report No. 1488* (23 March 1962), pp. 34-35.

49. Rashi Fein to Walter W. Heller, 21 November 1962, Heller Papers, Kennedy Library; Robert H. Atwell to Director, "Proposals for the President's Mental Health Program—A Report to the Interagency Group Appointed by the President," draft dated 1 November 1962, Daniel Patrick Moynihan to Boisfeuillet Jones, 21 August 1962, Brown Papers, NLM; Foley, *Community Mental Health Legislation*, pp. 39-41.

50. Anthony Celebrezze, Willard Wirtz, and J. Gleason to John F. Kennedy, 30 November 1962, White House Central Files, Box 338, Folder HE 1-1, Kennedy Library.

51. Feldman interview, vol. 14, pp. 13-15, 24-25, Bertram Brown interview, 6 August 1968, p. 24, Kennedy Library; "Message from the President of the United States Relative to Mental Illness and Mental Retardation," 88-1 Congress, *House Document No. 58* (5 February 1963), quotes from pp. 2-3.

52. 88-1 Congress, *Mental Illness and Retardation: Hearings before the Subcommittee on Health of the Committee on Labor and Public Welfare . . . Senate . . . March 5, 6, and 7, 1963* (Washington, D.C.: U.S. Government Printing Office, 1963), p. 191.

53. Gorman interview by Blain, p. 35; 88-1 Congress, *Mental Health: Hearings before a Subcommittee of the Committee on Interstate and Foreign Commerce House of Representatives . . . 1963* (Washington, D.C.: U.S. Government Printing Office, 1963), pp. 99-106, 341-42.
54. 88-1 Congress, *Mental Health. Hearings . . . House*, p. 97.
55. Grob, *From Asylum to Community*, pp. 231-33.
56. Public Law 88-164, *U.S. Statutes at Large*, 77 (1963): 282-99.
57. Robert Felix, "A Model for Comprehensive Mental Health Centers," *American Journal of Public Health*, 1964, *54*: 1965. See also Felix's "The National Mental Health Program," ibid., 1804-9, and "Community Mental Health: A Federal Perspective," *American Journal of Psychiatry*, 1964, *121*: 428-32.
58. Foley, *Community Mental Health Legislation*, chap. 4.
59. *Federal Register*, 29 (1964): 5951-56.
60. See Foley, *Community Mental Health Legislation*, pp. 89-98.
61. Stanley F. Yolles to Asst. Surgeon General for Plans, 16 November, 1964, NIMH Records, Miscellaneous Records 1956-67, Box 2, NA; Foley, *Community Mental Health Legislation*, pp. 107-10.
62. 89-1 Congress, *Research Facilities, Mental Health Staffing . . . Hearings before the Committee on Interstate and Foreign Commerce House of Representatives . . . 1965* (Washington, D.C.: U.S. Government Printing Office, 1965), pp. 28-59 (Yolles' quote from p. 58), 152, 168, 180-81, 213-28.
63. Public Law 89-105, *U.S. Statutes at Large*, 79 (1965): 427-30; *Federal Register*, 31 (March 1, 1966): 3246-48; Foley, *Community Mental Health Legislation*, pp. 113-16.
64. *New York Times*, 22 May 1989.
65. Donald G. Langsley, "The Community Mental Health Center: Does It Treat Patients?" *Hospital and Community Psychiatry*, 1980, *31*: 815-19. See also David F. Musto, "Whatever Happened to 'Community Mental Health?'" *Public Interest*, Spring 1975, *39*: 53-79.
66. Rosalyn D. Bass, "Trends Among Core Professionals in Organized Mental Health Settings: Where Have All the Psychiatrists Gone?" NIMH *Mental Health Statistical Note No. 160* (1981); Walter W. Winslow, "The Changing Role of Psychiatrists In Community Mental Health Centers," *American Journal of Psychiatry*, 1979, *136*: 24-27; Paul J. Fink and S. P. Weinstein, "Whatever Happened to Psychiatry: The Deprofessionalization of Community Mental Health Centers," ibid., 406-9; John A. Talbott, "Why Psychiatrists Leave the Public Sector," *Hospital and Community Psychiatry*, 1979, 30: 778-82.
67. See Howard H. Goldman, N. H. Adams, and C. A. Taube, "Deinstitutionalization: The Data Demythologized," *Hospital and Community Psychiatry*, 1983, *34*: 129-34; William Gronfein, "Incentives and Intentions in Mental Health Policy: A Comparison of the Medicaid and Community Mental Health Programs," *Journal of Health and Social Behavior*, 1985, *26*: 192-206; Charles A. Kiesler and A. E. Sibulkin, *Mental Hospitalization:*

Myths and Facts About a National Crisis (Newbury Park, California.: Sage Publications, 1987); and Morton Kramer, *Psychiatric Services and the Changing Psychiatric Scene, 1950-1985* (Washington, D.C.: U.S. Government Printing Office, 1977).

68. For a discussion of events since the 1970s, see Gerald N. Grob and Howard H. Goldman, *The Dilemma of Federal Mental Health Policy: Radical Reform or Incremental Change?* (New Brunswick, New Jersey: Rutgers University Press, 2006).

69. American Psychiatric Association, *Diagnostic and Statistical Manual of Mental Disorders* 3rd ed. (Washington, D.C.: American Psychiatric Association, 1980).

Radium and the Origins of the National Cancer Institute

David Cantor

Introduction

It is commonly supposed that the National Cancer Institute (NCI) began life in 1937 as a pure research organization, almost unsullied by its subsidiary functions of cancer control and prevention. Historians have shown that supporters of the 1937 Cancer Bill which led to the creation of the NCI strongly argued their case in terms of the need for research;[1] that the National Advisory Cancer Council (NACC), the NCI's advisory body, saw it as focused primarily on research;[2] and that basic and clinical research scientists took over the institute.[3] Most accounts of the history of post-1937 NCI thus tell the story of a research organization.[4] The general assumption is that research always dominated the NCI. An argument of this paper is that this assumption is quite mistaken. In its first fiscal year, the vast bulk of the NCI's money went not on research, but on routine therapy.

The point can be made by a focus on radium. The 1937 Act establishing the institute required the NCI to purchase radium, and Congress authorized the expenditure of $200,000 for this purpose, far exceeding the estimated expenditure for anything else in the appropriation of $400,000 for fiscal year 1938.[5] What must be recognized is that this radium was not intended for research.[6] Most of it was loaned to hospitals across the United States for the routine treatment of cancer, mainly for patients who otherwise would have been unable to afford the therapy. To put it another way, about half the budget of the NCI in its first year went on the routine treatment of indigent patients. The NCI was a New Deal program that used the resources of the federal government to alleviate the harsh conditions of the Great Depression on the poor.

I am not the first to argue that the NCI was a New Deal program. In her account of how the genetically standardized mouse came to play a central role in American biomedical research, Karen Rader notes Clarence Little's call in 1932 for a "New Deal for mice," by which he meant a New Deal for "mice researchers" or "research."[7] Little was the head of the Jackson Laboratory in Bar Harbor, Maine, then in financial difficulties, and his call had the objective not only of making federal support for cancer research a New Deal program, but also of creating a research market for the laboratory's strain of mice, and (against vivisectionist objections) of making mice a morally acceptable stand-in for humans in the cancer laboratory. In some ways, Little succeeded in his goals. The Jackson Laboratory's strain of mice became an important tool in NCI research, helping to secure the laboratory's economic viability.

But Little's vision of the New Deal as promoting cancer research was only one of many, and it was not the one that predominated in the first year of the NCI. Research–be it on mice, or on any other experimental material–obtained a smaller proportion of the NCI's budget than the 50 percent that went on radium. In short, the NCI embodied at least two different visions of the New Deal–one that sought to use the resources of the federal government to promote research into causes and cures of cancer, and one that sought to use the resources of the federal government to help indigent patients with cancer. It was this latter vision of the New Deal that won out in the first year of the NCI, and advocates hoped it would continue for many years with continued purchases of radium. These hopes were not realized, and research and training rather than radium therapy eventually came to dominate the programs of the NCI. But, for a while in the late 1930s, this outcome was not certain.

This paper seeks to explain why this was the case. My argument is that the radium loan program was, in part, the result of political maneuvers that sought to respond to congressional desires to do something for existing cancer patients, while averting the possibility that these desires might result either in the creation of a large cancer treatment center in the Washington, D.C., area, or in a subsidy of diagnostic or treatment centers across the country. Physicians and some supporters in Congress feared these possibilities would mark a further unwarranted expansion of government into the provision of health services, the Public Health Service (PHS) was reluctant to take on the responsibility, and researchers feared such outcomes would end their hopes that the NCI would be a research organization. Thus, while many disliked the idea of a radium loan program, they supported it so as to stop the other ideas of a proposed cancer hospital or subsidy. The first director of the NCI later recalled that in debates over the 1937 bill "the main question was whether to build another cancer hospital or whether to establish a National Institute, primarily devoted to cancer research,"[8] and he noted that the latter won out. I think it won out on the backs of the radium program, and ultimately of the vision of the NCI as providing care for the poor.

Radium Therapy

Discovered in 1898, by World War I radium had become an important supplement (and sometimes alternative) to surgery, the mainstay of cancer therapy. Often it was used in the form of a salt, packed in milligram quantities into tubes or needles that could be inserted into natural or artificial cavities of the body in or around the tumor. The salt could also be placed in applicators that were positioned on the surface of the body or tumor, arranged in such a way as to deliver a particular dose of radiation to the growth. Alternatively, several grams of radium might be collected in one place. This radium might be used to produce radon which would be collected in small containers, sometimes called "seeds," that were used in a similar way to the tubes or needles employed with the salt.[9] Several grams of radium might also be used at some distance from the body to produce a beam of gamma radiation in a manner akin to X-rays: the so-called "beam," "bomb," or "telecurie" therapy.[10]

Radium and radon therapy had complex relationships to surgery.[11] Some techniques required what was called a surgery-of-access to insert the tubes, needles, or "seeds" into the body. In addition, these and other techniques were often used in combination with surgery to counter pain and suffering in patients, to reduce "inoperable" tumors to operable size where they could be removed surgically, to help prevent recurrence of cancer after surgery, to attack cancer cells that had spread out from the original growth, or some combination of all of these. In 1931 James Ewing, the director of the Memorial Hospital in New York, referred to the emergence of "radium surgery" as a new branch of surgery that aimed to cooperate with radiation in the treatment of cancer, but not to attempt alone to cure the disease.[12] Seven years later, in 1938, he noted that "bloodless" methods such as X-rays and radium had replaced surgery in treatment of some types of cancer, especially of the skin, pharynx and uterus.[13]

As the foregoing suggests, use of radium was appealing to surgeons for several reasons: because it built upon their existing skills, because it extended the reach of surgery into otherwise inoperable conditions, and because it promised other means of improving the effectiveness of surgical interventions. But it also had another appeal. Surgeons constantly complained that patients delayed too long in seeking care, often arriving in the physician's office long after surgery could be effective.[14] Radium promised at least two ways of addressing this issue. First, it promised to tackle the consequences of delay by making advanced tumors more accessible to surgery. As has been noted, radium could reduce, to an operable size, tumors that had grown large during the period of delay, and it could kill cells that had spread out from the original cancer during this period. Second, radium promised to tackle the causes of delay by making medical interventions less frightening to patients. In the case of breast cancer, for example, cancer experts noted that part of the reason why people put off going to the physician was that they feared having to undergo a painful, mutilating operation that was popularly believed to be ineffective against cancer. Physicians acknowledged that radium therapy could be painful,[15] but did little publicly to discourage the popular belief that it was less painful and mutilating than surgery. Despite the need for a surgery-of-access, radium therapy was sometimes called surgery-without-the-knife, and before-and-after photographs routinely advertised cures by radium without the mutilation of surgery.

This is not to say that surgeons were unanimously in favor of radium. Some raised questions about its effectiveness compared to surgery or X-rays, some feared its harmful effects in the hands of inexperienced physicians, and some saw it as a threat to the reputation of cancer

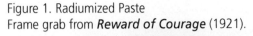

Figure 1. Radiumized Paste
Frame grab from *Reward of Courage* (1921).

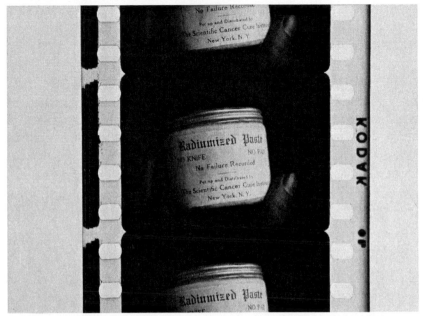

The emergence of radium as an alternative and supplement to surgery in orthodox practice was threatened by its use in alternative "quack" therapies. The American Society for the Control of Cancer (ASCC) attempted to discredit "quack" uses of radium by claiming that they were ineffective, and that quacks were motivated mainly by money, and bordered on the criminal. In the ASCC's educational movie *Reward of Courage* (1921), the fictional quack Morris Maxwell fraudulently attempts to sell Radiumized Paste as a cure for cancer and is eventually arrested for his efforts.

therapy, especially given its associations with quackery.[16] (Figure 1) Surgical enthusiasm for radium was thus initially patchy, with enthusiasts and doubters debating its effectiveness in different types of cancer, at different stages of tumor growth, in combination with other modalities, and in the hands of particular practitioners.

In the 1920s and especially the 1930s, these debates intensified as large numbers of physicians flooded into the field, deepening earlier concerns among cancer agencies about inexperienced physicians taking up the therapy without sufficient understanding of its dangers, or the complexities of dosage, filtration, and administration of treatment.[17] To these critics, some of the new radium enthusiasts were moved less by concern for their patients than by a desire for profit. As Daniel Quigley, the director of the Radium Hospital of Omaha, Nebraska, put it in 1929, targeting the growing tendency of physicians to rent radium:

> The proper use of radium requires the highest degree of skill and the greatest amount of experience, but the renting of radium puts it into the hands of the unskilled and dishonest. There can be only one motive in renting radium; that motive is the desire to get a fee and a fee to which obviously the doctor renting the radium is not entitled. He exploits his patients for a price, often causes death or disability on account of insufficient or bungling treatment, and causes all radium treatment to be cursed.[18]

For Quigley and others, commercial radium rental agencies were complicit in this problem, often issuing doctors with "full directions" for the use of radium in lieu of formal training.[19]

Criticism of the commercial motives behind radium renting also highlights growing concerns about quackery. For years anti-cancer organizations had warned the public to steer clear of quacks and to seek medical advice from a regular physician as soon as the possibility of cancer was identified. In these warnings, the public was advised that one way to distinguish a quack from a regular physician was his or her attitude towards money: Quacks were more interested in profit than patients. Amid the frenzy of physicians rushing to obtain radium in the 1920s and 1930s, cancer experts feared commercial motivations blurred this distinction, and led to exaggerated medical claims for radium therapy that were indistinguishable from those of quacks. Radium renters, like quacks, undermined patient trust by promising cures that they could not deliver, and risked patients' lives because they failed to understand the dangers of radium. Physicians pointed to quack cures that killed, like the infamous Radithor,[20] as signifying the dangers of quackery. But it was equally clear that inexperienced regular physicians could, as Quigley put it, cause death and disability.[21]

The Costs of Radium

The flood of physicians into radium therapy in the 1930s helped set the stage for the NCI's radium program. Radium was immensely costly, at one time the most expensive substance in the world, and physicians and medical institutions found it difficult to obtain sufficient amounts of the substance. Thus, while radium imports into the United States jumped dramatically after 1929–it was one of the few commodities not to be affected by the economic downturn, according to the U.S. Department of Commerce [22]–supply did not keep pace with medical demand. A 1931 survey undertaken by the Bureau of Mines estimated that the total radium for medical purposes available in the United States was 124.7 grams, a little over half the quantity the country needed.[23] A 1937 estimate suggests the situation had changed little. A report in the *Washington Post* noted that the United States had 115 grams of radium available for medical purposes, and that a further 125 grams would be needed.[24]

Despite the concerns about price, radium was in fact cheaper in the 1930s than in the late teens and early 1920s, and the price was continuing to fall.[25] Prices had peaked in 1914 when American production of the element began and fell substantially until around 1921, when the Belgians opened new sources of radium in their colony in the Congo. They came to dominate world supply, forcing an end to American production. However, demand for medical radium both in the United States and abroad, outstripped supply, and the rate of fall in price slowed following the beginnings of Congo production. To respond to accusations that they used their monopoly position to hike the price of radium, the Belgian radium suppliers highlighted the fall in prices and also the practical problems of production, for only a very small quantity of radium could be extracted from tons of the ore.[26]

In 1932 the near monopoly of the Belgians came to an end with the opening up of Canadian sources of radium. The rate of fall in the price of radium began to quicken until 1938, when an agreement to divide the world market and stabilize the price at $40,000 per gram was negotiated between the Belgians and Canadians. The price did in fact rise a little, but the manufacturers' desired price was not attained.[27] By the late 1930s, commentators hoped for further downward pressure on the price of radium from the introduction of high voltage X-ray machines (which produced rays of a similar wavelength to the gamma rays of radium) and from the newly developed cyclotron, a possible source of artificial radiation that might be substituted for radium.[28] The good news of lower prices was, however, tempered by the economic depression. Thus, while the price of radium dropped, hospitals and practitioners often found they were unable to purchase the substance.

Against this backdrop, the idea that the federal government might be involved in obtaining radium gained political and medical support. Government radium promised to improve supplies, lessen dependence on foreign radium companies, and improve the uneven distribution of radium across the nation. Most radium was concentrated in larger cities and cancer centers, mainly in the East and Mid-West. Many states had only a few milligrams of radium, and some of them had none.[29] There were vast swathes of the country, especially in the West, which had no radium for cancer treatment available within hundreds of miles.[30] Patients in these parts of the country were unlikely to obtain radium therapy without traveling a great distance. For some critics, this suggested that an increase in the supply of radium alone would not solve the problem. A fall in the price might mean that radium would simply go to places that already had a supply, exacerbating the uneven distribution of the element.[31]

But the growing support for federal involvement in the radium issue was not without opposition. Thus, when in 1934 Senator James Davis (R-Pennsylvania) introduced a bill into Congress allowing Belgium to pay $10,000,000 of its war debt in the form of radium, the surgeon-dominated American Radium Society (ARS) argued against the proposal, concerned that this would give the federal government significant influence over the specialty.[32] This radium was intended for distribution to hospitals and clinics, and, in the ARS view, it threatened to curb private enterprise, raised the spectre of greater federal competition with recognized practitioners, and threatened to exacerbate the problem of inexpert physicians entering the field. Despite anxieties about the growing numbers of quacks and inexperienced physicians using radium, the ARS preferred professional self-regulation to government regulation. The prospects of federal purchase of radium looked slim.

The Great Depression and Cancer

Three years later, the situation had changed. With millions of Americans unable to afford cancer services due to the economic depression, with hospitals and clinics continuing to find it difficult to obtain radium, with cancer mortality surpassing that of tuberculosis in the early 1930s, and with anti-cancer legislative initiatives by progressive Democrats in Congress, opposition to government involvement weakened. The door was opened to a greater role for federal agencies in cancer, and, ultimately, to the federal purchase of radium for therapy.

The door was opened, in part, by a very significant growth in cancer services that created more demand for radium. Encouraged by the American Society for the Control of Cancer (ASCC) and the closely-related American College of Surgeons (ACS), the numbers of cancer clinics began to boom.[33] In the early 1920s there were probably less than fifteen in the entire country.[34] However, following publication in 1930 of the ACS recommendations on standards for cancer services, this number rose dramatically.[35] By 1940 the number of clinics surveyed by the ACS was 490 with 345 approved. (See Table 1.) At the same time, state health departments also began to take a growing interest in cancer. In the 1930s, older control programs such as those in New York and Massachusetts[36] were joined by New Hampshire (1931), followed by Connecticut (1935), by Missouri, Illinois, and Georgia (1937), and by South Carolina and Vermont (1939). As Figure 2 indicates, by the 1940s several other states had the beginnings of an official anti-cancer program.[37]

Table 1. Clinics approved and surveyed by the American College of Surgeons, 1933-1940.

Year	Surveyed	Approved
1933	200	140
1934	239	181
1935	250	198
1936	246	210
1937	296	240
1938	332	272
1939	423	307
1940	490	345

Source: See sources listed in Table 2 for approved cancer clinics.
Note: This ACS list surveyed not only American but also Canadian and later a few Chinese and Cuban clinics–these clinics are included in the totals above.

Figure 2. State Cancer Control Programs in 1940.

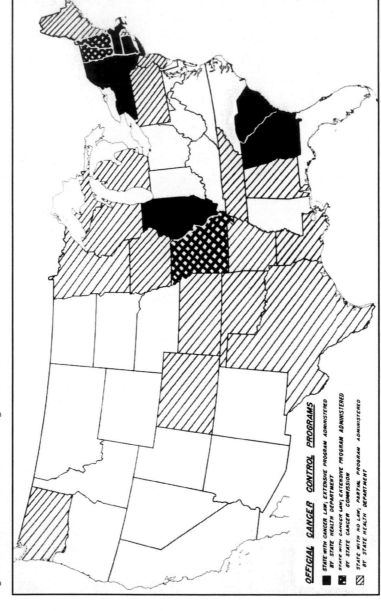

OFFICIAL CANCER CONTROL PROGRAMS

■ STATE WITH CANCER LAW, EXTENSIVE PROGRAM ADMINISTERED
  BY STATE HEALTH DEPARTMENT

▨ STATE WITH CANCER LAW, EXTENSIVE PROGRAM ADMINISTERED
  BY STATE CANCER COMMISSION

▧ STATE WITH NO LAW, PARTIAL PROGRAM ADMINISTERED
  BY STATE HEALTH DEPARTMENT

Source: Carl Voegtlin and R. R. Spencer, "The Federal Cancer Control Program," *Journal of the National Cancer Institute*, 1940, *1*: 5.

The burgeoning numbers of cancer clinics and services challenged opposition to the federal purchase of radium. With their budgets strained by hard economic times, many hospitals and state health departments found it very difficult to find the money for radium for such clinics, and so found themselves unable to compete in the frenetic market for the substance. Yet demand for radium continued to rise, fed by various education campaigns that informed the public that the only cure for cancer was early treatment by radium, X-rays, and surgery undertaken by a recognized physician.[38] In these circumstances it was often unclear what hospitals or state health departments should do to obtain radium. Occasionally, they began anti-cancer programs even in the absence of radium, perhaps in part to create political pressure for the substance.[39] But such strategies were risky. The pressure might not work, and patients would be left with nowhere to go, except perhaps to inexperienced physicians and quacks. Thus physicians were often reluctant to undertake campaigns until radium was available.[40] It was a double-bind: the absence of radium created pressure for campaigns to boost supplies, but the campaign could backfire and create demands that cancer programs could not meet.

Against this backdrop of growing anxieties about radium, and with the Belgian war-debt repayment scheme seemingly dead, Congress revisited plans for a cancer bill to authorize federal support for research and treatment. The Public Health Service had supported a small research program on cancer since August 1922, when the Surgeon General had assigned Joseph W. Schereschewsky to study the disease in a rented laboratory in the Department of Preventive Medicine at Harvard Medical School. But efforts to expand PHS support for research had faltered, and bills introduced into Congress in 1927, 1928, 1929 and 1930, did not pass into law.[41] Part of the reason for this failure was a lack of enthusiasm on the part of the PHS. This attitude changed with the appointment in 1936 of Thomas Parran as Surgeon General. As James Patterson notes, Parran had a particular interest in cancer: his wife had died of the disease, he had served on the ASCC, and he had a liberal, activist view of the government's role in public health.[42] The following year, Senator Homer Bone of Washington and Representatives Maury Maverick of Texas and Warren G. Magnuson of Washington, all progressive Democrats, introduced three cancer bills into Congress.[43] Parran was involved in shaping the Bone and Maverick bills, and perhaps Magnuson's as well.

Unlike the bills in the 1920s, the new bills were not restricted to research. Both Bone and Maverick were anxious to address the problems faced particularly by the poor, and both included the purchase and loan of radium for treatment in their bills. Bone seems to have introduced this measure on the recommendation of Parran, who argued against a broader proposal for a government subsidy to cancer diagnostic and treatment centers. Parran noted that the country was particularly lacking in an adequate supply of radium, that radium was particularly expensive ($30,000-$40,000 a gram), and that the country needed sixty to eighty additional grams. In his view, the public authorities were willing to take responsibility for the purchase and loan of radium, but not for the broader subsidy, which would involve considerable public expenditure.[44] Parran also made a case to Maury Maverick for the purchase and loan of radium.[45]

Political Compromise

The loan program thus entered the legislation as a means of addressing the national shortage of radium, and paradoxically of limiting the role of the newly activist Public Health Service in providing cancer services. But this still leaves one question: Why did the loan program constitute such a large percentage of the NCI's budget when a major justification for the creation of the NCI was that of research? The answer, I suggest, was the low status of cancer research as a field, and the inability of scientists to persuade Congress that the long-term benefits of laboratory research should win out over the immediate benefits of distributing radium.

Those who argued for federal support for cancer research often highlighted the poor status of the field in the country. It was, they claimed, undervalued. Philanthropic resources were insufficient to support cancer research, and there were not enough trained investigators in the field.[46] Pay was poor. The average wage of a cancer researcher with two to five years of experience was about that of a carpenter, and people were easily tempted by the better pay and prospects in industry. Moreover, the field was so technically complex, and the prospects of scientific advance so uncertain, that it was very unlikely a cancer researcher could make a name for himself or herself, and, even if he or she did, there was little in the way of a career structure by which they might advance. In 1932, Henry Sigerist, recently appointed to head the Institute of the History of Medicine at the Johns Hopkins University, recalled a German surgeon telling him: "If a great scientist at the end of a brilliant career wants to make a fool of himself, he takes up the problem of cancer."[47]

It was such problems that made cancer researchers particularly vociferous in their appeals for federal funding, but the problems also reveal the weakness of the researchers' position. By their own admission they could not promise results in terms of improvements in treatment for years, if ever, and so it was often quite unclear why, if federal money should be spent on cancer at all, it should not go to something like radium which promised immediate results in terms of relieving suffering. Put another way, part of the reason why research was not the main focus of the NCI was that its advocates were unable to promise results that might help already existing cancer patients. Improving cancer treatment for these patients had better political appeal in congress than nebulous promises of the future benefits of research.

Pleas for greater federal research funding were not helped by disputes among cancer experts over the value of fundamental research. For example, James Ewing argued in 1936 that in the past thirty years the major benefits to the cancer patient had come not from fundamental laboratory work, but from clinical research. Indeed, Ewing complained that the promotion of fundamental cancer research was sometimes carried out at the expense of practical steps to help patients: "the first step [he wrote] in the organization of cancer control in any community should be the provision of first-class clinical service, under cover of which one may pursue at his leisure, and without reproach, any number of interesting fundamental researches."[48] It was for this reason that, in evidence to a Joint Committee of Congress, he opposed the idea of federal support for research as: "merely another futile effort to discover the ultimate cause of cancer, which is an unsolvable problem."[49] Instead, he argued for the creation of a large central cancer institute in Washington designed mainly for the treatment of patients.[50]

As one of the most influential voices in cancer research, Ewing's criticism carried weight. With Bone and Maverick keen to do something for current cancer patients, and the American Medical Association (AMA) cautioning against federal government support for research on the grounds that it might paralyze private initiative,[51] Congress found that research alone was an insufficient political ground to support arguments for the federal funding of cancer. Attention, therefore, focused on measures that might have a quicker impact than fundamental research. The prospect was worrying to supporters of laboratory research. "I hope that the treatment feature will not be neglected," noted Clarence Little, then in the midst of his campaign to promote a New Deal for mice, in evidence to the Joint Committee, "but I hope also that it will not be overemphasized to a point where the pure research suffers, because the very scattered nature of that pure research makes it a very poor beggar, a very poor agent, to raise funds for itself." [52]

Ewing's proposal of a cancer treatment center seems to have persuaded some members of Congress. Thomas Parran noted later that Congress wanted to do something for the existing cancer patient. The specific proposal, he suggested, was that the Cancer Institute should be a central government cancer hospital. But Parran added ambiguously that the "implications of it were rather frightening,"[53] and, as a result, the law was drafted to authorize the purchase and loan of radium. This was a better means, he claimed, of treating people in institutions where radium was needed, and of developing improved methods for the use of radium. Parran did not elaborate what these frightening implications were, but it is likely that he felt the PHS would be reluctant to take responsibility for this hospital, just as he had noted earlier it would have been reluctant to take responsibility for a subsidy for cancer diagnostic and treatment services. It is also probable that politically powerful medical organizations such as the American Medical Association (AMA) and the ARS were opposed to proposals for a cancer hospital (as they would also have been opposed to the subsidy proposal) as an intrusion by the federal government into health provision.

The radium loan program, therefore, gained support in part as a political compromise. First, it promised to address Congress's desire to do something for present-day cancer patients (especially patients that could not afford care during the Depression) while avoiding a broader subsidy of diagnostic and treatment services or the creation of the hospital that Ewing desired.[54] Second, it also smoothed the path to congressional support for research. Despite anxieties that they might suffer if the Cancer Act supported treatment programs, cancer researchers gained Congress's backing as part of a mixed legislative package that included both research and treatment. It was the combination of the promise of long-term benefits from research and short-term benefits from radium that made the Cancer Act politically workable.[55]

Paradoxically, this mix of research and treatment may have put an end to an earlier idea that the radium might be used primarily for research. In circa 1936/1937, Schereschewsky had drawn up a memorandum that proposed a combined cancer research and treatment center, equipped with between eight and ten grams of radium.[56] But the loan program did away with this possibility of combining research and practice. (Perhaps it was too close to Ewing's suggestion of a cancer treatment hospital.) It also did away with another possibility that radium might be used for cooperative research among several institutions. Early plans for federal radium proposed to loan the salt to hospitals, research centers, and institutions across the country, not for routine therapy alone, but also for collaborative research—radium recipients would be required to join in research problems and cooperate with a cancer center in certain clinical problems.[57] While the 1937 Act allowed for the radium to be used for research, in practice only a tiny amount was used in this way.[58] Against a backdrop of concern that radium therapy was being sacrificed to research, the vast bulk of the radium went to routine therapy.[59]

The Radium Loan Program

The radium loan program might have begun life as a political compromise, but the NCI administrators who ran it saw it as much more. In their view, the program promised not only to improve the nation's supply of radium, but also to rationalize its distribution. It would coordinate federal, state and local anti-cancer programs, and ensure that only experienced or qualified individuals obtained government radium. In short, it promised to ensure that best-practice filtered down from leading centers, through to clinics and hospitals in far-flung corners of the country. NCI administrators also hoped to be able to use the government's purchasing power to obtain radium at lower than commercial price, and there was debate as to whether the NCI should put the purchase off until the price had fallen further.[60] In fact, following the government's acquisition of radium, the price rose, and the radium companies and the National Bureau of Standards began to predict further increases in the price of radium, in part because of increasing demand for the element, and because of the Belgian-Canadian agreement previously mentioned.[61] Rising prices prompted some to see the NCI not as a source of radium, but as a potential purchaser of their own surplus radium.[62]

The first loan was made to Sedgwick County Hospital, Wichita, Kansas, on 6 October 1938, and by 1940, 47 hospitals in 24 states and Hawaii had received radium.[63] The number had jumped to about 57 in 1943 (see Table 2 at pp. 121-24), not including the Marine Hospital in Baltimore to which the NCI allocated two grams of radium for a radon production plant.[64] As the name suggests, the program was a loan program. Hospitals that received radium were not given the radium; it remained the property of the NCI, and hospitals had to reapply each year to keep the radium on loan to them.[65] The NCI itself did not charge for the loan: hospitals that received radium agreed to obtain insurance for it, and not to charge their patients for its use, excepting some related nursing and medical costs. Occasionally, the NCI would visit the various hospitals for routine checks of the tumor clinics and the radium.[66] It also visited clinics to follow up complaints of poor practice. One such visit was in 1940 to the Sedgwick County Hospital.[67]

The vast bulk of the radium went not to elite cancer institutions, but to small city, county, and private hospitals, as well as to a sprinkling of university hospitals providing care for indigents.[68] Most of the hospitals that received radium were in the East, the South and the Mid-West (See Figure 3). Few hospitals west of Wichita received radium, excepting loans to Denver's Colorado General and St Luke's Hospitals, El Paso's City-County Hospital, Seattle's Swedish Hospital, the City County Hospital in Los Angeles, and the Queen's Hospital in Hawaii. If the program was intended to improve the distribution of radium throughout the country, it did not succeed. Although the loan program was an

Figure 3. Radium loans in 1940.

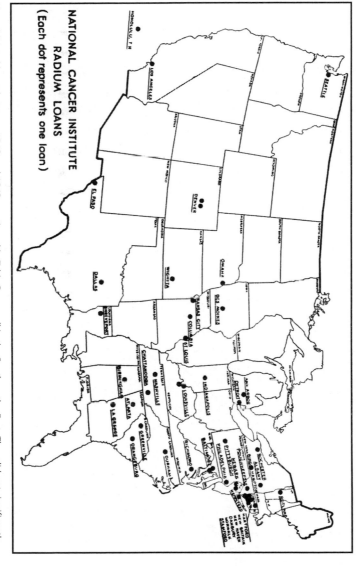

NATIONAL CANCER INSTITUTE
RADIUM LOANS
(Each dot represents one loan)

The additional loans between 1940 and 1943 mentioned in Table 2 were all in the South or the East. They did not significantly change the distribution of radium in the West.

Source: Carl Voegtlin and R. R. Spencer, "The Federal Cancer Control Program," *Journal of the National Cancer Institute,* 1940, 1: 6.

important element in state cancer control programs, many areas especially in the West remained without adequate medical radium.

As Table 2 indicates many hospitals that received radium between 1938 and 1943 had established tumor clinics in the 1930s, a significant number being formed in 1937/1939 shortly before the first loans of radium were sent out. As has been noted, creating cancer clinics could be an expensive undertaking because of the need to purchase X-ray, radium and laboratory equipment. Not all hospitals could obtain sufficient radium, and some could obtain none. Hospitals without radium had to send patients elsewhere for treatment,[69] or return them home,[70] and the absence of radium or X-ray equipment jeopardized recognition by the American College of Surgeons, which specified that tumor clinics must be equipped to properly treat patients with radium and X-rays.[71] Hospital administrators and physicians thus saw government radium as a way of easing the financial burden, expanding the range of services available for patients, and gaining ACS recognition.[72] Recognition by the ACS was not a prerequisite for an NCI loan. Eight hospitals did not have ACS-approved clinics prior to 1943, and others only obtained recognition after the loan was made (see Table 2).[73]

This is not to say that government radium was an unequivocal boon. The arrival of government radium was often reported in the local press, with the result that hospitals and clinics would suddenly find themselves inundated with new patients.[74] Growing numbers of patients could signify a welcome growth of public and medical awareness of the cancer problem.[75] But it also created demands for cancer services that hospital administrators and physicians feared they would be unable to meet. This could be a never-ending problem, with the acquisition of radium stimulating a new flow of patients, in turn creating demands for more radium and other cancer services, in turn promoting delay. Thus, the free radium from the NCI could be a temporary fix, and one that came with strings (such as particular qualifications of radium therapists) that hospitals could find difficult to meet.[76] But, despite these problems, hospital administrators were not reluctant to seek NCI radium, and demand rapidly outstripped supply.

If hospital administrators saw NCI radium as a means of improving cancer services, so too did state health administrators. Federal radium was an integral part of state cancer control programs established between 1937 and 1939, including those of Connecticut,[77] Missouri,[78] Georgia,[79] South Carolina,[80] and Vermont,[81] as well as older ones such as those of New York and Massachusetts. Like their hospital counterparts, state officials saw radium as a useful means of ensuring that cancer clinics were provided with a full range of therapeutic equipment.[82] The failure of some hospitals to secure government radium meant delay in establishing diagnostic or treatment clinics, and endangered these nascent state anti-cancer schemes. The director of the Georgia Department of Public Health made the point in 1938, fearful that one hospital's failure to secure government radium would undermine his efforts to establish a network of cancer centers across the state: "undue delay [he wrote to the NIH] in supplying this radium will materially affect the organization of additional treatment centers which we are endeavoring to establish in this State."[83] At first, each applicant hospital was required to have the approval of the official state boards of health and cancer commissions, where the latter existed.[84]

One Georgian state official argued that the growing importance of cancer as a public health issue meant that they were the ones most familiar with existing facilities in their states and best suited to judge where additional facilities should be established.[85] The point was endorsed by the NACC, which also hoped it would cement existing cooperative relations between the state health departments and the United States Public Health Service, and solve the practical problems of assessing the suitability of individual hospitals for a loan. The NACC wanted to ensure that loans were part of a coordinated effort by the state to deal with the cancer problem, and counter what Clarence Little saw as "immediate condemnation [from medical "men"] of even the idea that we should loan radium to any individual institutions."[86] But it was only a short term solution. Only a few state health departments had well-organized cancer control programs, and only a few of these included radiation therapy. One NCI official later noted that in consequence the requirement did not have a significant impact on the program.[87] The requirement for state approval was later dropped following the addition of qualified radiologists to the NCI's staff who served as consultants and advisors to the loan program, and with the growth of approval procedures by the various radiology organizations.[88]

In addition to the requirement for state approval, the NCI stipulated that only those with qualifications equivalent to those required for diplomates of the American Board of Radiology (incorporated in 1934) would be allowed to use the radium for treatment. "This is the highest standard that we know of in this country," explained Carl Voegtlin, the chief of the NCI, who went on to elaborate a legal rationale as well: "and it was adopted in order to protect ourselves against the possibility of lawsuits by persons who might be injured as the result of improper radium therapy."[89] However, Schereschewsky (who had now moved from Harvard to Georgia, where he was the acting director of cancer control for the state) worried that this recommendation might work against efforts to ensure that the radium was distributed to places that did not have it. In his view, the American Board of Radiology's qualifications were so strict that the creation of some outlying centers without such qualified radiologists would be unduly delayed, and would, as he put it, "seriously cripple cancer treatment facilities in the State."[90] By 1962, seven institutions had been denied a loan because their radiologists did not meet the qualifications of the Board.[91]

These issues highlight tensions between federal and state administrators over the radium loan program. The program might have begun as an effort to cement cooperative arrangements, but sometimes federal and state officials did not cooperate. Federal officials found state officials questioning how they ran the program. These officials queried federal decisions by which hospitals received or did not receive radium; federal decisions on the qualifications required of radium practitioners; and the federal decision that only indigent patients should receive government radium. Georgia makes the case again. The Georgian control scheme aimed to make cancer clinics available for both private and state-aided patients, and Georgian officials worried that federal rules dictated that, even where there was no other radium locally, paying patients would not be allowed to use NCI radium. Therefore they would be required to travel a considerable distance for treatment—a requirement that would probably result in delayed treatment.[92] The NCI's response is not recorded, but it does not seem to have changed its rules.

We do not know much about the technical use of radium: few records on this subject appear to have survived. However, the quantity of radium purchased by the NCI placed restrictions on the type of therapy that could be undertaken. Most radium was allocated in small milligram quantities, packed into standardized tubes and needles, apart from the two grams given to the Marine Hospital in Baltimore for radon production. Despite considerable discussion on the NACC, the Council decided not to allocate radium for telecurie or bomb therapy, the major technological innovation of the 1930s.[93] This required several grams of radium to produce a beam of radiation, and the NCI simply did not have enough to distribute for this purpose; not the eight to ten grams that Schereschewsky had requested for the proposed cancer research hospital, which would have been sufficient for a bomb.

Radium bombs would have tied up too much radium to allow the NCI to make the element widely available. Moreover, despite considerable enthusiasm for bomb therapy in Europe it was still regarded as an experimental technique on the American side of the Atlantic, and its superiority to newer supervoltage X-ray equipment was questioned, since the latter produced X-rays of similar wavelength to the gamma rays of radium. "The best testimony that Congress had," Thomas Parran told the NACC in answer to a question about the intention of Congress, "was that there was a deficiency in the amount of radium, that radium was a valuable agent for the treatment of cancer, and that more radium would save the lives of some patients. You would not be doing that in the next year whilst experimenting with the radium bombbs [sic], and there is a likelihood that in two or three years from now the price will be lower."[94]

Second, if the quantity of radium purchased by the NCI placed restrictions on the types of therapy that could be carried out, it also restricted the ways in which the NCI could influence the development of radiotherapy as a specialty. Comparison with the British system of radium distribution is worth mention here. The establishment in 1929 in Britain of a centralized national radium organization had resulted in the creation of one of the world's largest radium purchasing and supply organizations–the Radium Trust which purchased radium, and the Radium Commission which distributed it to hospitals. In 1931 the Trust ordered 24.9 grams of radium, and later obtained a further 20 grams on loan, with the option of purchase; quantities that dwarfed the 9.5 grams of radium purchased by the NCI for a much larger nation.[95] The

Commission used its control of radium to encourage the separation of radiotherapy from radio-diagnosis (this did not happen in the United States until the 1960s); to encourage the development of bomb therapy; to forge a common union between radium therapy and X-ray therapy, hitherto often quite separate specialties; and to make hospitals that wanted its radium appoint physicists, and adopt certain safety and practice standards.[96] The NCI quickly realized that it could not hope to emulate these efforts. After receiving a report on the British Radium Commission, the director of the NIH was moved to note in 1938: "the English are ahead of us in the development of a national plan for cancer control as far as the government is concerned."[97]

The End of a New Deal for Patients

The radium loan program began in 1938 with high hopes of a new future for radium therapy within the NCI. Indeed, at one time the prospect was that similar sums would be spent on radium in future years. The *Washington Post* reported in 1937 that the plan was for the federal government to spend $1,000,000 over a period of five years: ten grams a year at $20,000 a gram (less than Parran's estimated cost of the previous year) until the supply was increased to 50 grams.[98] But this plan never came about. Nineteen thirty-eight was the only year in which the use of radium constituted such a large part of the NCI's budget,[99] and while expenditure on cancer research boomed during the 1940s, the radium loan program soon disappeared from view, its budget so small that it barely figures in the NCI's accounts after 1940. All it cost was the salary of a part-time administrator, and $2,000 per annum which was transferred to the National Bureau of Standards to check the radium containers.

So why did it end? Part of the reason was the opposition of cancer researchers like Little, who saw in the radium program a danger that "their" institute might be turned into a treatment program for the poor.[100] It will be recalled that research alone had been insufficient justification for the creation of the NCI, and that researchers had piggy-backed on the appeal of radium therapy in Congress to get the 1937 Act passed. But having benefited politically from radium therapy, they now attempted to do away with it through the NACC: a body "seriously criticized for being made up of non-medical men on the one hand and pathologists on the other,"[101] as one NACC member noted. The initial efforts of its members, however, seem to have gone nowhere. At one point in its second meeting, the NACC tried to reduce the cost of the radium purchase to $10,000, prompting one later commentator to note: "Either it had not been made clear or the council lost sight of the fact that $200,000 of the Institute's appropriation for that year had to be spent for radium, or else not spent at all."[102]

Early efforts to get rid of the radium loan program might have been ineffective, but critics soon picked up on a broader anxiety about the program. Physicians and researchers had accepted the creation of the program as an alternative to even more worrying prospects, such as the creation of a federally funded cancer hospital or of a subsidy for diagnostic and treatment services, but, as soon as these problems were out of the way, critics began to focus attention on the radium program itself, fearful that this too might be the thin end of the wedge of socialized medicine. The *Washington Post's* suggestion that by 1942 the NCI might have about 50 grams of the element, would have given the institute enormous power over the development of radium therapy in the United States, and perhaps of cancer services more generally. Physicians could look across the Atlantic to Britain, where a government-controlled radium organization had effectively reshaped cancer services in that country by means of its control of a vast proportion of the nation's radium. American physicians were not enamored of the prospect of similar developments in the United States.

The opportunity to stop such a prospect came about with concerns that there were not enough hospitals and specialists that met the standards of equipment and skill set out by the NCI for a radium loan.[103] The result was that the NACC quickly agreed not to purchase any more radium in future years, and to focus attention instead on the question of medical training and education. To address this issue, the NACC appointed a committee on education, which met for the first time in January 1938, and effectively marked the beginning of the end of plans to expand the radium loan program. Schereschewsky's concerns that the high standards required of radium practitioners might undermine state efforts to obtain radium had come about, albeit not perhaps in the way he had anticipated.

The discussions that followed as recorded in the verbatim minutes of this committee show how questions of technical competency in the use of radium were intertwined with anxieties about the prospect of state medicine, the nature of specialization in cancer research, and the appropriate role of the federal government in cancer. While most speakers were willing to accept a role for the federal government in training physicians, they expressed deep misgivings about the prospect of state medicine, and about the impact of the federal government on the direction of medical specialization. The debate drifted off into a detailed discussion of training in cancer and the role of the federal government in this, laying the foundations of a new NCI program of clinical training in cancer. [104]

The NACC might have agreed not to purchase radium in future years, but this still left the question of what to do about the $200,000 appropriated for 1938. NACC opinion was a mix of political reluctance to support the loan program, and practical fears that the small hospitals to which they proposed to loan the radium would not have the staff or facilities to handle it safely and effectively. The result was that the NCI put off the purchase of radium while it worked out how to distribute the element, and determine whether it could ensure its competent and safe use. Ironically, this delay lead to a belated and somewhat reluctant support for the loan program as members calculated the political costs of not spending money on a project in which Congress was particularly interested. As one of the opponents of the radium program, Clarence Little, noted, there was a risk that the failure to purchase might endanger congressional support for other projects. "We have to depend on a certain amount of good will on the part of the Congress of the United States if the projects we have already started are to be continued let alone an expansion program,"[105] he noted with reference to plans to expand training and research.

Political calculations also ensured that the NACC continued to ask Congress for money for radium long after it had decided not to expand the program. The problem was, as the director of the NIH, Lewis R. Thompson, put it, that the budget line might disappear if they did not ask for money for radium. The purchase of radium had been in the first year's appropriation for the NCI, and if it was not included in subsequent years, the risk was that Congress might take away the money. Thompson explained: "The thing that occurs to them [members of Congress] always is, if you are not going to buy $100,000 worth of radium, let us take it off your appropriation."[106] This quandary put some members of the NACC into a difficult position. They did not want to lose the money, but they also worried, as Clarence Little put it, that a request for more money for radium "would open the doors to unnecessary political pressure which none of us wants."[107] The NCI had received more applications for radium than it could fill, and Congress was more interested in present cancer patients than in research. Little feared that the request for radium threatened plans to expand research funding.[108]

The consequence was an extended discussion on the NACC on how to include radium in the funding request to Congress in such a way as to allow the institute to spend the money on other projects. Any last hopes that the radium program might expand disappeared in this convoluted budgetary debate. A mix of medical and scientific opposition to government provision of cancer services, anxieties about the capacity of physicians to use government radium safely and effectively, and some deft political maneuvering, had destroyed hopes of using the resources of the federal government to help indigent cancer patients. Never again would such a large percentage of the NCI's budget be devoted to providing routine treatment. Instead, the NCI shifted resources to research and training. A different vision of the New Deal had won out. The vision of the NCI as providing free health care for the poor was dead.

Epilogue

What happened to the radium loan program? The vision of the NCI as providing free health care for the poor might have died in 1938, but the radium program did not die with it. Indeed, the number of radium loans increased to average between 52 and 54 hospitals per year for much of the early 1950s–this without any additional radium purchases. A 1962 report noted that between 1938 and 1962, the NCI received 114 applications for radium loans, from 109 institutions or hospitals, 75 of which were approved and 34 were not approved. Five additional loans were made to groups in the Public Health Service, one to a hospital and the remaining four to groups for research purposes.[109] We know the names of only two hospitals that were rejected, and of only 68 of the 75 hospitals that received radium.[110]

Despite the increase in loans, after 1940 the NCI gave little attention to the program beyond its routine administration. There were brief discussions of the program on the NACC in 1942 after Pearl Harbor (it was feared that enemy bombing might disperse the radium),[111] and in 1944 following the inclusion of the NCI into the NIH under the Public Health Service Act (it was feared the loan program might not be legal under an act that did not appear to allow for a treatment program: Lawyers confirmed that the program was legal).[112] In July 1947 the loan program–originally run from the NCI's Office of the Director–was transferred to the newly created Cancer Control Branch of the NCI, later renamed the Field Investigations and Demonstrations Branch.[113]

After 1947 the program continued quietly until the late 1950s, when the NCI became concerned about poor safety standards in many hospitals receiving radium.[114] The problem was not new. There had been concern about this issue in 1940 when a survey highlighted "rather startling" levels of radiation exposure in cancer clinics, [115] but the news was new to John Heller, the director of the NCI in the late 1950s. Fearful that the NCI would be criticized for not ensuring the safe use of the radium, Heller appointed an advisory committee to view the future of the program, which led to the radium being recalled, repackaged, and loaned out again under tighter rules.[116] Heller's successor, Kenneth Endicott (1960-1969), wanted to close the program down.[117] But, instead, in January 1961 he appointed a new committee to recommend standards for the allocation of radium, while in June 1961 another committee prepared a "Guide for Protection Against Radiations from Radium in Storage, Use, and Handling."[118] In part because of the tighter rules (and perhaps because now the NCI discovered it only had seven rather than nine and a half grams), the number of hospitals using radium seems to have dropped from 54/55 to about 45.[119]

After this flurry of interest, the program quietly disappeared from attention again. The last record I have of its existence is in 1966, so it probably came to an end in the late 1960s or 1970s.[120] We may never know precisely when it ended. The files were destroyed in 1988.[121]

Table 2. Hospitals receiving radium from the NCI, 1938-1943.

State	Institution	Location	Tumor Clinic Approved by ACS	Tumor Clinic Founded	Comments
Maryland/D.C.	NCI and the United States Marine Hospital	Washington and Baltimore	1941	c.1939[122]	(2 grams) Radium for the production of radon, and for research.[123]

State	Institution	Location	Tumor Clinic Approved by ACS	Tumor Clinic Founded
Alabama	Hillman Hospital†	Birmingham	1940-	TC:c. 1940.[124]
California	Los Angeles County General Hospital*†	Los Angeles	1935-	
Colorado	Colorado General Hospital University of Colorado (Bonfils Foundation Tumor Clinic)*†	Denver	1934 1937-	CC: 1926[125] TC: 1937[126]
	St. Luke's Hospital*†[127]	Denver	1933-	CC: 1931?[128]
Connecticut	Danbury Hospital*†	Danbury		In existence in 1939
	Grace Hospital*†	New Haven	1937-	In existence in 1935
	New Britain General Hospital†	New Britain	1939-	TC:1939[129]
	Norwalk General Hospital*†	Norwalk	1940-	IConf:1934[130]
	St. Francis Hospital*†[131]	Hartford	1933-	TG: 1935[132]
	Stamford Hospital*†	Stamford	1940-	TC: 1938[133]
Georgia	City-County Hospital*†	LaGrange	1942-	CC:1938[134]
	University Hospital?*	Augusta	1936-	
	Emory University Hospital†	Atlanta	1938-	CC?: 1937[135]
Territory of Hawaii	The Queen's Hospital*†[136]	Honolulu	1941-	CC: 1931[137]
Illinois	Cook County Hospital†	Chicago	1933-4 1941-	TC: 1938[138]
Indiana	Indianapolis City Hospital†[139]	Indianapolis	1936-	CC&W: 1938[140]
	Protestant Deaconess Hospital†	Evansville	1941-	CI: 1939[141]
Iowa	Broadlawns General Hospital†	Des Moines	1939-	
Kansas	Sedgwick County Hospital and Clinic*†[142]	Wichita	1939-40 (D) 1941-	TC/CC: 1937[143]
Kentucky	Norton Memorial Infirmary*†	Louisville	1933-	TC: 1932[144]
	St. Joseph's Infirmary†	Louisville	1933-	TC: 1932.[145]
Louisiana	Shreveport Charity Hospital*†[146]	Shreveport	1933-	TC: 1932
Maryland	Johns Hopkins Hospital*†[147]	Baltimore	1939 (D) 1939-[148]	
	University of Maryland Hospital*†	Baltimore	1933	OIc: 1930 [149]

Table 2. Hospitals receiving radium from the NCI, 1938-1943 (continued).

State	Institution	Location	Tumor Clinic Approved by ACS	Tumor Clinic Founded
Massachusetts	Worcester City Hospital†	Worcester	1934-5 1941-	TC: 1939[150]
Michigan	Mercy Hall Cancer Hospital†	Detroit		
	Receiving Hospital†	Detroit	1935-6 (D) 1937-	
	University of Michigan Hospital*†	Ann Arbor	1933-	
Missouri	Barnard Free Skin and Cancer Hospital*†[151]	St. Louis	1933-39 1940- (H)	
	Kansas City Municipal Hospital*†[152]	Kansas City	1936-	CC: 1938[153]
	Missouri Cancer Commission for the Ellis Fischel State Cancer Hospital*†[154]	Columbia	1940- (H)	Cancer Hospital opened 1940
	Fulton State Hospital*[155]	Fulton	1934-8 (D) 1939	TC/CC: 1933[156] Beds 1935/6[157]
Nebraska	University of Nebraska Hospital*†	Omaha	1938-	TC founded between 1935 & 1940
New Jersey	Newark Beth Israel Hospital*†	Newark	1933-	1929[158]
	Newark City Hospital*†[159]	Newark		1939/40 radiotherapy department.
New York	Albany Hospital*†[160]	Albany	1938-	
	Binghamton Hospital*†	Binghamton	1937-	
	Vassar Brothers Hospital*† (Duchess County Tumor Clinic)	Poughkeepsie	1939-	TC: 1939[161]
	Meadowbrook Hospital*†	Hempstead	1935-	TC: 1937[162]
	Strong Memorial Hospital (University of Rochester)*†[163]	Rochester	1933-	TC: c1930/1[164]
North Carolina	Charlotte Memorial Hospital†	Charlotte		
	Duke University Hospital*†	Durham	1939-	TC: 1935[165]
	North Carolina Baptist Hospital†[166]	Winston-Salem		TC: 1944[167]
Pennsylvania	Elizabeth Steel Magee Hospital†	Pittsburgh	1940-	
	Misericordia Hospital*†[168]	Philadelphia		Clinic planned 1933[169]
South Carolina	Greenville General Hospital†	Greenville		TC:c.1939/40[170]
	Tri-County Hospital†	Orangeburg		
Tennessee	The Baroness Erlanger Hospital*†	Chattanooga	1940-	?TC:1922[171] CC:1940[172]
	Nashville General Hospital*†	Nashville	1941-	TC: 1940[173]

Table 2. Hospitals receiving radium from the NCI, 1938-1943 (continued).

State	Institution	Location	Tumor Clinic Approved by ACS	Tumor Clinic Founded
Texas	Baylor University Hospital†	Dallas	1933-1942	TC: 1931[174]
	El Paso City-County Hospital† (El Paso Country Medical Society Tumor Clinic)	El Paso	1940-	Unknown
Vermont	Mary Fletcher Hospital†[175]	Burlington	1939 (D)	TC: 1939[176]
	Vermont State Cancer Commission for Use at the Rutland Hospital and the X-ray and Radium Institute†[177]	Rutland	1940-	TC: 1939[178]
Virginia	Medical College of Virginia*†[179]	Richmond	1937-	1937 a TC "in its infancy"[180] in existence. TC: 1939[181]
	University of Virginia Tumor Clinic†	Charlottesville	1934-	
Washington	Swedish Hospital*†[182]	Seattle	1933-	TI:c1932[183]
West Virginia	Mountain State Memorial Hospital†	Charleston	1933-	TC/CC: 1934[184]

SOURCES AND NOTES FOR TABLE 2

Radium Loans:

Sources

- "Radium Loans," *National Bulletin of the American Society for the Control of Cancer,* September 1939, *21(9)*: 11.

  * = hospitals recommended for loan in 1939 as listed in this article.

- Ora Marshino, "Administration of the National Cancer Institute Act, August 5, 1937, to June 30, 1943," *Journal of the National Cancer Institute*, 1944, *4*: 429-43, on p. 437.

  – Marshino notes that 55 loans were made during this period and that 49 were in effect on 30 June 1943. My own calculation is that 57 loans were made, not including the loan to the Baltimore Marine Hospital.

  † = hospitals which had received radium to 1943 as listed in this article.

- Endnotes.

ACS-Approved Clinics:

Sources:

"Cancer Clinics Approved to October 1, 1933," *Surgery, Gynecology and Obstetrics*, 1934, *58*: 517-19.

"Cancer Clinics Approved to October 1, 1934," *Surgery, Gynecology and Obstetrics*, 1935, *60*: 592-95.

And *Bulletin of the American College of Surgeons*, October 1935, *20, No. 3-A*: 86-91; 1936, *21*: 273-78; 1937, *22*: 351-57; 1938, *23*: 395-401; 1939, *24*: 434-41;1940, *25*: 661-69; 1941, *26*: 725-32; 1942, *27*: 372-79; 1943, *28*: 424-31.

Note: This column lists the date of first approval from 1933 (when the ACS issued its first list of approved clinics) to 1943 or earlier. Some clinics are approved and later removed from the list, hence multiple dates. A blank entry means that no ACS approved clinic existed at that institution from 1933 to1943. The ACS also included a category of "provisionally approved" clinics–these are included here, but are not identified.

Tumor Clinic Founded:

Sources: See endnotes.

Notes: This column lists the dates the tumor clinic was founded, if known. Some hospitals were serial founders of clinics; hence the multiple entries. Also, because records of the creation of all clinics have not been identified, there are some discrepancies between the dates in this column and the dates of approval. For example, Worcester City Hospital had an approved clinic before the founding of what must have been a new clinic in 1939.

Abbreviations:

TC= Tumor Clinic, Olc= Oncological Clinic, CC = Cancer Clinic, TI = Tumor Institute, CI = Cancer Institute, CW = Cancer Ward, TG = Tumor Group, TConf = Tumor conference.

D – Approved as a diagnostic clinic

H – Approved as a cancer hospital

The Johns Hopkins University was approved as an institution in which departments were carrying out approved cancer clinics.

Notes

Acknowledgments: The research for this paper was undertaken as part of my DeWitt Stetten, Jr., Memorial Fellowship in the History of Biomedical Sciences and Technology at the National Institutes of Health History Office. I am particular indebted to Victoria Harden, who helped me root out pertinent NCI archives and encouraged me to visit countless archives and libraries across the country to trace records of the radium loan program. I am also grateful to the many archivists and librarians who helped me locate these records; too many to acknowledge individually, but special mention should go to Judy Grosberg who helped me locate what records survived at the NCI. The paper also benefited from the support of Nancy Brun, then chief of the NCI's Information Resources Branch. Earlier versions of this paper were given at my DeWitt Stetten, Jr., Lecture at the NIH, 28 June 2001, and at the "Biomedicine in the Twentieth Century: Practices, Policies, and Politics" conference held at the NIH, 5-6 December 2005.

Note on sources: The NCI's archives are split in several sites, and the following abbreviations are used: NCI archives (refers to archives listed in the NCI's LION database); NCI records (refers to archives obtained through the records managers, Ressa Nichols and Karen Hubbard); National Archives (refers to NCI archives held at the National Archives at College Park). The creation of a cancer clinic and the arrival of government radium were often reported in local papers. I relied on newspaper clippings files maintained by local city and county libraries and some hospitals and university centers to identify these reports, and most newspaper citations are from these files. Newspapers are generally cited by the name and date that is given in the clippings file, for example the St. Louis *Globe-Democrat*, is listed here as the St. Louis *Globe*. The libraries from which the clippings are taken are generally not cited here unless they are non-local.

1. Karen A. Rader, *Making Mice: Standardizing Animals for American Biomedical Research, 1900-1955* (Princeton, New Jersey: Princeton University Press, 2004). The speeches collected by William A. Yaremchuck provide a good example of such arguments. William A. Yaremchuk, *The Cancer War: The Movement to Establish the National Cancer Institute, 1927-1937* (Published by Yaremchuk, 1977).

2. James T. Patterson, *The Dread Disease: Cancer and Modern American Culture* (Cambridge, Massachusetts: Harvard University Press, 1987), pp. 131-35.

3. Lester Breslow, Daniel Wilner, Larry Agran, et al., *A History of Cancer Control in the United States, with Emphasis on the Period 1946-1971*, 4 vols., prepared by the History of Cancer Control Project, UCLA School of Public Health, pursuant to Contract no. N01-CN-55172 (Bethesda, Maryland.: Division of Cancer Control and Rehabilitation, National Cancer Institute; Dept. of Health, Education, and Welfare, Public Health Service, National Institutes of Health, 1977). The bills that eventually formed the Cancer Act also prioritized research–see U.S. Congress, Senate, *Cancer Research: Joint Hearings Before a Subcommittee of the Committee on Commerce, Senate and Subcommittee of the Committee on Interstate and Foreign Commerce*, Senate and Subcommittee of the Committee on Interstate and Foreign Commerce, 75th Congress, 1st Session, 8 July 1937 (Washington, D.C.: U.S. Government Printing Office, 1937), pp. 2-6.

4. Stephen P. Strickland, *Politics, Science and Dread Disease: A Short History of United States Medical Research Policy* (Cambridge, Massachusetts: Harvard University Press, 1972), chap. 1.

5. The wording of the item in the deficiency appropriation act covering the institute's appropriation (H. R. 8245) was as follows: "National Cancer Institute: For carrying into effect the provisions of section 7 (b) of the National Cancer Institute Act, approved August 5, 1937, fiscal year 1938, $400,000, of which $200,000 shall be available for the purchase of radium." In 1937, the director of the NIH estimated that expenditure for 1938 would be:

Expenses of the National Advisory Cancer Council		$ 10,750
Pulmonary cancer study		27,000
Purchase of radium and X-ray equipment		220,250*
Miscellaneous comprising:		
Est. San Antonio (Jackson)	$ 4,000	
Est. Baltimore (Gey)	6,000	
Pub. Health Methods	33,330	
All other expenses	96,670	
(including grants-in-aid, training of specialists, and fellowships)		
Total miscellaneous	$140,000	140,000
Total		**$400,000**

*$22,250 for X-ray equipment

L. R. Thompson, "Memorandum for the Executive Director, National Advisory Cancer Council," 5 November 1937, AR-3711-000030, NCI archives. It should be noted that the Cancer Act also authorized an appropriation of $750,000 for building and equipping the NCI building in Bethesda, but this was a one-off appropriation. H.R. 8245 was the first of the annual appropriations for support of the NCI's activities. A copy of the act is in AR003910, NCI archives.

6. Noka B. Hon, "National Cancer Institute Radium Loan Program," 1 October 1962, AR-6210-001741, NCI archives.

7. Rader, *Making Mice*, chap. 4.

8. "NCI Historical Materials, Vol. V. Report by Dr. Carl Voegtlin on Early Cancer Research of the Public Health Service," p.12. AR-6000-5166, NCI archives.

9. The Chicago-based physician Frank Edward Simpson, director of the eponymous Simpson Radium Institute, also referred to another less common therapeutic use of radon: the use of radium deposits, the decayed products of radium emanation (labeled RaA, RaB, RaC, RaD, RaE and RaF) that were deposited on the walls of the radon container when the emanation sealed in the container decayed. Frank Edward Simpson, *Radium Therapy* (St. Louis, Missouri: C. V. Mosby, 1922), pp. 114-15.

10. For discussions of radium therapy apparatus and methods of applying radium, see Simpson, *Radium Therapy*, pp. 109-15. See also American Institute of Medicine for the United States Radium Corporation, *Radium: Abstracts of Selected Articles on Radium and Radium Therapy* (New York: United States Radium Corporation, 1922), pp. 153-60; Ira I. Kaplan, *Practical Radiation Therapy* (Philadelphia and London: W. B. Saunders, 1931), pp. 122-24; Ira I. Kaplan, *Radiation Therapy: Its Use in the Treatment of Benign and Malignant Conditions* (New York: Oxford University Press, 1937), pp. 15-16; A. J. Delario, *A Handbook of Roentgen and Radium Therapy* (Philadelphia, F. A. Davis Company, 1938), pp. 59-70. Radium therapy was also the subject of motion pictures demonstrating therapeutic techniques, including two by Max Cutler available at the National Library of Medicine, Bethesda, Maryland: Max Cutler, *Radium Treatment of Carcinoma of the Cervix* (Produced by Chicago Film Laboratory, Chicago, Illinois: Petrolager Laboratories, 1938); Max Cutler and Jack M. Everett, *Radium Treatment of Mouth Cancer: Dental Vulcanite Moulds Used in the Application of Radium* (Produced by Chicago Film Laboratory, Inc., 1938).

11. For surveys of the relations between surgery and radium therapy, see David Cantor, "Cancer Control and Prevention in the Twentieth Century," *Bulletin of the History of Medicine*, 2007, *81*: 1-38, esp. pp. 12-14; John Pickstone, "Contested Cumulations: Configurations of Cancer Treatments through the Twentieth Century," *Bulletin of the History of Medicine*, 2007, *81*: 164-96, esp. pp. 171-81. For a history of radium and cancer in Canada, see Charles Hayter, *An Element of Hope: Radium and the Response to Cancer*

in Canada (Montreal: McGill-Queens University Press, 2005). Hayter's book includes a valuable account of the various ways in which radium was used in the interwar years.

12. James Ewing, *Causation, Diagnosis and Treatment of Cancer* (Baltimore: Williams and Wilkins, for the Wayne County Medical Society, Detroit, Michigan, 1931), p. 71.

13. James Ewing, "Cancer as a Public Health Problem," in *A Symposium on Cancer* (Madison: University of Wisconsin Press, 1938), pp. 73-77, esp. p. 76.

14. Robert A. Aronowitz, "Do Not Delay: Breast Cancer and Time, 1900-1970," *Milbank Quarterly*, 2001, *79*: 355-86.

15. Ewing, *Causation, Diagnosis and Treatment of Cancer*, p. 70.

16. Spencer R. Weart, *Nuclear Fear: A History of Images* (Cambridge, Massachusetts: Harvard University Press, 1988). An indication of the scale of efforts to sell various radium impregnated waters, airs, pastes, salves and other substances is provided in the O. Henry short story, *A Tempered Wind* (1908), in which a character, discussing a proposed marketing program, indicates the prominence of radium advertisements: "we want our ads., in the biggest city dailies, top of the column, next to editorials on radium and pictures of the girl doing health exercises." O. Henry, "A Tempered Wind," in *41 Stories by O. Henry*, selected by Burton Rafael (New York: Signet Classic, 1984), pp. 162-78, quote on p.172.

17. Joseph C. Bloodgood, "The Importance of the Trained Radiologist in Every Cancer Clinic," *Surgery, Gynecology and Obstetrics*, 1932, *55*: 676. See also, "Warns on Hiring Radium," *New York Times*, 17 June 1934, p. N2. On efforts to develop standards of radiation dosage and safety, see Daniel Paul Serwer, *The Rise of Radiation Protection: Science, Medicine and Technology in Society, 1896-1935* (Informal Report BNL 22279, Brookhaven National Laboratory, 1976).

18. Daniel Thomas Quigley, *The Conquest of Cancer by Radium and Other Methods* (Philadelphia: F. A. Davis, 1929), p. 219.

19. Quigley, *Conquest of Cancer*, p. 220. Simeon T. Cantril, "A Primer of Radiation Therapy," *Radiation Therapy: A Supplement to the Staff Journal of the Swedish Hospital, Seattle, Washington from the Tumor Institute*, February 1940, *No. 1*: 3-6, p. 3. Cantril takes this point from Harry Sturgeon Crossen and Robert James Crossen, *Diseases of Women* (St. Louis, Missouri: C. V. Mosby, 1935), pp. 685-86. (Note that in his 1940 article Cantril misdates the Crossen and Crossen volume, and provides the wrong page numbers.)

20. Roger M. Macklis, "The Great Radium Scandal," *Scientific American*, August 1993, *269 (2)*: 94-99. Roger M. Macklis, "Radithor and the Era of Mild Radium Therapy," *Journal of the American Medical Association*, 1990, *264*: 614-18.

21. The dangers of radium would also have been highlighted to the public by the contemporary scandal over the radium dial painters. See Claudia Clark, *Radium Girls: Women and Industrial Health Reform, 1910-1935*

(Chapel Hill: University of North Carolina Press, 1997). For a comparison of different national approaches to radiation protection, see Serwer, *Rise of Radiation Protection.*

22. "Importations of Radium," *Journal of the American Medical Association,* 1934, *103*: 1161.

23. Of the 124.7 grams, the report noted that hospitals owned about 85.8 grams, physicians had 33,286.93 mg, and laboratories and companies had 5,545.42 mg. It estimated that a further 117.4 grams were needed for medical purposes. R. R. Sayers, "Radium in Medical Use in the United States," *Radiology,* 1933, *20*: 305–10, p. 308. This is a reprint of R. R. Sayers, *Radium in Medical Use in the United States* (Department of Commerce, United States Bureau of Mines Information Circular, I.C. 667, October 1932). See also, "Radium in the United States," *Journal of the American Medical Association,* 1932, *99*: 1609. This is reprinted in part in "Radium in the United States," *Bulletin of the American Society for the Control of Cancer,* December 1932, *14 (12)*: 3. For other estimates of the quantity of radium in the country, see John W. Cox's estimate of 80 grams in Herbert L. Lombard, "State-Aided Cancer Clinics in Massachusetts," *Surgery, Gynecology and Obstetrics,* 1931, *52*: 536-41, on p. 540. Reprinted as John Cox, "The Present Status of Cancer Treatment Facilities in the United States," *Bulletin of the American Society for the Control of Cancer,* May 1931, *8 (5)*: 1-2 & 8, p. 2. And there is an ASCC estimate of 85,228 mg. owned in quantities of 75 mg. and over in the United States. "Radium Owned by Hospitals and Physicians," *Journal of the American Medical Association,* 1931, *96:* 2057.

24. Christine Sadler, "'Conquer Cancer' Adopted as Battle Cry of the Public Health Service," *Washington Post,* 8 August 1937, p. 2. In 1939 it was estimated that there were 133 grams of radium in use in the country. According to a report by the ASCC, public health experts estimated that there should be 2 grams for every million people, or at least 260 grams for the entire country. See, "Radium Loans," *National Bulletin of the American Society for the Control of Cancer,* September 1939, *21(9)*: 11.

25. The best accounts of the history of radium production are Edward R. Landa, "The First Nuclear Industry," *Scientific American,* November 1982, *247(5)*: 180-93, and Edward R. Landa, "Buried Treasure to Buried Waste: The Rise and Fall of the Radium Industry," *Colorado School of Mines Quarterly,* Summer 1987, *82(2)*: i-viii + 1-77.

26. See, for example, Union Minière du Haut Katanga, *Radium: Production– General Properties–Therapeutic Applications–Apparatus* (Brussels: Union Minière du Haut Katanga, n.d. probably late 1920s/early 1930s), pp. 12-18.

27. Landa, "First Nuclear Industry," p. 189.

28. National Advisory Cancer Council (hereafter NACC) meeting, 9 November 1937, pp. 99-100, Record Group 443, Box 6, National Archives, College Park, Maryland.

29. Sadler, "Conquer Cancer," p. 2.

30. In 1932, R. R. Sayers noted that five states reported no radium in hospitals and that one state, Wyoming, had no radium available for medical purposes at all. Sayers, "Radium in Medical Use in the United States," p. 308.

31. A. U. Desjardins, "Radium in the United States," *Journal of the American Medical Association*, 1932, *99*: 2133-34. Reprinted in Arthur U. Desjardins, "Radium in the United States," *Bulletin of the American Society for the Control of Cancer*, March 1933, *15(3)*: 6.

32. Carl R. Bogardus, "Intersociety, Government, and Economic Relations," in *Radiation Oncology*, vol. 3 of *X-ray Centenary History volumes of the American Radiological Society*, ed. R. A. Gagliardi and J. F. Watson (Virginia: Radiology Centennial Inc., 1996), pp. 201-29, at p. 218. "Bill Asks Radium for War Debt," *New York Times*, 9 March 1934, p. 22. For the position of the Union Minière du Haut Katanga on radium war-loan repayment see "Radium Firm Leans to Exchange on Debt," *Washington Post*, 10 March 1934, p. 15.

33. On the ASCC campaign in the 1920s to promote clinics, see Ella Hoffman Rigney, "The American Society for the Control of Cancer, 1913-1943 (continued)," *Bulletin of the American Cancer* Society, 1944, *26*: 134-142, on p. 136. This campaign continued into the 1930s, and the ASCC undertook cancer surveys in numerous states to encourage the development of services, including Kansas, Iowa, Minnesota, Missouri, Colorado, and Nebraska. For an example of one survey, see Frank Leslie Rector, "A Report of a Survey of Nebraska," *Nebraska State Medical Journal*, 1935, *20*: 409-42.

34. Ella Hoffman Rigney notes that by 1925 there were 15 permanent cancer clinics: Huntington Memorial Hospital, Boston, Massachusetts; New York State Institute for Malignant Disease, New York; Barnard Free Skin and Cancer Hospital, St. Louis, Missouri; Columbus Cancer Clinic, Columbus, Ohio; Blodgett Memorial Hospital, Grand Rapids, Michigan; Albert Stein Ward (Grady Hospital) for Cancer and Allied Diseases, Atlanta, Georgia; Memorial Clinic and Cancer Institute of the Hospital of the University of Minnesota, Minneapolis, Minnesota; Memorial Hospital, New York Skin and Cancer Hospital, and New York City Cancer Institute, all in New York, New York; Pittsburgh Skin and Cancer Foundation, Pittsburgh, Pennsylvania; American Oncologic Hospital and Philadelphia General Hospital, Philadelphia, Pennsylvania; Rochester Clinic of the New York State Branch of the American Society, Rochester, New York; and the Cancer Clinic of the Women's Welfare Association, Washington, D.C. Rigney, "American Society for the Control of Cancer, 1913-1943," p. 137.

35. American College of Surgeons, "Organization of Service for the Diagnosis and Treatment of Cancer. Recommended by the Committee on the Treatment of Malignant Diseases of the American College of Surgeons," *Surgery, Gynecology and Obstetrics*, 1930, *51*: 570-74. For later attempts to link the NCI's radium program to the development of cancer clinics, see Ludvig Hektoen in "Discussion of Symposium on Cancer Clinics in General Hospitals," *Radiology*, 1943, *40*: 561.

36. Lombard, "State-Aided Cancer Clinics in Massachusetts."

37. Clifton R. Read, "State Cancer Programs," *Bulletin of the American Society for the Control of Cancer*, August 1938, *20(8)*: 8. For a survey of state cancer control programs in 1940, see NCI, USPHS, "A Résumé of State Cancer Control Programs," February 1940, Department of Public Health, Bureau of Administration, Administrative Files of the State Health Office, 1933-1940, SG 7110, Folder "United States Public Health Service 1940," Alabama Department of Archives and History, Montgomery, Alabama.

38. On public education efforts in the 1930s, see Patterson, *Dread Disease*; Aronowitz, "Do Not Delay;" Breslow et al., *History of Cancer Control in the United States*; Barron H. Lerner, *The Breast Cancer Wars: Fear, Hope and the Pursuit of a Cure in Twentieth-Century America* (New York: Oxford University Press, 2003); Kirsten E. Gardner, *Early Detection: Women, Cancer, and Awareness Campaigns in the Twentieth-Century United States* (Chapel Hill: University of North Carolina Press, 2006).

39. Faced with a shortfall in money that prompted the closure of all its clinics, in 1940/1941, the state of South Carolina continued to carry out cancer education programs, perhaps in the hope of creating demand for these clinics and for radium, and so pressuring the state legislature for funding. *Sixty-Second Annual Report of the State Board of Health of South Carolina, 1 July 1940-30 June 1941*, p. 142.

40. See, for example, "Report of the Cancer Committee," *Transactions of the Forty-Ninth Annual Meeting of the Medical Society of Hawaii. Reorganized 1925, as the Hawaii Territorial Medical Association*, 1939, pp. 5-8.

41. For an unpublished history of cancer legislation and of pre-1937 involvement of the federal government in cancer research, see the anonymous document that begins "This chapter tells of the growing concern in Congress about cancer during the 1920's, culminating in establishment of the National Cancer Institute in 1937; and a brief outline of cancer research in the PHS from 1922 to 1937," (no date), AR-0000-000188, NCI archives. Note that the 1930 bill S.4531 focused on cancer control as well as research

42. Patterson, *Dread Disease*, p. 128.

43. On Maverick, see Judith Kaas Doyle, "Out of Step: Maury Maverick and the Politics of the Depression and the New Deal" (Ph.D. dissertation, University of Texas at Austin, 1989); Richard B. Henderson, *Maury Maverick: A Political Biography* (Austin: University of Texas Press, 1970). There is no book-length biography of Bone, but see the notes provided with the finding aid for his papers at Washington University, St. Louis, http://www.lib.washington.edu/specialcoll/findaids/docs/papersrecords/BoneHomer3456.xml (accessed 6 July 2007). On Magnuson, see Shelby Scates, *Warren G. Magnuson and the Shaping of Twentieth-Century America* (Seattle: University of Washington Press, 1997).

44. Thomas Parran to Homer T. Bone, 18 March 1937, AR-3703-002326, NCI archives.

45. Thomas Parran to Maury Maverick, 28 December 1936, AR-3612-002276, NCI archives.

46. See, for example, the comments by Francis C. Wood in NACC meeting, 9 November 1937, pp. 46-49. Francis Carter Wood, "Cancer Research Found Seriously Handicapped," *New York Times*, 4 April 1937, p. 72. "Cancer: The Great Darkness," *Fortune*, March 1937, *15 (3)*: 112-14, 162, 164, 167-68, 170, 172, 174, 176, 179.

47. Henry E. Sigerist, "The Historical Development of the Pathology and Therapy of Cancer," *Bulletin of the New York Academy of Medicine*, 1932, *8*: 653.

48. James Ewing, "The Practical Results of Modern Cancer Research," *Journal of the Medical Society of New Jersey*, 1937, *34*: 667-72, quote on p. 672.

49. James Ewing, in U.S. Congress, Senate, *Cancer Research: Joint Hearings*, p. 53.

50. See also James Ewing to L. R. Thompson, 11 June 1937, AR-3700-002244, NCI archives.

51. Olin West representing the American Medical Association, in U.S. Congress, Senate, *Cancer Research: Joint Hearings*, pp. 63-70.

52. Clarence Little, in U.S. Congress, Senate, *Cancer Research: Joint Hearings*, p. 56.

53. Thomas Parran, in NACC meeting, 9 November 1937, p. 50.

54. Perhaps it was for this reason that Ewing was opposed to the radium program. James Ewing, in U.S. Congress, Senate, *Cancer Research: Joint Hearings*, p. 53.

55. Note also the comment by the Secretary of the Treasury that, without both research and facilities for early diagnosis and treatment, any campaign against cancer would only be "partly successful." Secretary of Treasury to Clarence F. Lea, Chair, House of Representatives Committee on Interstate and Foreign Commerce, n.d. probably 1937, AR-3700-003251, NCI archives.

56. J. W. Schereschewsky, "Memorandum Relative to the Desirability of Establishing a Combined Cancer Treatment and Cancer Research Center in the Public Health Service," no date, AR-2900-000058, NCI archives. Schereschewsky retired from Harvard in November 1937 and moved to Georgia. NACC meeting, 9 November 1937, p. 86. For a biography of Schereschewsky, see H. B. Andervont, "J. W. Schereschewsky: An Appreciation," *Journal of the National Cancer Institute*, 1957, *19*: 331-33.

57. Dudley Jackson to Maury Maverick, 19 April 1937, in "NCI Historical Materials, Vol. 4, Exhibits to Accompany Vols. I, II, and III, Copies 1 and 2," Exhibit 29, AR005165, NCI archives.

58. The 1937 Act in fact allowed the radium to be used "for the study of the cause, prevention, or methods of diagnosis or treatment of cancer, or for the treatment of cancer," but it was treatment rather than research or study that dominated the use of radium. See the copy of the act in "NCI Historical Materials, Vol. II," AR-6000-005163, NCI archives. For

exceptions, note the report that Strong Memorial Hospital in Rochester, New York, obtained 200 mg. of radium, worth about $6,000 for cancer treatment and research. "Hospital Gets $6,000 in Radium," *Democrat and Chronicle* (Rochester), 26 September 1939.

59. For example, at a time when Grace Hospital in New Haven, Connecticut, had no radium, an article in the hospital journal bemoaned the huge sums given to cancer research while so little was given to routine radium therapy. "Radium Valueless Unless Funds Are At Hand for Cancer Cure: Lack of Radium Supply for Cancer Treatment Deplored," *The Grace Hospital News*, August 1937, *1 (6)*: 4.

60. NACC meeting, 9 November 1937, pp. 99-101.

61. The Canadian Eldorado Radium Company told Winthrop K. Coolidge in 1939 that within a year or two the price of radium could rise to $35,000 per gram. The Japanese were purchasing radium steadily, several institutions in the United States had substantial appropriations for its purchase, and supplies were limited. Coolidge also reported that Dr. Curtis at the National Bureau of Standards also expected the price to rise, though he did not venture an opinion as to how high it might go. Winthrop K. Coolidge to Howard A. Kelly, 31 May 1939, Howard A. Kelly papers, Box 7, Folder, "Radium 1939," Alan Mason Chesney Medical Archives, The Johns Hopkins Medical Institutions, Baltimore, Maryland. On the Belgian-Canadian agreement, see Landa, "First Nuclear Industry," and Landa, "Buried Treasure to Buried Waste."

62. For example, the Citizen's Hospital in Talladega, Alabama, wanted to sell the government 50 mg. of radium, Claude Sims to J. N. Baker, 20 January 1939, and J. N. Baker to Claude Sims, 23 January 1939. Department of Public Health, Bureau of Administration, Administrative Files of the State Health Office, 1939, SG 7106, Folder "United States Public Health Service 1939," Alabama Department of Archives and History. Also, Howard A. Kelly, the physician who established the Kelly Hospital in Baltimore, was advised to try the NIH when he considered selling radium in 1939. Charles L. Parsons to Howard A. Kelly, 7 June 1939, Box 7, Folder, "Radium 1939," Alan Mason Chesney Medical Archives, The Johns Hopkins Medical Institutions.

63. Hon, "National Cancer Institute Radium Loan Program," p. 4. A 1939 press release noted that 8.5 grams of radium were allocated to 35 hospitals in 1939. Later a further 13 were allocated in 1940, suggesting the one hospital had already dropped out, possibly the Fulton State Hospital in Missouri. On the original loan, see the U.S. Public Health Service press release B-3006, 21 July 1939, in RG 26-2-3, "U.S. Public Health Service Records," Georgia Department of Archives and History, Morrow, Georgia. On the second loan, see "Radium Loans," *Bulletin of the Greenville County Medical Society*, 1940, *3*: 108-9.

64. The NCI established a clinical cancer research center in the U.S. Marine Hospital at Baltimore, Maryland, under Dr. John E. Wirth. This center was a cooperative project between the Hospital Division of the Public Health Service and the National Cancer Institute. It aimed to bring in all cancer patients east of the Mississippi River who were eligible for treatment in the U.S. Marine Hospitals.

65. See the folder, "Radium, Use of NCBH (1941-1956)," Dorothy Carpenter Medical Archives, Wake Forest University Baptist Medical Center, Winston-Salem, North Carolina.

66. For details of one visit to all hospitals in 1942, see Leonard A. Scheele to James N. Baker (State Health Officer, Alabama), 31 December 1940, Department of Public Health, Bureau of Administration of the State Health Office, 1941, SG 7111, Folder "United States Public Health Service through Miscellaneous 1941 National," Alabama Department of Archives and History. Scheele noted that he and the physicist Mr. Dean Cowie would visit each of the hospitals.

67. NACC meeting, 24 June 1940, pp. 6 & 23, RG 443, Box 7, National Archives. The NACC worried that the complaint about Sedgwick was motivated by local rivalries. In the same meeting, another complaint prompted the NCI to consider a visit to the Nashville General Hospital.

68. Very few records survive regarding the application process for a radium loan. One exception is that of the application by the University of Arkansas Hospital in Class 20DB8, Box 7, Record Group, "College of Medicine Dean's Office," Folder, "Cancer Tumor Clinic, Minutes of Faculty Meetings, 1939-1941," University of Arkansas for Medical Sciences Archives, Historical Research Center, UAMS Library, Little Rock, Arkansas. This was a late application, begun in 1940, and the university did not get the radium until after 1943; hence its absence from Table 2.

69. Shortly before it acquired NCI radium, the New Britain General Hospital in Connecticut noted that a lack of radium meant it had to send patients elsewhere. Paul D. Rosahan, "Summary of Experiences with Malignancies at New Britain General Hospital, 1929-1938," *Journal of the Connecticut State Medical Society*, 1939, 3: 405.

70. For example, in 1936/1937 Shreveport Charity Hospital's O. K. Allen tumor clinic noted that because of its limited facilities it had had to return patients to their homes and have them appear at a later date for treatment. "The most serious handicap which remains is the lack of enough X-ray Therapy equipment and Radium to enable us to dispose of all cases without delay." *Report of Shreveport Charity Hospital for the Biennial Period, 1936-1937*, p. 18.

71. American College of Surgeons, "Organization of Service for the Diagnosis and Treatment of Cancer. Recommendations by the Committee on the Treatment of Malignant Diseases, American College of Surgeons," *Surgery,*

Gynecology and Obstetrics, 1930, *51*: 570-74. The rules for recognition were printed each year with the list of approved clinics; see the citations for approved clinics in Table 2. Thomas H. Russell, "Report of the Committee on Tumor Study," *Proceedings of the Connecticut State Medical Society*, 1934, 142nd Annual Meeting: 47- 50, p. 47.

72. Deborah Kraut in a private communication suggests that administrators at Newark Beth Israel Hospital may have applied for a loan as part of a broader effort to reform the hospital. In 1936, Abraham Lichtman, the incoming hospital president at Beth Israel, initiated changes consistent with what had been implemented at Brooklyn Jewish: physicians who were operating their own practices within the hospital and "paying" an overhead, were given the opportunity to become hospital staff–or leave. The laboratory chief was terminated and replaced, the anesthesia division reorganized, and the physician who was delivering his personal bills to the patients' beds during their recovery from an operation was reprimanded. Subsequently, his name disappeared from the rolls. As a committee was formed to review the radiation therapy program that same year, Dr. M. Friedman, who owned the radium used by the hospital, was nudged out, and ultimately left, taking his needles with him. On Newark Beth Israel Hospital, see Alan M. Kraut and Deborah A. Kraut, *Covenant of Care: Newark Beth Israel and the Jewish Hospital in America* (New Brunswick, New Jersey: Rutgers University Press, 2007).

73. These were Danbury Hospital, Connecticut; Mercy Hall Hospital, Detroit, Michigan; Newark City Hospital, New Jersey; Charlotte Memorial Hospital, North Carolina; North Carolina Baptist Hospital, Winston-Salem, North Carolina; Misericordia Hospital, Philadelphia, Pennsylvania; Greenville General Hospital, South Carolina; and Tri-County Hospital, Orangeburg, South Carolina.

74. The problem had begun before the creation of the NCI, when hospital and state authorities found that clinics were a magnet for indigent patients, which led to more demands for more expensive equipment that threatened to overwhelm resources. For example, following the opening of a clinic at the City Hospital in Worcester, Massachusetts, there was an increase in X-ray treatment, amounting to some 45 percent more than the previous year. The numbers of patients increased again in 1941 by 145, so that a total of 297 patients had come under the supervision of staff members interested in cancer. See *Annual Report of the Trustees of the City Hospital of the City of Worcester for the Year Ending December 31, 1939*, 1940, p. 5; *Annual Report of the Trustees of the City Hospital of the City of Worcester for the Year Ending December 31, 1941*, 1942, p. 3. Similarly, Los Angeles County General Hospital reported an increase of 19 percent in 1937/1938 in the total work load of the Radiology Service, with striking increases in therapeutic exposures and radiation treatments (X-rays and radium), being 20 percent and 27 percent respectively. See County of Los Angeles,

Department of Charities, *Los Angeles County General Hospital, Annual Report for the Fiscal Year ended June 30, 1938*, p. 49. See also the comments of James Ewing in NACC meeting, 14 February 1938, p. 542, RG 443, Box 6, National Archives.

75. For example, in 1937 the Indianapolis City Hospital noted that its tumor or cancer clinic had increased its average daily attendance over the past year, due to referrals by doctors in other clinics of suspicious malignant lesions, and also due to the follow-up work being done. Patients, it argued, were becoming more conscious of the need for periodical examinations and were cooperating better than in the past. The City Hospital opened a new cancer clinic in 1938, financed with a philanthropic gift of $100,000 that offered free diagnosis and treatment to the poor. The NCI's loan of radium in 1940 was part of this broader hospital effort to expand cancer services. See *Annual Report of the City Hospital, Indianapolis, Indiana, for the Year ending December 31, 1937*, p. 31; Hester Anne Hale, *Caring for the Community: The History of Wishard Hospital* (Indianapolis: Wishard Memorial Foundation, 1999), p. 79; "City Hospital Given Radium Worth $7000," *Indianapolis News*, 18 March 1940, pt. 2, p. 1.

76. One hospital in Waycross, Georgia, was turned down for a loan because the hospital did not have a qualified radiotherapist to handle the radium. The local medical society protested this decision, because the local physician had installed, at his own expense, a deep X-ray therapy machine, and because following the reopening of the clinic, X-ray cases had gone elsewhere. Kenneth McCullough (Secretary, Ware County Medical Society) to T. F. Abercrombie (Director, Georgia Department of Public Health), 13 November 1939; T. F. Abercrombie to Kenneth McCullough, 18 November 1939; R. Mosteller (Director, Cancer Control, State of Georgia) to Kenneth McCullough, 20 November 1939; T. F. Abercrombie to Dr. B. H. Minchew (Waycross, Georgia), 28 November 1939; B. H. Minchew to T. F. Abercrombie, 4 December 1939, all in Public Health Director Correspondence Files, Record Group 26, Sub-Group 2, Series 3, Georgia Department of Archives and History.

77. Connecticut was one of the most successful states in acquiring federal radium, with six hospitals in receipt of radium by 1943, more than any other state. On cancer control in Connecticut, see Charles L. Larkin, "Cancer Problem in Connecticut," *Journal of the Connecticut State Medical Society*, 1936, *1*: 15-17; Charles L. Larkin, "Cancer Organization in Connecticut," in Tumor Committee of the Connecticut State Medical Society, *Cancer: A Handbook for Physicians* (Hartford, Connecticut: Connecticut State Department of Health, 1939), pp. 12-18; Herbert F. Hirsche, "The Connecticut State Tumor Program," *Connecticut State Medical Journal*, 1940, *4*: 468-70.

78. The loans to the Barnard Free Skin Hospital, the Kansas City General Hospital, the Ellis Fischel State Cancer Hospital, and the Fulton State

Hospital were part of a broader attempt to create a cancer control program in Missouri eventually based around the Ellis Fischel Hospital which opened in 1940. The origins of this scheme can be traced in *Second Biennial Report of the Board of Managers of the State Eleemosynary Institutions to the Fifty-Third General Assembly of the State of Missouri for the Two Fiscal Years beginning January 1, 1923, and Ending December 31, 1924* (Jefferson City: State of Missouri, 31 December 1924), p. 13; *Seventh Biennial Report of the Board of Managers of the State Eleemosynary Institutions to the Fifty-Eighth General Assembly of the State of Missouri for the Two Fiscal Years beginning January 1, 1933, and Ending December 31, 1934* (Jefferson City: State of Missouri, 31 December 1934), pp. 39-40; *Eighth Biennial Report of the Board of Managers of the State Eleemosynary Institutions to the Fifty-Ninth General Assembly of the State of Missouri for the Two Fiscal Years beginning January 1, 1935, and Ending December 31, 1936* (Jefferson City: State of Missouri, 31 December 1936), pp. 31-32; *Ninth Biennial Report of the Board of Managers of the State Eleemosynary Institutions to the Sixtieth General Assembly of the State of Missouri for the Two Fiscal Years beginning January 1, 1937, and Ending December 31, 1938* (Jefferson City: State of Missouri, 31 December 1938), pp. 27-28. All these reports are available in a Box titled "Reports of Eleemosynary Institutions," Missouri State Archives, Jefferson City, Missouri. On Fulton, see Richard L. Lael, Barbara Brazos, and Margot Ford McMillen, *Evolution of a Missouri Asylum: Fulton State Hospital, 1851-2006* (Columbia: University of Missouri Press, 2007).

79. The loans to the City-County Hospital in La Grange, the Emory Hospital in Atlanta, and the University Hospital in Augusta, were part of a broader effort by the state health department to establish a network of cancer clinics and hospitals across Georgia. All three hospitals had established tumor clinics shortly before the NCI program. The Georgia scheme is discussed in the body of this paper.

80. Loans to Greenville General and Tri-County Hospitals were part of a South Carolinian anti-cancer crusade that was established under the state's 1939 cancer act. Greenville and Tri-County were two of nine hospitals in South Carolina which agreed to accept state-aid patients under the state board of health's plan for the treatment of indigent cancer patients which began operation on 1 May 1940. Under this plan, the state board of health would pay for hospital care and the use of X-rays and radium in diagnosis and treatment and physicians were to give their services free of charge. The plan was evolved in accordance with a law submitted by the cancer commission of the South Carolina Medical Association and passed by the legislature. See "Cancer Control in South Carolina," *Bulletin of the Greenville County Medical Society*, 1939, 2: 115; "General Hospital to Treat Needy Cancer Victims with State Aid," *Greenville Piedmont*, 30 April 1940, p. 9; General Assembly in June 1939, *Acts and Resolutions of the General Assembly*

of the State of South Carolina, Regular Session of 1939, First Part of Forty First Volume of Statutes at Large, pp. 464-65.

81. On the impact in the southern part of the state of the NCI loan of 90 mg to the Vermont Cancer Commission at Rutland, see *First Annual Report of the Vermont State Cancer Commission for the Year Ending June 30, 1940,* p. 5.

82. In Alabama, a loan to Hillman Hospital in Birmingham took place against concern about limited supplies of radium in the state and the impact this had on broader attempt to develop cancer services. Hillman itself had obtained its first radium–50 grams from its Lady Board of Managers– in 1939 amid concerns that it had been forced to borrow radium from local doctors. See "Grain of Radium is Given Hillman to Treat Cancer," *Birmingham News,* 11 July 1938; "Hillman Will Be Given Its Own Radium," *Birmingham Post,* 9 July 1938; "Hillman Hospital Gets Money for Radium," *Birmingham News Age Herald,* 1938. These clippings are from Collection MC51, Folder 140H, UAB archives, University of Alabama at Birmingham. The articles differ as to whether the hospital obtained 50 or 60 mg. "Hillman Gets First Radium," *Birmingham Post,* 1 November 1938, Collection MC28, Folder 1.14, UAB archives. The Hillman Hospital created its first tumor clinic in 1940, the year it also obtained government radium See, for example "Hillman Keeps Pace with Medical Advances," *Birmingham Post,* 7 May 1941, p. 7.

83. T. F. Abercrombie to R. R. Spencer (Executive Assistant, NIH), 22 March 1938, U.S. Public Health Service Records (Report Files), Record Group 26, Sub-Group 2, Series 3, Georgia Department of Archives and History.

84. "Radium Loan Regulations," *Bulletin of the American Society for the Control of Cancer,* December 1938, *20 (12):* 9. Hon, "National Cancer Institute Radium Loan Program." Raymond Kaiser and Rosalie Peterson, Memorandum, 1959, "Activities of the Field Investigations and Demonstrations Branch," p. 12. RG 443 Accession Number 73-556, FRC Box 20/2, National Archives; Folder: "Organization (NCI–Field Investigations & Demonstrations Branch) (Formerly: (CA. Control Br.)" (Unprocessed box marked with NIH-NCI-OD and NN3 443-95-011), National Archives.

85. T. F. Abercrombie to R. R. Spencer, 22 March 1938. The point was echoed by the acting director of cancer control in Georgia. See J. W. Schereschewsky to Dr. L. R. Thompson (Director, NIH), 30 May 1938. Both in U.S. Public Health Service Records (Report Files), Record Group 26, Sub-Group 2, Series 3, Georgia Department of Archives and History.

86. Clarence Little in NACC meeting, 25 July 1938, p. 120, RG 443, Box 6, National Archives.

87. Hon, "National Cancer Institute Radium Loan Program," p. 3.

88. "Radium Loan Regulations," p. 9; Hon, "National Cancer Institute Radium

Loan Program;" Kaiser and Peterson, Memorandum, 1959, "Activities of the Field Investigations and Demonstrations Branch," p. 12.

89. Carl Voegtlin to Dr. S. P. Cromer (Dean of the School of Medicine, University of Arkansas), 9 April 1941, in Class 20DB8, Box 7, Record Group "College of Medicine Dean's Office," Folder, "Cancer–Tumor Clinic. Minutes of Faculty Minutes, 1939-1941," Historical Research Center, University of Arkansas Medical Sciences Archives. The University of Arkansas was in the process of applying for NCI radium. In this letter, Voegtlin asked whether the gynecological surgeon and radium therapist, Dr. Glenn Johnson, who was to handle the radium at the University of Arkansas, had the equivalent qualification of the diploma of the ABR. Johnson did not have the diploma, and this request led the Dean of the College of Medicine to write several letters to physicians asking for statements that Johnson's qualifications were equivalent to this qualification. For similar concerns about the liability of the government for the mishandled radium, see comments by L. R. Thompson, in NACC meeting, 25 July 1938, p.125.

90. J. W. Schereschewsky to Dr. L. R. Thompson (Director, NIH), 30 May 1938 in U.S. Public Health Service Records (Report Files), Record Group 26, Sub-Group 2, Series 3, Georgia Department of Archives and History. The Georgian solution was that the state would be responsible for maintaining minimal standards at centers, by appointing a consulting radiologist who would standardize treatment at the various centers in Georgia. For concern that the federal regulations for providing free radium treatment might be a problem for the clinic at Augusta, see G. T. Bernard to T. F. Abercrombie, 25 July 1939, Public Health Director Correspondence Files, Record Group 26, Sub-Group 2, Series 3, Georgia Department of Archives and History.

91. Hon, "National Cancer Institute Radium Loan Program," p. 4.

92. J. W. Schereschewsky to Dr. L. R. Thompson (Director, NIH), 30 May 1938, U.S. Public Health Service Records (Report Files), Record Group 26, Sub-Group 2, Series 3, Georgia Department of Archives and History.

93. Hopes of obtaining radium for a bomb to be located at Memorial seem to have died in February 1938. See comments by Ewing and Little in NACC meeting, 14 February 1938, p. 533, RG 443, Box 6, National Archives.

94. NACC meeting, 9 November 1937, p. 99.

95. F. G. Spear and K. Griffiths, *The Radium Commission: A Short History of its Origin and Work, 1929-1948* (London: HMSO, 1951), p. 36, n. 2. The NACC noted that the British were purchasing 15 grams of radium in 1937. See NACC meeting, 14 February 1938, p. 504.

96. Spear and Griffiths, *Radium Commission*; David Cantor, "The Definition of Radiobiology: The Medical Research Council's Support for Research into the Biological Effects of Radiation in Britain, 1919-1939" (Ph.D. dissertation, Lancaster University, 1987); Caroline Murphy, "A History of

Radiotherapy to 1950: Cancer and Radiotherapy in Britain, 1850-1950" (Ph.D. dissertation, University of Manchester, 1986).

97. NACC meetings, 14 February 1938, pp. 501-2 and 28 April 1938, p. 498, in RG 443, Box 6, National Archives.

98. Sadler, "Conquer Cancer," p. 2.

99. Hektoen noted that the appropriation for 1938 was the same as for the previous year, but that there was no requirement to use the money for particular purposes. Ludvig Hektoen, "The National Cancer Institute Act," *Bulletin of the American Society for the Control of Cancer*, October 1938, *20 (10)*: 1-3, on p. 2.

100. On Little's opposition to the distribution of radium for treatment, see NACC meeting, 9 November 1937, p. 93. He preferred that the radium be used for research.

101. Comments of R. R. Spencer in NACC meeting, 3 January 1939, p. 89, RG 443, Box 7, National Archives.

102. Comments probably by Ora Marshino, "NCI Historical Materials, Vol. III," AR-6000-005164, NCI archives. The NACC was advised by the Director of NIH, L.R. Thompson, that the $200,000 allocated to radium could be reduced. See NACC meeting, 9 November 1937, p. 34. He later noted that legal counsel said that unless the $200,000 was spent on radium the money would revert. NACC meetings, 14 February 1938, pp. 501-2 and 28 April 1938, p. 613, RG 443, Box 6, National Archives.

103. NACC meeting, 3 October 1938, pp. 114-21, RG 443, Box 6, National Archives.

104. Meeting of Committee on Cancer Service, and Training of Cancer Specialists, Memorial Hospital, New York City, 8 January 1938, AR-005168, NCI Archives.

105. NACC meeting, 14 February 1938, p. 535.

106. NACC meeting, 3 October 1938, p. 111.

107. NACC meeting, 3 October 1938, p. 113.

108. On radium applications and congressional interest in present cancer patients, see comments by Ludvig Hektoen and Francis C. Wood, NACC meeting, 3 October 1938, pp. 100 and 110.

109. Six of the seventy-five hospitals that received radium terminated their original contracts, and reapplied for a second loan, all of which were approved. Thirty-four institutions remained in the program until all the contracts were terminated in 1962 at the time of reorganization. Hon, "National Cancer Institute Radium Loan Program."

110. For an example of a hospital that wanted NCI radium but did not obtain any, see the discussion about the Juanita Coleman Colored Hospital in Demopolis, Alabama. It is unknown why the hospital did not receive government radium, or even if its application got beyond the state health office: J. N. Baker to A. H. Bobo, 27 January 1939, and A. H. Bobo to J. N. Baker, 23 September 1939 in Department of Public Health, Bureau

of Administration, Administrative Files of the State Health Office, 1939, SG 7106, Folder "United States Public Health Service 1939,"Alabama Department of Archives and History.

111. NACC meeting, 19 January 1942, pp. 97-104, RG 443, Box 8, National Archives.

112. See the following correspondence: Ora Marshino to Dr. R. R. Spencer, 19 October 1944; R. R. Spencer to Surgeon General, 20 October 1944; Charles W. Staub to Asst. Surgeon General, L. R. Thompson 9 November 1944; Ora Marshino to Dr. R. R. Spencer, 21 December 1944; Ora Marshino to Dr. R. R. Spencer, 10 February 1945; R. R. Spencer to Ora Marshino, 12 February 1945. All in NCI records: File titled "Legal (Legal Decisions–NCI Act 1937-1947)" (As of 30 October 2000, this file was due to be transferred to the National Archives.)

113. Kaiser and Peterson, Memorandum, 1959, "Activities of the Field Investigations and Demonstrations Branch," p. 12.

114. The problem emerged when radiologists at the various hospitals began to ask to exchange radium appliances on loan to them for sizes more suitable to their needs. These requests prompted a survey of the use of radium which revealed a huge variation among the hospitals in the frequency of testing for leakage, contamination, and uniformity of distribution of the radium in the containers. See Hon, "National Cancer Institute Radium Loan Program," p. 5 ff. For a discussion of how the National Bureau of Standards handled NCI radium, see the following documents regarding the renewal of the contract in 1959: A. V. Austin to Director, NCI, 13 June 1958; N. B. Hon, "Contract for Radium Handling," 5 September 1958; Scott W. Smith to N. B. Hon, 22 September 1958; Owen W. Scott, "Agreement for Radium Handling by National Bureau of Standards," 3 October 1958; H. K. Painter to A. V. Austin, 8 October 1958: All in AR-5810-001739, NCI archives.

115. NACC meeting, 24 June 1940, pp. 7-25, RG 443, Box 7, National Archives. Quotation at p. 8. This survey was not of clinics to which the NCI had loaned radium, but members of the NACC saw implications for its own program.

116. The committee was headed by Eugene Pendergrass: Hon, "National Cancer Institute Radium Loan Program," p. 8. For other documents, see N. B. Hon, "Study and Correction of Radium Loan Program," 12 June 1959, AR-5906-001750, NCI archives; Eugene P. Pendergrass to Noka B. Hon, 25 June 1959, AR-5906-001757, NCI archives; N. B. Hon, "Cost and Schedule of Conversion of the Radium Loan Program," 6 August 1959; "Conversion of Unusable Radium," 10 September 1959; R. G. Temple, "Conversion of Unusable Radium," 19 October 1959; Chief, Property and Supply Section, SMB, "Conversion of Unusable Radium," 23 October 1959, AR-5910-001751, NCI archives; Noka B. Hon and Owen W. Scott, "Surrender of Radium for Conversion and for Salvage,"

25 January 1960, AR-6001-001749, NCI archives. Contract #SA-43-ph-3081 with the Canadian Radium and Uranium Corporation in the amount of $73,189.05, to handle the technical work of reconditioning the radium loaned to hospitals, dated 20 April 1960 is available in AR-6004-001744, NCI archives.

117. Kenneth M. Endicott to Eugene P. Pendergrass, 12 October 1960; Eugene P. Pendergrass to Kenneth M. Endicott, 17 October 1960, AR-60101-001760, NCI archives.

118. In January 1961, the NCI's director invited a group of experts to serve on a joint committee to recommend standards for allocation of radium. Chaired by Dr. M. M. Copeland, the committee comprised Drs. Harry M. Nelson, Justin J. Stein, James P. Cooney, Noka B. Hon, Eugene P. Pendergrass, Arnie Arneson, Robert Gorson, Robert J. Shalek, and met on 9 February 1961 at the American College of Surgeons, in Chicago, Illinois. In June 1961 another committee produced a "Guide for Protection Against Radiations from Radium in Storage, Use, and Handling." Prepared in accordance with the recommendations of the National Committee on Radiation Protection Handbook No. 73, and in consultation with an ad hoc committee with representatives of the Cancer Committee of the American College of Surgeons. The NCI staff was assisted by: Dr. E. P. Pendergrass, Antolin Raventos, John Hale, J. Robert Andrews, Wendell G. Scott, Lauriston Taylor and Noka B. Hon. "Highlights Relating to National Cancer Institute Personnel And Programs: 1910-1973," January 1984, AR-0000-000358, NCI archives. See also Hon, "National Cancer Institute Radium Loan Program."

119. Hon, "National Cancer Institute Radium Loan Program," p. 15.

120. William L Ross, "Cancer Control Branch Activities. A Report to the National Advisory Cancer Council," November 1966, p. 3. In RG 443. Accession Number 73-556, FRC, Box 1 of 2 (Unprocessed box marked with NIH-NCI-OD and NN3-443-95-011), file "Organization 2-1 (Cancer Control Branch Program)," National Archives.

121. Karen Hubbard (NCI) email to David Cantor (OD) Cc: Ressa Nichols (NCI) Subject: Records Request. Sent: Thursday, September 14, 2000, 9:33 AM. "We checked our records again and have come to the conclusion that the documents you requested have indeed been destroyed. There is a hand written notation that says "disposal authority 10/88" next to decryption on the form. Sorry to say, but I guess those records are gone."

122. Ernest R. Bryan, "The Tumor Clinic of the Baltimore Marine Hospital," *Public Health Reports*, 1940, *55*: 2195-99.

123. Ora Marshino, "Administration of the National Cancer Institute Act, August 5, 1937, to June 30, 1943," *Journal of the National Cancer Institute*, 1944, *4*: 429-43, on p. 437.

124. "Hillman Keeps Pace with Medical Advances," *Birmingham Post*, 7 May 1941, p. 7.

125. "Free Cancer Clinic Announced at Colorado General Hospital," *Denver Post*, 4 July 1926, p. 9.

126. "Bonfils Foundation Provides Fund for Free Tumor Clinic," *Denver Post*, 6 October 1937.

127. "Are You Sure You Haven't Cancer?" *Rocky Mountain News*, 24 February 1946, p. 32.

128. "Are You Sure You Haven't Cancer?" *Rocky Mountain News*.

129. Rosahan, "Summary of Experiences with Malignancies at New Britain General Hospital," p. 405.

130. William Stone in "Seventh Meeting of the Association [of Connecticut Tumor Clinics] held at Norwalk Hospital, Norwalk, December 15, 1937," *Journal of the Connecticut State Medical Society*, 1938, *2*: 144-47, p. 144.

131. L. P. Hastings (Chairman) and C. J. McCormack (Medical Secretary), "Report of Tumor Committee," in *Forty-Second Annual Report of St. Francis Hospital. Hartford, Conn., Conducted by Sisters of St. Joseph, Year 1939* (Hartford, Connecticut: Calhoun Press, 1940), p. 27. (Copy in St. Francis Hospital and Medical Center Archives, Hartford, Connecticut.)

132. Louis P. Hastings (Chairman), "Report of Tumor Group Committee," in *Thirty-Eighth Annual Report of St. Francis Hospital, Hartford, Conn., Conducted by Sisters of St. Joseph for the Year 1935* (Hartford, Connecticut: Calhoun Press, 1936), p. 54. (Copy in St. Francis Hospital and Medical Center Archives.)

133. "Stamford Hospital Grows From Tiny Unit in 49 Years," *Tercentenary Edition, Stamford Advocate*. Stamford Hospital archives, A 380, Stamford, Connecticut.

134. Glenda Major, *Paid in Kind: The History of Medicine in Troup County, 1830-1930* (LaGrange, Georgia: Troup County Historical Society, 1989), p. 224. "Callaway to Head New Cancer Clinic in Troup Hospital," unattributed clipping dated 19 June 1938, in Dr. and Mrs. Enoch Callaway Collection, 1906-1975, MS 62, Box 5, "Callaway, Enoch, Dr. Scrapbook," Troup County archives, LaGrange, Georgia. The article "Cancer Clinic Helping Curb Nation's Most Dread Disease," *LaGrange Daily News*, 4 June 1952, pp. 1 & 6, suggests that a clinic was founded in 1923. However, this may be a reference to an earlier clinic founded by Dr. Enoch Callaway for the relief of indigent patients—this clinic treated cancer patients but may not have specialized in cancer. See Major, *Paid in Kind*, pp. 223-24.

135. "New Cancer Facilities," *Journal of the American Medical Association*, 1937, *109*: 880.

136. On the original loan, see the Minutes of the 2 October 1939 Meeting of Board of Trustees of the Queen's Hospital. My thanks for this reference to Leilani Marshall, Reference Librarian/Archives, Mamiya Medical Heritage Center, Hawaii Medical Library, Honolulu.

137. *Seventy-Second Annual Report of the Queen's Hospital* (to 31 December 1931) (Honolulu: Hawaii Printing Company, 1932), p. 23.

138. John G. Raffensperger, ed., and Louis G. Boshes, assoc. ed., *The Old Lady on Harrison Street: Cook County Hospital, 1883-1995* (New York: Peter Lang, 1997), p. 175.

139. "City Hospital Given Radium Worth $7000," *Indianapolis News*, 18 March 1940.

140. Hale, *Caring for the Community: The History of Wishard Hospital*, p. 79.

141. "Treat Cancer Here in Fall," n.d. (probably July 1939), Clippings file, Protestant Deaconess archives. "Local Hospital Chosen as Site of Cancer Clinic," *Evansville Courier*, 7 July 1939.

142. "Cancer Clinic Gets $6,000 in Radium," *Wichita Beacon*, 14 November 1939.

143. The clinic opened on 3 April 1937. "Cancer Clinic Gets $6,000 in Radium," *Wichita Beacon*.

144. T. C. Carroll, "Cancer Clinics in Kentucky," *Bulletin of the [Kentucky] Department of Health*, March 1946, *18 (8)*: 554-55, p. 554.

145. The clinic opened 19 May 1932. "Outline of a Procedure Followed by the Tumor Clinic of St. Joseph's Infirmary, Louisville, Ky," *Bulletin of the American Society for the Control of Cancer*, February 1933, *15 (2)*: 6. "St. Joseph Infirmary Dedicates Cancer Unit," *Courier-Journal* (Louisville), 15 August 1948. Carroll, "Cancer Clinics in Kentucky," p. 554.

146. On the original loan, see "Monthly Staff Meeting, Hospital News, Etc.," *Shreveport Charity Hospital Review*, 1940, *1*: 1.

147. According to a letter from the NCI to Senator Bone, the Johns Hopkins Hospital had had no radium of its own by 1939. It had relied on radium emanations and radium from private owners. Anon. to Homer T. Bone, 16 February 1939, AR002321, NCI Archives.

148. Note that while the Johns Hopkins cancer clinic only achieved recognition in 1939, the Howard A. Kelly Hospital (founded 1904) had an ACS recognized clinic from 1933 to 37.

149. J. Mason Hundley, Jr. and Grant E. Ward, "Oncological Clinic of the University of Maryland," *Bulletin of the School of Medicine, University of Maryland*, 1939, *23*: 169-74

150. *Annual Report of the Trustees of the City Hospital of the City of Worcester for the Year Ending December 31, 1939*, 1940, p. 5. Note that whereas the 1939 report uses the term "establishment" to describe the formation of the clinic, the 1941 report claims that it was "reorganized" in 1939. *Annual Report of the Trustees of the City Hospital of the City of Worcester for the Year Ending December 31, 1941*, 1942, p. 3.

151. Hospital Association annual meeting minutes, A series of the Barnard record group, 22 January 1940. My thanks to Paul Anderson, archivist of the Washington University Medical School, for this information.

152. "Barnard Hospital to Accept Radium Loan," *Globe* (St. Louis), 1 September 1939. Untitled clipping from *Kansas City Star*, 22 July 1939, Kansas City (Missouri) Public Library, Special Collections, Newspaper Clippings File.

153. Untitled clipping from *Kansas City Star*, 2 October 1938, Kansas City (Missouri) Public Library, Special Collections, Newspaper Clippings File. On the clinic, see also Mary Cecile Sutton, "A History of the Kansas City, Missouri, General Hospital" (Master's thesis, University of Chicago, 1946), pp. 42-43. Copy available in University of Missouri, Kansas City, Health Sciences Library.

154. "Barnard Hospital to Accept Radium Loan," *Globe* (St. Louis), 1 September 1939.

155. "Barnard Hospital to Accept Radium Loan," *Globe* (St. Louis).

156. *Seventh Biennial Report of the Board of Managers of the State Eleemosynary Institutions to the Fifty-Eighth General Assembly of the State of Missouri for the Two Fiscal Years beginning January 1, 1933, and Ending December 31, 1934* (Jefferson City: State of Missouri, 31 December 1934), pp. 39-40 (Missouri State Archives: Box titled "Reports of Eleemosynary Institutions").

157. *Eighth Biennial Report of the Board of Managers of the State Eleemosynary Institutions to the Fifty-Ninth General Assembly of the State of Missouri for the Two Fiscal Years beginning January 1, 1935, and Ending December 31, 1936* (Jefferson City: State of Missouri, 31 December 1936), pp. 31-32 (Missouri State Archives: Box titled "Reports of Eleemosynary Institutions").

158. I am grateful to Deborah Kraut who found this information in the material on the Beth Israel Hospital in the archives of the Jewish Historical Society of Metrowest. According to an article in the *Jewish Chronicle*, 13 December 1929, p.1, the clinic opened 9 December 1929.

159. *Annual Report of the Newark City Hospital (Department of Public Works) City of Newark, New Jersey, for the Year Ending December 31, 1939*, p. 11.

160. "Hospital Gets Radium", *Philadelphia Evening Bulletin*, 25 September 1939; "Uncle Sam Lends Radium," *Philadelphia Evening Bulletin*, 24 October 1939.

161. *Vassar Brother Hospital, Poughkeepsie, N.Y., Annual Report for the Year Ending December 31, 1938*, pp. 11-12.

162. Earle G. Brown, "Aftercare for Cancer Cases in the University of Michigan School of Public Health," in *Proceedings of Inservice Training Course on Cancer Services for Health Directors and Public Health Nurses. January 26, 27 and 28, 1948* (Ann Arbor, Michigan: University of Michigan School of Public Health, 1948), pp. 103-9, on p. 105

163. "Hospital Gets $6,000 in Radium," *Democrat and Chronicle* (Rochester), 26 September 1939.

164. Report of the Dean of the School of Medicine and Dentistry, *Annual Reports of the President and Treasurer to the Board of Trustees of the University of Rochester, August, 1931* (Rochester, New York: The University, 1931), p. 141.

165. *The First Twenty Years: A History of the Duke University Schools of Medicine, Nursing and Health Sciences, and Duke Hospital, 1930-1950* (Durham, North Carolina: Duke University Press, 1952), p. 17. See also "Educational Service Stressed by Duke Hospital," *Durham Herald-Sun*, 21 July 1940, Section 1, p. 5.

166. Correspondence on this loan is in "Radium, Use of NCBH (1941-1956)," Dorothy Carpenter Medical Archives, Wake Forest University Baptist Medical Center.

167. A tumor clinic supported by the Forsyth County Unit of the ACS Field Army was established 4 April 1944. Gertrude Jones, *North Carolina History of the American Cancer Society* (Raleigh, North Carolina: North Carolina Division of the American Cancer Society, 1966), pp. 8-9. A photograph of a plaque commemorating this event is in *The Gray and White Matter* (published by students of the Bowman Gray School of Medicine of Wake Forest College and North Carolina Baptist Hospital School of Nursing, Winston-Salem, North Carolina, 1947), p. 13. The clinic is also mentioned in Wake Forest College, The Bowman Gray School of Medicine, *Report on the First Five Years of Operation and Recommendations to the President, Advisory Council and Board of Trustees*, 30 June 1945, pp. 37-41, Dorothy Carpenter Medical Archives, Wake Forest University Baptist Medical Center.

168. "Hospital Gets Radium," *Philadelphia Evening Bulletin*, 25 September 1939. "Uncle Sam Lends Radium," *Philadelphia Evening Bulletin*, 24 October 1939.

169. Sister M. Francis de Sales (Superintendent) to his Eminence the Cardinal, the Right Reverend Bishop and to Members of the Board of Directors of the Misericordia Hospital, "Annual Report of the Misericordia Hospital for 1933," in Cardinal Dougherty Collection, Group 80.00, Shelf G-5, Box 1, file 80.8588, Philadelphia Archdiocesan Historical Research Center, Philadelphia, Pennsylvania.

170. A 1938 report fails to mention the existence of a cancer clinic, but one in 1940 notes that a cancer clinic meets at 4 p.m. on Wednesdays, by appointment only. "Procedures for Admissions of Charity in General Hospital," *Bulletin of the Greenville County Medical Society*, 1938, *1*: 117 & 122-24; "Clinic Schedule at Greenville General Hospital," *Bulletin of the Greenville County Medical Society*, 1940, *3*: 127.

171. "Tumor Clinic Rated Among Best," *Chattanooga Times*, 4 March 1959.

172. Wanda V. Poole and Susan S. Sawyer, *The Baroness Collection: Erlanger Medical Center, 1891-1991* (Chattanooga, Tennessee: Erlanger Medical Center, 1993), p. 142. "Erlanger's New Cancer Clinic Gets Approval," *Chattanooga News-Free Press*, 20 October 1940.

173. Margaret Sanders, "Aged and Despairing Victims Get New Hope, Life in Modern Miracle," *Tennessean* (Nashville), 8 August 1943.

174. Charles L. Martin, "The Value of Tumor Clinics," *Southern Medical Journal*, 1938, *31*: 1255-61, p. 1257.

175. *Second Annual Report of the Vermont State Cancer Commission for the Year Ending June 30, 1941*, p. 13.

176. This clinic was created 1 July 1939: *First Annual Report of the Vermont State Cancer Commission for the Year Ending June 30, 1940*, pp. 3-4, 11-12.

177. *First Annual Report of the Vermont State Cancer Commission for the Year Ending June 30, 1940*, p. 5.

178. This clinic, like that of the Mary Fletcher clinic, was created 1 July 1939: *First Annual Report of the Vermont State Cancer Commission for the Year Ending June 30, 1940*, pp. 3-4, 13.

179. "Hospital Gets Radium," *Philadelphia Evening Bulletin*, 25 September 1939. "Uncle Sam Lends Radium," *Philadelphia Evening Bulletin*, 24 October 1939. H. A. Cowardin to O. F. Northington, 8 June 1956, "Tumor Clinic," Sanger Historical Files, Special Collections and Archives, Tompkins-McCaw Library, Virginia Commonwealth University, Richmond, Virginia.

180. H. A. Cowardin to O. F. Northington, 8 June 1956, "Tumor Clinic," Sanger Historical Files, Special Collections and Archives, Tompkins-McCaw Library, Virginia Commonwealth University.

181. H. A. Cowardin to O. F. Northington, 8 June 1956. See also *Bulletin of the Medical College of Virginia, Session 1938-39*, 15 June 1939, *36 (12)*: 11, and "Director's Report. Hospital Division. July 1, 1937 to June 30, 1939," *Bulletin of the Medical College of Virginia*, September 1939, *34 (13)*: 10.

182. "Radium to be Furnished to Local Hospital," *Seattle Times*, 23 July 1939.

183. "Seattle to Have $150,000 Radium, X-ray Institute," *Seattle Times*, 8 July 1932. See also "Dr. Padelford's Remarks at Ceremonies Opening High Voltage X-ray Laboratory," and two undated reports one beginning "Gov. Clarence T. Martin…" and the other entitled "The Governor," Unpublished Manuscripts, Tumor Institute Clippings Book, Swedish Hospital Archives, Seattle, Washington.

184. *The Birth of a Medical Center: A History of CAMC* (Charleston, West Virginia: Published for the CAMC Foundation by Pictorial Histories Publishing Company, 1988), pp. 35-36. The hospital began to mention this clinic directed by J. Ross Hunter in its advertisements in 1938. See *West Virginia Medical Journal*, November 1938, *34 (11)*: xxiii. It was named "Mountain State Hospital Memorial Cancer Clinic" in 1939; see, for example, the advertisement in *West Virginia Medical Journal*, December 1939, *35 (12)*: xv. Ross Hunter had had a supply of radium of his own which he advertised in the directory of physicians in limited practice; see, for example, *West Virginia Medical Journal*, March 1935, *31 (3)*: xxxiii.

Transplant Nation: The NIH and the Politics of Heart Transplantation in the 1960s

Susan E. Lederer

On 28 December 1967 Donald Fredrickson, director of the National Heart Institute (NHI), presided over an extraordinary three-hour meeting. This meeting did not take place in Bethesda at the National Institutes of Health (NIH). Instead Fredrickson and top administrators at the NHI invited fourteen eminent American surgeons from around the nation to a VIP conference room at Chicago's O'Hare Airport.[1] This group of American physicians, thirteen of them grantees of the National Heart Institute, included experts in the fields of cardiovascular surgery, extra-corporeal circulation, heart transplantation, the transplantation of other organs, and the immunology of transplantation. The NHI paid their travel expenses to attend the meeting; the institute did not pay the expenses of the South African surgeon who also attended the meeting. Although Christiaan Barnard had received research funding from the NHI, his travel expenses to the meeting were paid not by the American health agency but by the Columbia Broadcasting System. The network brought the South African surgeon to the United States to appear on a television program about Barnard's world famous heart transplant, the so-called Cape Town miracle.[2]

Christiaan Barnard's transplantation of a human heart from one person to another captured the world's imagination. It also stimulated Donald Fredrickson to convene the meeting in the Chicago airport. As the NHI administrators explained to the surgeons, they sought to assess "how the first case of human cardiac transplantation would affect the plans that the American investigators might have for the extension of this experimental method to human application, especially in the United States."[3] They were also confounded by the fact that the operation took place in a remote South African hospital, rather than in a surgical suite in Palo Alto, California, Richmond, Virginia, Houston, Texas, or New York City. Given the ambitious American research programs, Fredrickson and his administrators, as well as the assembled American surgeons, had assumed that the first such transplant operation would be an American triumph, the result of the partnership between cardiovascular surgeons and the National Heart Institute, which had funded much of the basic research to make such transplants possible.

Figure 1. Meeting group convened by Donald Fredrickson at O'Hare Airport, 28 December1967.

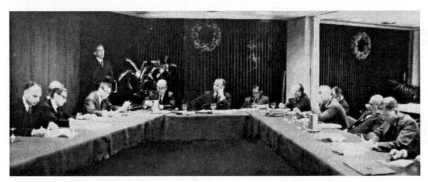

Photograph courtesy of the NLM.

It was small comfort to such American heart transplanters as Norman Shumway, who many believed would perform the world's first heart transplant, that American surgeons would quickly eclipse the South Africans in performing the surgeries. In the weeks and months that followed what *Time* magazine dubbed "the ultimate operation," American surgeons led the world in performing heart transplants.[4] In 1968 surgeons in South Africa performed two heart transplants; American surgeons performed fifty-four. In 1969, as evidence of the high mortality associated with cardiac transplantation mounted, American surgeons performed thirty-four heart transplants, South African surgeons performed four. By 1972, American surgeons accounted for 132 of the world total of 202 heart transplants, and for twenty-two of the twenty-six survivors of the transplant procedure.[5] This paper explores how and in what ways national and international politics affected the visibility, funding, and continuation of heart transplants in the 1960s.

The idea that the heart, like the kidney and lung, could be transplanted was hardly novel in the 1960s.[6] In the first decade of the twentieth century, French surgeon Alexis Carrel's development of a technique to join together arteries and veins prompted popular discussion about the movement of a heart from one body to another. In 1912, journalist Carl Snyder described how Carrel not only "transported kidneys" from one animal to another, but also introduced the heart of a small dog into the neck of a larger animal, thereby having done "probably what has never been done before, all poetry and fancy to the contrary–made two hearts to beat as one!"[7] In the 1930s, Carrel worked closely with American aviator Charles Lindbergh at the Rockefeller Institute of Medical Research in New York on a device to maintain organs outside the body. Inspired by the desire to aid his sister-in-law whose damaged heart could not be surgically repaired, Lindbergh worked closely with Carrel to create a Pyrex perfusion pump, which could then be used to maintain organs– kidneys, thyroid glands, and hearts–outside the body. The elaborate glass apparatus and the enormous fame of Charles Lindbergh attracted considerable attention in the popular press, which quickly dubbed the pump "the glass heart."[8] Despite such early enthusiasm, there remained formidable obstacles to organ transplantation, and to heart transplantation in particular, including the challenge of immunosuppression to prevent acute rejection of the transplanted tissue.

In the postwar era, the development of the heart-lung machine by John H. Gibbon at Jefferson Medical College in Philadelphia facilitated new surgical operations in which the heart was successfully stopped and re-started.[9] In 1955, surgeon Charles Bailey at Philadelphia's Hahnemann Hospital successfully sutured a second heart, an auxiliary heart, in a dog. When his portrait appeared on the cover of *Time* magazine in March 1957, Bailey, who was performing four open heart surgeries a week, informed the reporter that heart transplants were "only a matter of time."[10] When the chair of surgery at Stanford University Medical Center announced in 1959 that the first heart transplants were being performed (in animals), the center was deluged with requests from the press.[11] Over the course of the next decade, predictions about the imminent transplantation of a human heart continue to stud the popular press.

Cardiac research programs at Stanford University and the University of Minnesota intensified optimism that human heart transplantation could be accomplished. At Stanford University, surgeons Norman Shumway and Richard Lower performed heart transplants on hundreds of dogs, developing a technique with which to sever the great vessels and reattach the arteries of the donor heart, and which was "consistently productive of living animals after orthotopic transplantation of the heart."[12] After Lower left Stanford to pursue a heart transplant research program at the Medical College of Virginia (MCV), Shumway and his other colleagues at Stanford published extensively on surgical techniques and immunosuppressive regimens for their canine recipients of heart transplants.

In January 1964 James Hardy and his surgical team at the University of Mississippi Medical Center in Jackson, Mississippi, used the Shumway-Lower technique when they performed the first heart transplant. Hardy was the first surgeon to remove a beating human heart with the intention of replacing it with another. His patient, however, did not have a human donor. Hardy removed the heart from a chimpanzee, named Adam, and implanted the organ into the body of a 68-year-old man who was pronounced dead two hours after receiving the chimpanzee organ.[13] Hardy had purchased two chimpanzees from Tulane surgeon Keith Reemstma, who was having extraordinary success with kidney xenografts, a reminder of the extent to which transplantation has always existed within a confluence of artificial organs, animal organs, and living and dead human donors.[14] Reemtsma transplanted chimpanzee kidneys into thirteen patients, including an African American man from New Orleans, Jefferson Davis, who lived for two months with the organ. Another of Reemtsma's chimpanzee kidney recipients lived almost nine months, which even in a period of crude immunosuppression prompted greater confidence in transplant surgery.[15] Hardy and Reemstma's novel surgeries were made possible by grants from the National Heart Institute.

Alongside the research efforts with human heart transplantation, the NHI, with the approval of Congress, established in 1964 the artificial heart program. Although "absurdly underfunded and overly ambitious," as Muriel Gillick has noted, expectations ran high that an artificial heart would be available in a mere five years.[16] Eminent cardiac surgeon Michael DeBakey received a $2.5 million grant from the NHI to create a mechanical heart as a replacement for a non-functioning human heart. DeBakey's heart surgeries received considerable public attention. In 1963 the Houston surgeon agreed to a live satellite television broadcast of a heart valve operation. By 1965 he had appeared on the cover of *Time* magazine and in the press after treating such celebrity patients as the Duke of Windsor, who survived the surgery on his abdominal aneurysm, and actress Jeanette MacDonald, who did not survive (DeBakey told reporters, her heart was already failing badly when she arrived in Houston.)[17] In 1966 he invited a photographer from *Life* magazine into the operating room at Methodist Hospital to record the placement of a left ventricular bypass device. Although the operation was hardly a complete success (the patient died within 48 hours) millions of *Life*'s readers saw the ten-page color photo-essay on DeBakey and the development of the artificial heart.[18]

On 20 November 1967 American newspapers reported that the transplantation of the human heart was not far off. In a rare interview in the *Journal of the American Medical Association*, the usually reticent Shumway signaled that his team was ready to move from experimental trials on dogs to a clinical trial with a human patient. "The way is clear," Shumway announced, "for trial of human heart transplantation." Although "the ideal donor and recipient" had not been available at the same time at the Stanford Medical Center, Shumway and his team remained confident that they could provide appropriate care to a patient with a cardiac transplant.[19] Advance copies of Shumway's interview were sent to American newspapers, which quickly seized upon the surgeon's remarks and overwhelmed the Stanford media office. As the science correspondent for the *San Francisco Chronicle*, David Perlman, noted, where surgeons once sought secrecy about such innovative surgeries, the Stanford surgeon publicly predicted the arrival of the heart transplant: "A decade ago, if such an operation was in the offing, it would be a medical secret as closely guarded as the atomic bomb. No surgeon would talk about it until the first one was a proven success."[20]

Shumway's decision to go public with the announcement that human heart transplantation was imminent was influenced by his express desire to prepare the public for some of the realities of heart transplants: "What is needed is to acquaint the public with the necessity of using relatively fresh human tissue for transplantation." At the same time, Shumway expressed optimism that public awareness of heart transplant would create support for the procedure: "People are becoming more interested in the possibility of heart transplantation. If they surmise that it is possible, they soon will demand that it be done."[21] The Stanford surgeon later acknowledged that he and his team had been ready to attempt a heart transplant in October 1967, but had lacked an appropriate heart donor.

At the Maimonides Medical Center in Brooklyn, surgeon Adrian Kantrowitz also believed that the way was clear for trials of human heart transplantation. With funding from the National Heart Institute, the surgeon and his associates had performed extensive surgeries on animals seeking to develop a treatment for severe cardiac problems. Like Shumway's group at Stanford, the Brooklyn group performed some 300 experiments on adult dogs and puppies. These animal experiments had allowed refinements in surgical technique for removing the heart from the donor's body, for placing the donor heart in the recipient's body, and for some experience in managing the rejection process of the foreign tissue. In May 1966, more than a year prior to Shumway's announcement, Kantrowitz identified a male infant born at Maimonides Hospital as an appropriate candidate for a heart transplant. The Brooklyn surgeon selected an anencephalic infant, recently transferred to the hospital, as a donor. When the anesthesiologist objected to removing the still-beating heart from the brain-impaired infant donor, the surgeons were forced to wait for the heart to stop. This delay rendered the heart unusable for transplantation and the transplant was cancelled.

In November 1967, Kantrowitz identified another potential infant heart transplant recipient. In the months between these two infant heart transplant candidates, Kantrowitz and his team had sent word out to obstetricians asking to be notified about births of anencephalic infants who might be considered as potential heart donors. On 4 December 1967, a "grossly malformed" and anencephalic infant was transferred to

Maimonides. Although the donor heart could not catheterized, the surgeons determined that the donor and recipient had compatible blood types and no major tissue incompatibility (the surgeons employed the irradiated hamster test for lymphocyte histocompatability).[22] Three days after Barnard's historic human heart transplant in Cape Town, South Africa, Kantrowitz and his surgical team removed the heart from the anencephalic infant, cooled the body of their infant patient, removed the child's malformed heart and replaced it with the heart of the other infant. The infant patient lived for several hours before the heart stopped working.

Announced on 6 December 1967, Kantrowitz's infant heart transplant received far less attention than the announcement three days earlier that South African surgeon Christiaan Barnard had transferred the heart of Denise Darvall into the chest of Louis Washkansky. As the news of this first human heart transplant flashed around the world, media outlets scrambled to cover details of the surgery, the surgeon, the donor, and the recipient. Reporters chronicled virtually every aspect of Louis Washkansky's experience with the new heart, including the first words he spoke to the nurses, how many sips of water he drank, the details of his diet, and after eighteen days, his dying and death. The young surgeon Christiaan Barnard received even more sensationalized and adulatory attention from the press:

> His handsome, photogenic face graced the covers of maga-
> zines around the world from *Time* to *Der Spiegel*. He was
> photographed with Gina Lollobrigida, signed a contract
> with CBS, had a private audience with the Pope, was flown
> on a U.S. Air Force jet so he could barbecue with President
> Johnson, and gathered up prizes and awards.[23]

Hailed as a miracle worker, path breaker, pioneer, and savior, Barnard ignited an international media frenzy.[24]

In the late December airport conference, NHI director Donald Fredrickson acknowledged what everyone present already knew–that American-sponsored research had made possible the historic human heart transplant performed in Cape Town. Indeed, one of the first things Fredrickson did following the meeting was to document the nature and extent of the support that the NHI had provided for Barnard. Jerome C. Green, the associate director for the NHI's extramural programs, confirmed that University of Minnesota surgeon Owen Wangensteen had telephoned the NHI in April 1958 requesting that Barnard receive funds to continue the research on heart valves that he had conducted during his visit to Minnesota. In May 1958 the NHI approved Wangensteen's request for $3,500 for equipment and $3,500 for personnel.[25] During his extended stay at the surgical research laboratory in Minnesota, Barnard had impressed Wangensteen, who facilitated Barnard's visits to the Mayo Clinic where he observed the operations of surgeon John Kirklin, one of the December conference attendees. With financial support from Wangensteen, Barnard visited Houston where he met surgeons Denton Cooley and Michael DeBakey (another December conference attendee). Cooley welcomed the South African and allowed him to observe his technique; DeBakey, according to Barnard, was far less cordial to the younger South African surgeon.[26] During his stay in Minneapolis, Barnard learned to operate the heart-lung machine, assisting with the open-heart surgeries performed by C. Walton Lillehei. In 1958 as he prepared to return to South Africa, the NHI, at Wangensteen's request, provided the funds to enable Barnard to purchase the heart-lung bypass machine that would "allow the Groote Schuur to be the first hospital in all Africa to perform cardiac surgery with cardiac bypass."[27] With the specialized devices from medical faculty at Minnesota, including Richard Dewall, who provided the bubble oxygenator which Barnard shipped to Cape Town, Barnard began practicing heart surgery on dogs.

In 1966, Barnard applied for a training course in the department of surgery at the Medical College of Virginia. Surgeon David Hume, a leading renal transplant surgeon and chair of the department of surgery, had recruited Richard Lower, Norman Shumway's protégé from Stanford, to create a heart transplant research program. In Richmond, Barnard assisted with kidney transplants and learned to manage patients in the post-operative period in an effort to stave off the rejection of foreign tissue. Hume allowed Barnard to visit surgeon Thomas Starzl at the Veterans Administration Hospital in Denver where Starzl pursued liver transplantation and sought to manage tissue rejection.

Barnard apparently was able to attempt novel therapies in Richmond, including using a baboon to aid a patient in liver failure. Barnard proposed to get a baboon, cool the animal down, wash out its blood with water, then fill the animal with blood of the same type as the young man in liver failure. Barnard then discovered "that America has almost everything, but it is very low on baboons."[28] After several telephone calls, he acquired one which was shipped by air freight to Richmond, and Barnard proceeded to perform the washout and blood in procedure, which the animal endured. Surgeon David Hume reminded him about the "hidden danger" of such a procedure. "Suppose the patient wakes up to find he's practically in bed with a baboon—what next?" Barnard admired what he called "the precious mixture of knowledge and faith" that he had come to expect in the "best of the Americans."[29] He was less enthusiastic about the international press who pursued the political dimensions of transplantation in an apartheid society.

When Barnard returned to South Africa in 1966, he began a kidney transplant program. Almost immediately he confronted some of the realities of practicing surgery under apartheid. His first patient, a white South African woman named Edith Black, received a kidney from a young man with massive brain injury from an automobile accident. Although the South African newspapers celebrated the surgical effort, reporters outside of South Africa made much of the fact that white Edith Black received a "black kidney" from a "colored youth." At the same time as he pursued a kidney transplant program, Barnard remained focused on the real prize, the transplantation of the heart.[30]

At the Groote Schuur Hospital in Cape Town, he established a research laboratory where he and his team performed forty-eight heart transplants in dogs. Barnard claimed that in 90 percent of the cases, the transplanted heart began to beat regularly. He was prepared to extend the procedure to human patients.

> It was a technique built on that developed by Shumway and Lower who had experimented on more than three hundred dogs. The body of their work was formidable—especially in the studies of rejection. Adding their findings to ours, I could see little sense in continuing the further sacrifice of

animals. Scientific inquiry consisted in this: the use of knowledge to go on to further knowledge.[31]

Barnard claimed that his series of forty-eight dogs, together with the hundreds of animals from the laboratories of Shumway, Lower, and other American researchers, was sufficient to try the procedure in human patients. Barnard knew about Norman Shumway's November 20th announcement that the Stanford surgeons were ready to attempt a transplant once they had an appropriate donor and recipient.

Although Barnard later denied that he had been determined to win the race to transplant the first human heart, he readily acknowledged that political considerations had influenced his decision making in December 1967. Sensitive to the treatment that Barnard's patient Mrs. Black received for her "black kidney," Velva Schrire, the chief of cardiology at the Groote Schuur Hospital in Cape Town, and Barnard concurred that a "young Bantu man" with "severe heart disease" would not be an acceptable recipient. "Dr. Schrire and I," Barnard recalled, "decided that we would not use a black recipient or a black donor for the first transplant in case we, as South Africans, were accused of 'experimenting' on black people."[32] Instead Barnard's first transplant recipient was a "54 year old Caucasian groceries dealer," Louis Washkansky.[33]

Being "Bantu" or "colored" in the South African racial caste system apparently did not deter one's potential as a heart donor. Indeed, the first potential heart donor for Louis Washkansky was identified as "a colored youth," who was struck by a car. The youth's blood and tissue type were compatible with those of the recipient, and Washkansky was prepped for the surgery (his chest and belly shaved). During the hours the surgeons waited to receive permission from the donor's family, however, the boy's condition deteriorated and the heart was no longer acceptable for the transplant. Barnard was more fortunate with the second potential heart donor for Louis Washkansky. Denise Darvall, a white South African woman, became a candidate when she was struck by an automobile and sustained serious brain injury. Her father authorized the use of both her heart and her kidneys for transplantation. Sensitive to the racial dynamics of heart transplantation in an apartheid society, both the New York Times and Life magazine explicitly identified one of the recipients of Darvall's kidney as a ten-year-old "colored boy."[34] Louis Washkansky lived for eighteen days with the heart of Denise Darvall before he died from pneumonia. But the public and professional interest in heart transplantation remained high. As physician Michael Crichton remarked in May 1968, the advances in cardiac transplantation had "probably received more publicity in the mass media than any other single development in the history of medicine."[35]

At the December meeting in the O'Hare airport, the American heart surgeons, including Michael DeBakey, Adrian Kantrowitz, and Norman Shumway among others, agreed that management of the post-operative course of the transplanted heart–the immunobiology of transplantation–was the most critical area for future research, that what was needed was a "fundamental understanding of the immunological problem."[36] Perhaps not surprisingly, the American surgeons expressed concern about the lack of financial support from the NHI for cardiac transplantation. Several surgeons noted that grant applications for transplantation had not fared well in Study Section reviews, but they were optimistic that Barnard's first human heart transplant would encourage a more favorable reception from the study section. The experience with the transplanted heart and the problem of cardiac antigenicity would result, some surgeons noted, in the development of grant proposals and protocols that would receive greater consideration.

The National Heart Institute administrators reminded the surgeons that grants involving cardiac transplantation continued to be funded by the institute. Even though Donald Fredrickson, the NHI director, continued to champion a totally implantable mechanical heart and to regard a heart transplant as a way "to complement rather than replace" an implantable heart, he reminded the surgeons that in the fiscal year 1966, the NHI supported 64 grants in the general area of heart transplantation, which had a total monetary value of some $1.3 million dollars.[37] Moreover, another institute (the National Institute of Allergy and Infectious Diseases) was also supporting research in the development of tissue typing, which represented an additional investment in the field of cardiac transplantation. One of the requests from the NHI administrators was an estimate from the surgeons of the cost of an individual transplant and the cost to sustain a research program related to heart transplantation. The surgeons estimated that a heart transplant would cost $20,000 (but this estimate did not include post-operative care beyond the first few days). They offered estimates of the funds needed to support ongoing animal experiments, ranging from $200 to $1,200 per dog experiments, and expressed the need for an additional $150,000 per year to support research into the fields of cardiovascular surgery, extracorporeal circulation, and transplantation biology.[38] This represented a substantial American investment in heart transplantation. Who would reap the benefits of such investment?

There were no doubt many people who shared the surprise of the American president Lyndon Baines Johnson that such a surgical innovation as heart transplantation would take place in far-off South Africa rather than in the United States. Following the O'Hare meeting, on 30 December 1967, the press reported that Christiaan Barnard and his wife Louwtjie visited the President and First Lady Lady Bird Johnson at their ranch in Texas.[39] Not only did Barnard enjoy a "copter spin" at the Texas ranch, he touched off a minor diplomatic incident by describing Johnson, who had suffered a major heart attack in 1955, as looking "worried and tired."[40] In his autobiography, Barnard recalled that the President asked him how it had happened that the first human heart transplant occurred in a nation as small as South Africa. It was made possible, Barnard acknowledged, by "the generosity of the American government," and the support he received from such American surgeons as Owen Wangensteen, Richard Lower, and David Hume.[41] Barnard certainly realized that many Americans believed that he had deliberately "jumped the gun" to get ahead of the American surgeons, to be the first to transplant a human heart.[42]

Barnard benefited not only from American expertise and American investment in heart transplantation; he also benefited from the more permissive climate of South African surgery. Whereas the American heart transplanters, especially Norman Shumway, had sought to prepare the lay public about the ethical and legal implications of removing the heart of one person to implant it into another person, Barnard preferred to act. In South Africa, physician Raymond Hoffenberg recalled, "the removal of the heart did not arouse such feelings of abhorrence; there was less likelihood of criticism that this would, in fact, 'kill' the donor.

Fewer questions would have been asked and there would have been less accountability had the operation failed."[43] But Barnard did not fail, and with his second transplant achieved even greater success, despite the ongoing political issues.

On 2 January 1968, upon his return to Cape Town, Barnard and his team at Groote Schuur transplanted the heart of Clive Haupt into the chest of Philip Blaiberg, a fifty-eight-year-old white, Jewish dentist. Blaiberg lived for 593 days with the heart removed from the body of the young man, but not before igniting a furor over who would serve as donors and who would benefit as recipients of transplanted hearts. In the South African racial system codified under apartheid, Clive Haupt was not a white man; instead he was labeled as "Cape Colored." As the reporter for the *Washington Post* explained, "Cape Coloreds are persons of varied racial background. They are usually a mixture of European, Hottentot, Asian, and Black African Stock."[44] In the apartheid system, Cape Coloreds were regarded as lower than whites, but of higher status than those South Africans identified as "Bantu."[45]

The racial dynamics of this surgery prompted worldwide comment. In England, a South African diplomat was quoted to the effect that the transplant of Clive Haupt's heart did not alter Philip Blaiberg's status as a white man under South African law.[46] In Uganda, the Deputy Foreign Minister, Vincent Rwamaro, expressed fears that a black African might be "dragged from his house to a hospital and his heart pulled out to save a dying white man." Apprehensive that blacks would serve as "spare parts for whites," Rwamaro insisted that white South Africans regarded black South Africans as less than human.[47] Still, for the South African government and leaders of South Africa, the transplants, which catapulted Barnard on to the world stage, represented a source of national pride, an "affirmation of the country as a first world contender among technologically capable developed countries."[48]

In the United States, where some Americans continued to resent Barnard as a usurper of the heart transplant, the news of his second and successful transplant also resonated with a different kind of national politics, the politics of racial discrimination and the civil rights movement.[49] Some American commentators welcomed the news of the Haupt donation as a sign of social progress: "the acceptance of the heart of a colored donor by a white patient, or the heart of a woman by a man, is a lesson in ethics as well as physiology…. The dying South African accepted the heart of a colored man as eagerly as he would have the heart of a white man, and not even the most bigoted Afrikaners said a word."[50] Others were more skeptical. If black Africans in South Africa had few international outlets to voice their protest over the racial politics of the transplant enterprise, African Americans publicly questioned Barnard's policies. In a letter to the *New York Times*, for example, Ellen Holly called for Barnard to use the organs of a white man to save a black man's life, noting "All I know is that, as a black, if I lived in South Africa, I would be terrified at the prospect of going into a white South African hospital with a major illness. I also know that because of the inadequacies of the bush hospitals I might have no other choice."[51]

The African American press expressed pleasure over the conundrums created by the transplant and the "supreme irony" that Haupt would be the "first colored man in South African history to have his heart eventually rest in a white grave while the rest of his body is buried in a black grave."[52] The editors of *Ebony* noted with evident pleasure how the transplant would enable the Cape colored man's heart to go places that Haupt himself had not been permitted to enter. "Haupt's heart will ride in the uncrowded train coaches 'For Whites Only' instead of in the crowded ones reserved for blacks. It will pump extra hard to circulate the blood needed in a game of tennis where the only blacks are those who might tend the heavy rollers to smooth the courts. It will enter fine restaurants, attend theaters and concerts and live in a decent home instead of the tough slums where Haupt grew up."[53] But the editors cautioned that the use of a black person's organs to save a dying white man in South Africa also raised fears that the practice would not remain in South Africa. "Many black people today in both the United States and South Africa," the editors noted, "fear hospitals because they believe that white doctors use black patients only for experimentation."[54]

In the wake of the Barnard transplants, surgeons around the world began performing the procedure. The veneration of the transplant surgeon became a source of national pride. In London, for example, when the cardiac surgeon Donald Ross performed a heart transplant procedure, he was photographed waving a Union Jack flag and with a poster proclaiming "we're backing Britain."[55] That these surgeons were engaged in an international contest, what one reporter labeled a "kind of rivalry in medical athletics," was echoed by another editorialist who asked: "Are we now engaged in a gruesome kind of medical Olympic Games?"[56] In the United States, the image of an international athletic competition was reinforced by the language adopted by physician Theodore Cooper, who succeeded Donald Fredrickson as the director of the National Heart and Lung Institute. In 1969, when Cooper addressed a Maryland Academy of Sciences Symposium on the medical and moral aspects of organ transplantation, he began with heart transplantation, or "what could be referred to as the box score for cardiac transplantation." His scoring system credited American surgeons: "Since December 1967, 130 transplants have been performed on 128 people in 20 different countries. It may be of interest to you that 73 of that first 131 were done in the United States and 58 abroad. The cumulative survivors are 35, 18 in the United States and 17 abroad."[57]

Among the American surgeons who received credit for upping the box score, author Lee Edson singled out Denton Cooley, the heart surgeon, "always introduced as the man with the largest number of transplants on his belt." Perhaps it was the language of box scores and notches on the belt that also prompted Edson to describe the Stanford surgeon as "tall, lean-faced, almost Marlboro-country like," when he quoted Shumway's concession that "the box score for heart transplantation] isn't good...that is, if you're keeping tally.[58]

By May 1969 the United States had also experienced some of the racial politics provoked by the South African transplants. In January 1968, Stanford surgeon Norman Shumway performed the world's fourth heart transplant; his patient, Mike Kasperak, lived fifteen days before he died. In Houston, Texas, surgeon Denton Cooley joined the transplant race in May 1968 (Cooley would go to move hearts into seventeen patients in the remaining months of 1968, including a sheep-to-human heart transplant). In Richmond, Shumway's former colleague Richard Lower was also eager for the opportunity to translate his research into clinical practice. In May 1968 surgeons at the Medical College of Virginia in Richmond had identified a potential recipient–Joseph Klett,

Figure 2. Theodore Cooper presented the "box score" for cardiac transplantation in 1969, noting the American lead in both the number of transplants performed and the number of survivors.

MORTALITY: HEART TRANSPLANTS
TOTAL RECIPIENTS=129 as of 5-1-69

PATIENTS	OPERATIVE DEATHS (0–1 MONTH)	LATE DEATHS (1–6 MOS)
● FIRST 72	44% (32 OF 72)	55% (22 OF 40)
● NEXT 48	48% (23 OF 48)	NOT YET AVAILABLE

HEART TRANSPLANT SURVIVAL

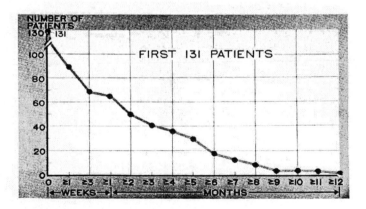

Source: Alfred M. Sadler and Blair L. Sadler, eds., *Organ Transplantation–Current Medical and Medical-legal Status: The Problems of an Opportunity* (Bethesda, Maryland, National Institutes of Health, 1969), p. 19.

a retired executive, with ongoing heart problems. But where would they get the necessary heart?

They located the organ in the body of Bruce O. Tucker, a fifty-four-year-old African American man and a longtime employee at a Richmond egg-packing plant. After a severe fall onto concrete, Tucker had been brought by ambulance to the MCV. He was unconscious, and alone; he was unaccompanied by friends and relatives. At the MCV, he underwent a craniotomy to relieve the pressure in his brain. He was placed on a respirator, which kept him "mechanically alive." The following afternoon, Tucker was evaluated by a neurologist who offered the opinion that it was "very likely" that Tucker's condition was "irreversible" when he had been admitted the evening before. He received both anesthesia and oxygen to maintain his organs. When he was removed from the respirator, the surgeons waited for his breathing to stop. They called for the medical examiner to pronounce him available for organ harvest. Both his heart and kidneys were removed for transplant into other patients.[59]

The members of Bruce Tucker's family were not consulted about the decision to remove his heart and kidneys. His brother, William Tucker, did not learn from the surgeons or from the hospital staff that his brother's heart had been removed. The family was not informed that Tucker had been declared one of the "unclaimed dead;" this pronouncement made his body, under Virginia state law, available for medical use. Tucker and another brother, Grover Tucker, discovered their brother's role in transplant history from the undertaker, who received the body for burial. The surviving Tuckers were especially distressed by the identification of their loved one as "unclaimed." They were disturbed at how quickly Bruce Tucker's status mutated from dead person to "unclaimed dead." African Americans had long-standing and well-justified fears about the medical appropriation of black corpses.

In fact, Virginia law required a 24-hour waiting period for family or friends to come forward to claim a deceased loved one. Amidst the exigencies of the transplant-race, however, surgeons disregarded the waiting period. Such a delay would have made Tucker's organs unusable for transplant. Within one hour of the state medical examiner's pronouncement that he was "unclaimed dead," surgeons made the incision into his chest to remove his heart.[60] Angered by these events, William Tucker retained a young African American lawyer, L. Douglas Wilder, and brought two lawsuits. One lawsuit sought $100,000 from the three MCV surgeons Richard Lower, David Hume, and David Sewell, and from Dr. Abdullah Fatteh, a Virginia state medical examiner, on the grounds of "wrongful death, deprivation of property rights, insubstantial due process and 'mutilation' of the body without consent." The other, a federal suit made possible by recent 1960s legislation, sought $900,000 dollars in U.S. District Court for deprivation of civil rights.[61]

Tucker's attorney Douglas Wilder explicitly identified race as a critical issue in the MCV heart transplant. A person accorded higher status in the community, charged Wilder, would not have been treated in the manner accorded Bruce Tucker. The hospital "pulled the plug because he was poor and black, a representative of the faceless masses."[62] Against the backdrop of Virginia race politics, before the case came to trial, Wilder, who also served as the first black state senator in Virginia since Reconstruction, successfully opposed a bill in the 1970 Virginia state legislature that would have legalized the removal of organs for transplantation without permission from the family of the deceased. Wilder called on a traditional wisdom in the African American community about so-called night-doctors, who abducted black children for use in medical experiments. "They're not going to be taking the hearts of any white mayors," Wilder noted, "You know whose hearts they're going to be taking. If this bill passes, it's going to be so that black mothers will tell their children, 'Don't go walkin' down by the Medical College at night or the student doctor's gonna get you.'"[63]

William Tucker did not prevail in his lawsuit; an all-white, all-male jury deliberated little over an hour before they absolved the surgeons of wrongdoing and accepted a novel medical definition of death based on the loss of brain function.[64] But it seems clear that racial considerations influenced Richard Lower and his surgical team at the MCV when they performed another heart transplant in August 1968. Unlike Christiaan Barnard, who publicly announced that a black African would be the recipient of a heart transplant but then continued to perform the procedure on whites, the MCV surgeons did transplant a heart into an African American recipient. Although initially reticent to release the details in order "to protect the privacy of the organ donors and their families," the hospital announced in August, 1968 that a forty-three-year-old man had received the heart of a seventeen-year-old gunshot victim.[65] Unlike the Tucker transplant, both the donor and recipient in the August transplant were African American. In subsequent news reports the recipient was identified as Louis B. Russell, Jr., an elementary school teacher from Indianapolis. Russell became the thirty-fourth transplant recipient, when he received the heart of Clarence Robert Brown, who had been shot in the back of the head with a small caliber pistol following an argument in a Virginia restaurant.[66] A Richmond radio station broke the news of the identity of the donor.[67] Although newspapers outside the Richmond area did not identify the donor's race, a front-page story in the *Richmond Times-Dispatch* described the gunshot victim as "Brown, a Negro."[68] When the parents of the boy expressed the desire to meet Russell, the MCV arranged transportation for the family to the Richmond hospital where Russell was convalescing.[69] Russell went on to become one of the longest surviving heart transplant patients in the early cohort of recipients; he survived six years with the transplanted heart. After his death in November 1974, the American Heart Association created the Louis B. Russell, Jr., Memorial Award in 1976, to encourage greater outreach to minority and low-income communities.[70]

From all accounts, the transplant of an African American heart into an African American recipient was unusual in the first decade of cardiac transplantation. Certainly there were fears expressed about the unequal benefits and burdens. As NHI director Theodore Cooper noted, the executive board of the National Capitol Civil Liberties Union in January 1969 had expressed concern that the majority of donor organs came from minority groups and "the majority of organ recipients have been from the more fortunate and indeed the white population." Acknowledging the difficulty in determining racial and ethnic origins, Cooper pronounced such allegations as "false and totally unfounded."[71] Only a year earlier, in the wake of the enormous media attention accorded to heart transplants, the American College of Chest Physicians' Committee on Heart Transplantation recommended greater responsibility in media reporting of heart transplants, including the stipulation that all donors remain anonymous.[72] This proposal was rejected by W. Montague Cobb, editor of the *Journal of the National Medical Association*, who insisted that this endorsement of anonymity was premature. Cobb cited the practice of declaring some dead persons as "unclaimed" as a particular area of concern. "Minority and impoverished groups," Cobb explained, "would be the most likely to be affected by the policy of anonymity. Therefore, any approval of such a policy should be withheld until all aspects of the situation have been publicly explored in depth."[73] In 1970, Cyril Jones, a professor of surgery at the Downstate Medical Center in Brooklyn, New York, cited a report from the American Civil Liberties Union's ad hoc committee on civil liberties and organ transplantation, which claimed that among the first 100 heart transplants, there were 64 black donors but only one black recipient.[74] The registry of heart transplants maintained by the American College of Surgeons-National Institutes of Health offered a different picture. In 1970 the ACS-NIH registry recorded heart transplants by the race of the donor and the recipient. Whites served as donors in 110 cases and 113 white patients received hearts. Hearts were obtained from seven black donors, one "Oriental," and four individuals identified as "other." Nine blacks received a heart, as did one "Oriental." Only one "other" patient received a heart transplant.[75]

In the late 1960s the successful transplantation of the heart prompted unprecedented popular attention as a "medical miracle" and "the ultimate operation" in vanquishing the menace of heart disease, a major killer in developed countries. But the heart transplants also represented a political operation, especially for the nation of South Africa whose rigid policy of apartheid increasingly provoked international criticism and controversy. Barnard's successful appropriation of the "winner's spoils" in performing the first heart transplant created political tensions at the National Heart Institute, which had invested in the surgical research programs that made Barnard's triumph possible. As Donald Fredrickson explained in his memorandum to NIH director James Shannon, "in anticipation of increasing public and congressional inquiry" into the status of the National Heart Institute's grantees who had yet to perform heart transplants, it was "imperative that the Institute be completely up to date on plans and progress in this area."[76] Moreover, some of the political tensions provoked by Barnard's transplants–especially using black hearts in white patients–resonated with American racial politics and the specter of medical inequality in matters of life, death, and second lives.

Notes

1. "Specialists Voice Mixed Reaction to Heart Transplantation and its Future," *Journal of the American Medical Association,* 1968, *203*: 39-41.
2. "Heart-Transplant Surgeon Will Appear on C.B.S. TV," *New York Times,* 9 December 1967, p. 77. For Barnard, see his own autobiographies: Christiaan N. Barnard, *One Life* (New York: Macmillan Company, 1970), and Chris Brewer, ed., *Chris Barnard: The Second Life,* (Cape Town, South Africa: Vlaeberg Publishers, 1993). See also Chris Logan, *Celebrity Surgeon: Christiaan Barnard-A Life* (Jeppestown: Jonathan Ball Publishers, 2003), and Donald McRae, *Every Second Counts: The Race to Transplant the First Human Heart* (New York: G. P. Putnam's Sons, 2006).
3. Summary of the Conference on Cardiac Transplantation, December 28, 1967–O'Hare Airport, Chicago, Illinois, Fredrickson Papers, National Library of Medicine (NLM), Bethesda, Maryland.
4. "The Ultimate Operation," *Time,* 15 December 1967, *79*: 64-66.
5. Advisory Committee to the Registry, "ACS/NIH Organ Transplant Registry: Third Scientific Report," *Journal of the American Medical Association,* 1973, *226*: 1211-16.
6. For the transplant imaginary, see Susan E. Lederer, *Flesh and Blood: A Cultural History of Transplantation and Transfusion in Twentieth-Century America* (New York: Oxford University Press, forthcoming 2008).
7. Carl Snyder, "Carrel–Mender of Men," *Colliers,* 1912, *50*: 12-13; "Are the Parts of the Human Body Interchangeable?" *Current Opinion,* 1920, *68*: 359.
8. A. Scott Berg, *Lindbergh* (New York: G. P. Putnam's Sons, 1998), pp. 336-37.
9. Nicholas L. Tilney, *Transplant: From Myth to Reality* (New Haven, Connecticut, and London: Yale University Press, 2003), pp. 166-67.
10. "Surgery's New Frontier," *Time,* 25 March 1957, *69*: 66-72.
11. Norman E. Shumway, "Thoracic Transplantation at Stanford," in *Thoracic Transplantation,* ed. Sara J. Shumway and Norman E. Shumway (Cambridge, Massachusetts: Blackwell Science, 1995), p. 33.
12. Norman E. Shumway, Edward B. Stinson and Eugene Dong, Jr., "Cardiac Homotransplantation in Man," *Transplantation Proceedings,* 1969-70, *1*: 739.
13. James D. Hardy and Carlos M. Chavez, "The First Heart Transplant in Man: Developmental Animal Investigations with Analysis of the 1964 Case in the Light of Current Clinical Experience," *American Journal of Cardiology,* 1968, *22*: 772.
14. David K. C. Cooper and Robert P. Lanza, *Xeno* (New York: Oxford University Press, 2000), pp. 33-34.
15. McRae, *Every Second Counts.*
16. Muriel R. Gillick, "The Technological Imperative and the Battle for the Hearts of America," *Perspectives in Biology and Medicine,* 2007, *50*: 276-94, on p. 279.

17. "Windsor Leaves Hospital," *New York Times,* 1 January 1965, p. 13, and "Jeanette MacDonald Rites Scheduled for Next Week," *New York Times,* 16 January 1965, p. 27. For DeBakey, see Thomas Thompson, *Hearts* (New York: McCall Publishing Company, 1971), pp. 128-30.

18. R. Bailey and A. Kerr, "Patient's Gift to the Future of Heart Repair, *Life,* 6 May 1966, *60*: 84-92.

19. "Way is Clear for Heart Transplant," *Journal of the American Medical Association,* 1967, 202: 31-32.

20. McRae, *Every Second Counts,* p. 178.

21. "Way is Clear for Heart Transplant," pp. 31-32.

22. Adrian Kantrowitz, Jordan D. Haller, Howard Joos, Marcial M. Cerruti, and Hans E. Carstensen, "Transplantation of the Heart in an Infant and an Adult," *American Journal of Cardiology,* 1968, *22*: 782-90.

23. W. David Gardiner, "The Heart is a Lonely Hunter," *Ramparts,* June 1969, *7*: 34-38, on p. 37; Logan, *Celebrity Surgeon,* pp. 147-54.

24. Gail Moloney and Iain Walker, "Messiahs, Pariahs, and Donors: The Development of Social Representations of Organ Transplants," *Journal for the Theory of Social Behaviour,* 2000, *30*: 203-27; Ayesha Nathoo, "The Transplanted Heart: Surgery in the 1960s," in *The Heart,* ed. James Peto (New Haven, Connecticut: Yale University Press, 2007), pp. 156-70.

25. Jerome C. Green to Carolyn Caspar, Memorandum dated 19 January 1968, Fredrickson papers, NLM.

26. Barnard, *One Life,* pp. 199-205.

27. Barnard, *One Life,* p. 214.

28. Barnard, *One Life,* p. 246.

29. Barnard, *One Life,* p. 247.

30. Barnard, *One Life,* pp. 248-52.

31. Barnard, *One Life,* p. 249.

32. Brewer, *Chris Barnard,* p. 25.

33. Christiaan N. Barnard, "Human Cardiac Transplantation: An Evaluation of the First Two Operations Performed at the Groote Schuur Hospital, Cape Town," *American Journal of Cardiology,* 1968, *22*: 584-96, on p. 584.

34. Margaret Lock, *Twice Dead: Organ Transplants and the Reinvention of Death* (Berkeley: University of California Press, 2002), p. 80.

35. J. Michael Crichton, "Heart Transplants and the Press," *The New Republic,* 25 May 1968, *158*: 28-34.

36. Summary of the Conference on Cardiac Transplantation, December 28, 1967.

37. "Specialists Voice Mixed Reaction to Heart Transplantation and its Future," *Journal of the American Medical Association,* 1968, *203*: 39-41.

38. Summary of the Conference on Cardiac Transplantation, December 28, 1967.

39. Brewer, *Chris Barnard,* pp. 33-34.

40. "Heart Surgeon Visits Johnson and takes Copter Spin at Texas Ranch," *New York Times,* 30 December 1967, p. 8.

41. Barnard, *One Life*, p. 209.
42. Raymond Hoffenberg, "Christiaan Barnard: His First Transplants and Their Impact on Concepts of Death," *British Medical Journal*, 2001, *323*: 1478-80, on p. 1479.
43. Hoffenberg, "Christiaan Barnard," p. 1479.
44. "Another Heart Transplant," *Washington Post*, 3 January 1968, p. A1.
45. Peter Lynch, "'Cape Colored' Clive Haupt's Heart Lives in White Dentist," *Atlanta Daily World*, 6 January 1968, p. 6.
46. "No Legal Significance," *New York Times*, 3 January 1968, p. 32.
47. *The People* (Uganda), 6 January 1968, p. 17.
48. Alexandria Niewijk, "Tough Priorities: Organ Triage and the Legacy of Apartheid," *Hastings Center Report*, 1999, *29*: 42-50, on p. 43.
49. See Susan E. Lederer, "Tucker's Heart: Racial Politics and Heart Transplantation in America," in *A Death Retold: Jesica Santillan, the Bungled Transplant, and Paradoxes of Medical Citizenship*, ed. Keith Wailoo, Peter Guarnaccia, and Julie Livingston (Chapel Hill: University of North Carolina Press, 2006), pp. 142-57.
50. "Surgical Show Biz," *The Nation*, 22 January 1968, *206*: 100.
51. Ellen Holly, "Transplant Abuse," *New York Times*, 29 September 1968, p. E11.
52. "Only His Heart Crosses Over Racial Barrier," *Chicago Tribune*, 4 January 1968, p. C2.
53. "The Telltale Heart," *Ebony*, March 1968, p. 118.
54. "The Telltale Heart," *Ebony*, March 1968, p. 118.
55. Hoffenberg, "Christiaan Barnard," p. 1479.
56. Moloney and Walker, "Messiahs, Pariahs, and Donors," p. 211.
57. Alfred M. Sadler and Blair L. Sadler, eds., *Organ Transplantation–Current Medical and Medical-Legal Status: The Problems of an Opportunity* (Bethesda, Maryland: National Institutes of Health, 1969), p. 18.
58. Lee Edson, "The Transplantation of the Species," *Esquire*, December 1969, *72*: 169-71, 320-21, on p. 169.
59. Abdullah Fatteh, "A Lawsuit that Led to the Redefinition of Death," *Journal of Legal Medicine*, July/August, 1973, *1*: 30-34.
60. Robert M.Veatch, *Transplantation Ethics* (Washington, D.C.: Georgetown University Press, 2000), pp. 43-44.
61. "Seeks $1 Million in Mixed Heart Transplant Case," *Jet*, 11 June 1970, *38*: p. 15.
62. "Civil Rights Questions Nag After Transplant Death Trial," *Medical World News*, 16 June 1972.
63. "Heart Snatch Case," *Richmond Afro-American*, 3 June 1972, pp. 1-2. For "night doctors," see Patricia A. Turner, *I Heard It Through the Grapevine: Rumor in African-American Culture* (Berkeley: University of California Press, 1993), pp. 67-70.
64. "Jury Rules in Favor of the Heart Team," (Richmond) *Journal and Guide*, 3 June 1972, p. 16.

65. "Man, 43, Receives a Heart Transplant at Virginia College," *New York Times*, 25 August 1968, p. 50.

66. See "Heart Donor's Killer Sought by Police," *Washington Post*, 29 August 1968, p. E18, which does not include mention of race. For identification of Russell by name (but not race) the following day, see "Latest Heart Patient, 43, Fed Day After Transplant," *New York Times*, 26 August 1968, p. 8.

67. "34th Heart Transplant Aired," *Washington Post*, 25 August 1968, C2.

68. Beverley Orndorff, "Heart Transplant Performed at MCV," *Richmond Times-Dispatch*, 25 August 1968, p. 1. In the numerous articles that appeared subsequently about Russell's successful transplant, the race of the donor is not mentioned. The only place where the race of the Russell's donor was identified was in the *Times-Dispatch* article. My thanks to Jodi Koste for helping to locate this item.

69. "Teacher with Transplanted Heart Returns to Classroom," *Jet*, 27 February 1969, 46-52.

70. Diana Christopulos, *Time, Feeling and Focus: A Newly Designed Culture: The Evolution of the American Heart Association, 1975-1997* (Dallas, Texas: American Heart Association, 2000). The first recipient of the award was a black nurse from Los Angeles, Winifred Ray Carnegie, 1977. Press Release, American Heart Association, 28 January 1977, AHA materials, Dallas, Texas.

71. Sadler and Sadler, *Organ Transplantation*, p. 26.

72. For support of "donor secrecy," see "Proceedings of the International Committee on Heart Transplantation," *Chest*, 1969, *55*: 64-66.

73. "Withholding Names of Organ Transplant Donors," *Journal of the National Medical Association*, 1968, *60*: 523.

74. Cyril J. Jones, "Medical Ethics and Legal Questions in Human Organ Transplantation," *Journal of the National Medical Association*, 1970, *62*: 8-13, 24; and in the same issue, Charles Carroll, "The Ethics of Heart Transplantation," *idem*, pp. 14-20, 24.

75. Registry Data, Richard Lower Papers, Box 6, folder: Transplant Registry, Archives, Tompkins-McGaw Library, Medical College of Virginia, VCU, Richmond, Virginia.

76. Donald Fredrickson to NIH Director [James Shannon], 18 December 1967, Fredrickson papers, NLM.

Mobilizing Biomedicine: Virus Research Between Lay Health Organizations and the U.S. Federal Government, 1935-1955[*]

Angela N. H. Creager

The mobilization of American scientists during World War II brought a generation of researchers into a new relationship with the United States government. Their notable contributions to the Allied war effort inspired widely held expectations that researchers could be marshaled to fight other enemies, particularly those responsible for dread diseases. Within a decade, public funding became the principal source of support in the United States for basic and clinical medical research. Yet the federal government's role in realizing these expectations did not follow inevitably or immediately from the organization of scientists in the war effort. Voluntary health agencies played a critical–and largely unexamined–role in adapting the example of the scientific mobilization from World War II to peacetime. This essay examines how these philanthropies helped catalyze changes in the funding patterns for life scientists in the early postwar period, during which time the term "biomedicine" came into common parlance.[1]

Conventional interpretations of the legacy of World War II for science tend to focus on scientists and politicians as the brokers of postwar policy. Accordingly, the historiography features Vannevar Bush's vision for government-sponsored research and the debates it sparked over the proper role of the state in the affairs of science, which delayed establishment of the National Science Foundation (NSF) until 1950.[2] The contentious politics over military versus civilian control of atomic energy meant that anxieties about national security figured heavily in debates concerning the government's role sponsoring research, particularly for physical scientists.[3] Yet while politicians, newspaper editors, and scientists debated postwar science policy, voluntary health organizations were already enrolling biomedical scientists in a "war against disease." The fundraising campaigns of these philanthropies conveyed the benefits of continuing mission-oriented science after the war–and help explain why U.S. taxpayers were, by the late 1940s, willing to foot the bill. The picture that emerges suggests that lay activities and mass culture had more of a role in contributing to science policy than is often acknowledged.[4]

The field of virus studies provides a useful prism for viewing the effects of these developments. From the earliest discoveries of viruses at the turn of the century, these filterable agents were identified in a wide range of hosts, including humans, animals, and plants, making the field important to both medicine and agriculture. The spectacular successes of chemical experimentation on viruses, particularly in the 1930s, drew the interest of biologists as well. The importance of virus research to lay health organizations, of course, derived from the fact that viruses were implicated in many dread diseases–influenza, polio, encephalitis, and even cancer. Organizations such as the National Foundation for Infantile Paralysis (NFIP) and the American Cancer Society (ACS) supported laboratory research not only on human pathogens, but also on other viruses, in the hope of uncovering knowledge and methods applicable to those responsible for human diseases. In doing so, these two philanthropies sponsored a cohort of outstanding biologists at the forefront of biochemistry, microbiology, genetics, and biophysics as well as virology; many of these lines of investigation and achievements were consolidated into the emerging field of molecular biology in the 1950s. More generally, national voluntary health agencies played a key role in channeling political sentiments towards large-scale federal patronage of laboratory research in the name of conquering disease. Although scientists voiced concern that any mode of "directed" research funding would limit the freedom of scientific investigation, the ultimate scale of public patronage for biomedicine left much autonomy to scientists, underwriting basic research nominally related to health.

Voluntary Health Agencies Prior to World War II

As noted by an American Foundation report in 1955, national voluntary health associations are "largely a twentieth century development in organized philanthropy."[5] Each society developed efforts to address a single disease or health condition, encompassing public education, subsidies of treatment and, over time, medical research. Those founded in the first two decades of the century brought community leaders and physicians together to work on preventing disease through education and early intervention. The National Tuberculosis Association (NTA; today's American Lung Association), founded in 1904, reflected the Progressive Era's recourse to public education and scientific intervention. As James Patterson has noted, the association's effectiveness "relied in part on arousing fear of the disease...[by providing saloonkeepers with] exhibits of tuberculous lungs in formaldehyde and big painted skeletons show-ing the damage done by the disease."[6] Similarly, the American Society for the Control of Cancer (ASCC), founded in 1913, emphasized public education and early surgical treatment of cancer, and the members of this society were largely physicians.[7]

National health associations relied on annual fund drives rather than a subscribing membership to support their activities. For example, the Christmas Seal sales of the NTA raised substantial sums of money in the 1920s, over $4.25 million in 1923 alone.[8] These drives appealed to "large numbers of small purchasers" and the majority of these funds remained in local chapters to support their efforts in hygiene and prevention.[9] In 1915, the NTA created a Committee on Research, but its disbursements of grants did not begin until after World War I, and even then funding remained small-scale.[10] Annual campaigns such as the Seals sales not only raised money, but also secured national awareness of the disease and an army of volunteers committed to the cause.[11] Other benevolent societies imitated the NTA's fundraising approach, even issuing their own seals.[12]

The NTA was the most visible and wealthiest of many such organi-zations founded to fight specific diseases or health problems, including mental hygiene, infant mortality, blindness, hearing loss, crippled children, heart disease, and cancer.[13] In 1917 the Rockefeller Foundation's Inter-national Health Board, in a report critiquing the fragmented grassroots approach to improving public health, counted 57 voluntary groups wholly or partly engaged in health work. The Rockefeller Foundation's president, George Vincent, in an article entitled "Teamplay in Public Health," proposed consolidating these various organizations into one.[14] Not surprisingly, the Rockefeller Foundation's own Board, with its vast funding and popular hookworm campaign in the South, provided his preferred example of effective philanthropy.[15] The lay health philanthropies aimed not to fund medical science (in contrast to some of the Rockefeller Foundation's efforts) but to disseminate it, through education campaigns and clinics.

However, beginning in the 1930s, voluntary health organizations began to develop a new relationship with laboratory researchers. Mouse geneticist Clarence Cook Little became head of the ASCC and shifted the focus of its educational efforts from the public to doctors themselves, promoting the value of medical research against cancer to physicians.[16] The leadership of the ASCC was instrumental in using magazine articles to build popular support for the passage of the 1937 congressional bill that established the National Cancer Institute, providing the first federal extramural grants to medical scientists. Many doctors remained skeptical of the government's new role as a patron of medical investigation; the editor of the *Journal of the American Medical Association* warned of "[t]he danger of putting the government in the dominant position in relation to medical research."[17] In reality, the New Deal's benefits for medical research were small-scale. Roosevelt did upgrade the research activities of the Public Health Service, including limited grants to university researchers, but in 1938, even after the passing of the National Cancer Institute Act, the National Institute of Health's research appropriation was only $2.8 million, barely over 10 percent of the research funds of the Agriculture Department.[18]

Roosevelt's impact on the state of medical research was not limited to his formal activities as President. The National Foundation for Infantile Paralysis, founded in 1938 by Roosevelt and cooperating lawyers and businessmen, targeted research as the key to conquering polio.[19] As President Roosevelt declared at the outset, "the new foundation...will make every effort to ensure that every responsible research agency in this country is adequately financed to carry on investigations in the cause of infantile paralysis and the methods by which it may be prevented."[20] Among the committees established in 1938 to implement the NFIP's agenda were two concerned solely with supporting research.[21] The Committee on Research for the Prevention and Treatment of After-Effects made grants advancing understanding of the clinical management of polio.[22] The other committee, the Committee of Scientific Research, supported virus research almost exclusively; it was renamed the Committee on Virus Research by 1940.[23]

Thomas M. Rivers, a virologist at the Rockefeller Institute for Medical Research, served as chair of the Committee of Scientific Research, Paul de Kruif acted as secretary, and three other researchers sat on the committee along with three NFIP administrators, including the president, Basil O'Connor.[24] These scientific advisers recommended that the philanthropy target research on all viruses rather than restricting its efforts to poliomyelitis, as part of an effort to develop comparative approaches to controlling the disease.[25] More significantly, because the NFIP's predecessor, the President's Birthday Ball Commission, had been associated with the disastrous Brodie-Park and Kolmer polio vaccine trials of 1935, the new foundation was motivated to eschew further vaccine trial programs in favor of fundamental laboratory research on viruses.[26] From its first meeting in 1938, the Committee held as one of its principal objectives to advance understanding of the "nature of the virus," as epitomized by Wendell Stanley's recent chemical purification and characterization of tobacco mosaic virus (TMV).[27] Thus, in addition to grants for research on chemotherapy, pathology, pathogenesis, nutrition, and immunology, the Committee awarded grants for fundamental virus research.[28] The Committee on Research targeted work in several areas, ultimately including "bacterial virus infection, growth, mutation, and genetics; the chemical and physical structure and properties of TMV; the molecular structure of proteins and especially nucleic acids; and the growth of animal viruses in tissue cultures of mammalian cells."[29] By supporting a broad portfolio of laboratory research, the NFIP sought a long-term and comprehensive solution to the polio problem, establishing a pattern for other health agencies to follow.

World War II and Postwar Science Policy

As historians of science since A. Hunter Dupree's classic study of "The Great Instauration" have noted, the organization of scientific research for war offered new and attractive possibilities to both the public and researchers of how scientists might contribute to peacetime society.[30] In his influential 1945 manifesto *Science–The Endless Frontier*, Vannevar Bush advocated the initiation of federal government funding of basic research in universities and institutes to ensure public welfare, national security, and advances in medical care. Although historians of science have tended to view the consequences of Bush's vision in terms of the natural (and especially physical) sciences, the continuities with the wartime mission were most evident in medical research: Bush urged that life science be supported to fight the "war against disease" in peace.[31] The Committee on Medical Research of the Office for Scientific Research and Development (OSRD) took credit for having funded four of the most dramatic medical advances during the war: antibiotics, DDT, improved anti-malarial drugs, and plasma fractionation products.[32] As historian of medicine Richard Harrison Shryock observed in 1947,

> The war has stimulated public interest in research. Newspaper editors demand funds for studies of the more dreaded diseases, pointing out that medical scientists now "labor against inexcusable odds." ... Public enthusiasm for continuing a war-scale program in medical research has even been carried to a point somewhat disturbing to medical leaders. There is some fear that legislators, fired by the achievements of the Committee on Medical Research, will assume that solutions for all present problems can be promptly provided by similar methods.[33]

Public demand for scientific solutions to medical needs was high, a sentiment not lost on politicians.[34]

Despite this popular motivation to continue some kind of mutually beneficial partnership between government and scientists after the war, translating this vision into coherent national policy proved politically difficult in the late 1940s. As Daniel Kevles has shown in his classic article,

Bush's report was an essentially conservative response to Senator Harley Kilgore's proposed legislation for a public research foundation: "Kilgore wanted a foundation responsive to lay control and prepared to support research for the advancement of the general welfare; Bush and his colleagues wanted an agency run by scientists mainly for the purpose of advancing science."[35] Debates over the nature and range of a government foundation for the support of research delayed the establishment of the National Science Foundation until 1950. Many scientists objected to legislation that gave politicians or bureaucrats control over the selection of research topics and projects, fearing this would interfere with the freedom of scientific inquiry.[36]

For experimental biologists, these political deliberations were fraught for other reasons. As Stephen Strickland and Harry Marks have demonstrated, considerations of federal funding for biomedical research were part of larger debates about government involvement in health care and medical education.[37] The Public Health Service Act of 1944 enlarged the authority of the agency to "pay for research to be performed by universities, hospitals, laboratories, and other public or private institutions" beyond the area of cancer investigations; the Division of Grants Research was soon expanded to assimilate unfinished OSRD contracts.[38] However, critics of the Public Health Service (many in private medical schools) vigorously opposed interference by the federal government in medical research and education.[39] Officials at the National Institute of Health (NIH), the Public Health Service's research arm, had to defend the legitimacy of government funding to medical scientists at the same time as they had to protect "their new authority to conduct a broad extramural program" from being assimilated into a new national research agency.[40]

In the years immediately after World War II, in the midst of these political contentions, voluntary health organizations took the lead in launching the research-based "war against disease."[41] In particular, two health agencies advanced their causes by funding research on a large scale by the conclusion of World War II. The ACS (formerly ASCC) began funding medical research at the end of the war after lay activists took control of the organization.[42] In the 1940s, the dreaded polio epidemics provided the other obvious and immediate context for the extension of military language and research organization to the domain of bio-medical research. The NFIP publicized the value of disease-related research at university laboratories in its yearly fundraiser, the March of Dimes.[43] (The organization now goes by that name.) The fact that voluntary associations such as the NFIP and ACS were not governmental agencies meant that critics of federal support of research did not see in these "directed" research programs the specter of socialism, even if they were being conducted in the name of the public.

During the demobilization period, the NFIP was poised to attract many medical researchers who had been working on war projects to initiate investigations pertinent to polio. An upsurge in NFIP research grants included an increase in support for biophysical virus research. In 1946, the NFIP granted the University of Southern California and Yale University School of Medicine sufficient funds to acquire an ultracentrifuge and an electron microscope respectively.[44] The Committee on Virus Research's overall appropriations grew from $304,000 in 1945 to over $1.26 million in 1946.[45] With the increased resources, the NFIP expanded its research funding further into basic research, often centered on viruses but encompassing current biochemical topics such as vitamin analogues, nucleic acid synthesis, and carbohydrate metabolism.[46] The enlarged grants program reflected the remarkable success of the March of Dimes campaigns, which brought in $6.5 million in 1943, $12 million in 1944, and $19 million each in 1945 and 1946, record amounts despite the economic constraints of the war. As John Storck has commented, "In fund raising the results that were achieved from January, 1942, through January, 1945, were nothing less than spectacular."[47]

The 1945 March of Dimes campaign drew on the recent experience of war mobilization and its civilian institutions. The campaign booklet for that year advised communities to form union-management committees to obtain contributions from employees and management from the existing war production committees. Among the many public relations efforts suggested to local chapters were radio "interviews with ex-polios, especially those engaged in war work."[48] The wartime mobilization of scientists provided an ongoing metaphor for the significance of research in the fight against polio. In 1947, the NFIP entitled one summary of its sponsored research "Weapons of Defense":

The challenge of epidemics and their aftermath claimed much of our attention in 1947. These were dramatic front-line activities designed to minimize the weight of the polio attack. Meanwhile, behind the scenes, the year-round job of forging new defensive weapons continued without interruption as twenty-four branches of science prosecuted their relentless search for answers to the mystery of polio virus under National Foundation sponsorship.[49]

The NFIP fundraisers were also savvy in choosing effective solicitation venues; like the Red Cross, the March of Dimes relied increasingly on movie theaters as points of collection.

Cancer fundraising was similarly popular and also made substantial funding available to biologists. The ASCC was undergoing a transformation during the war years, as businessmen and advertising executives, led by philanthropist Mary Lasker, took over control of the board from conservative doctors and began fundraising in earnest for research.[50] The organization was renamed the American Cancer Society in 1946. From an annual budget of $102,000 in 1943, the transformed society brought in $10 million in 1946. Convinced of the necessity for "fundamental scientific research directed toward a solution of the cancer problem," the ACS arranged for the National Research Council to administer a grants program through a newly established Committee of Growth.[51] While the NRC had previously helped disburse funds from private sources (most notably the Rockefeller philanthropies), the collaboration with a voluntary health organization represented a significant new commitment.[52] As Frank Jewett, president of the National Academy of Sciences, wrote Karl Compton (president of MIT) in the summer of 1946, "one of the big jobs which the Medical Division of the NRC has taken on is that of scientific advisor to the American Cancer Society and administrator of its research programs."[53]

The NRC Committee on Growth was given $3,500,000 to disburse in 1947-1948, through Divisions of Chemistry, Physics, Biology, and Clinical Investigations.[54] Six panels were organized within the Division of Biology, among them a Panel on Viruses, inspired by evidence in animal models that tumors were virus-induced, and a Panel on Milk Factor to further investigation of the virus-like agent responsible for mammary tumors in mice.[55] Thus the ACS as well as the NFIP targeted fundamental virus research for funding, while supporting a broader portfolio of scientific approaches. Beyond virus researchers, ACS grant recipients included dozens of prominent biologists and biochemists, including George Beadle, Erwin Chargaff, Milislav Demerec, Sterling Emerson, Martin Kamen, Carl Lindegren, and Salvador Luria.

Campaigns to raise research funds in the fight against cancer found a responsive citizenry. In the summer of 1946 Memorial Hospital in New York collected more than $3 million from "over 20,000 individual contributors representing a wide cross-section of the general public," to be used "for the purpose of initiating an attack upon the problem of cancer on a much greater scale than ever before attempted."[56] The cancer crusades, like those against polio, represented their research activities by reference to the wartime mobilization of scientists. The ACS report summarizing the Committee of Growth's activities in 1945-1946 described "a technique of coordinated research developed under the forced draft of war and now used in peacetime to answer a widespread demand for the control of cancer."[57]

Given the ambivalence of many scientists about continued involvement after the war in "mission-oriented" work, it is perhaps not surprising that tensions surfaced between scientific leaders and lay activists over the cancer research funds. Early in 1947, James A. Adams, chair of the Executive Committee of the ACS, wrote Lewis Weed of the NRC expressing concerns over whether the Committee on Growth's grant recipients were advancing the research cause against cancer. The Executive Committee had decided that "the American Cancer Society must employ a small staff for the purposes of checking upon the results of the research" funded through the NRC Committee on Growth.[58] As Adams explained to Jewett, "we feel we would not be carrying out our obligation to the public, if we did not carry out our responsibility as a policy making body who will, in the end, be responsible by the public for results."[59] Jewett found the prospect of ACS oversight very disturbing, as he felt that the scientists at the NRC were best equipped to evaluate any research results supported through the program. The disagreement touched on a nerve; the degree to which government bureaucrats might dictate the course of scientific research by holding the purse strings had also surfaced in congressional debates over establishing a federal research foundation.[60] In the end, the ACS was not content to have the NRC make all of the decisions regarding its research funding; while the grants-in-aid program controlled by the Committee on Growth continued, the ACS also began making its own grants for institutional and developmental research.[61] It should be noted that many scientists felt that it was worth accommodating the lay leaders for the sake of generous research funds. As E. B. Wilson wrote A. N. Richards about the situation, "Where there is so much apparent friction I suppose personal contacts are desirable in addition to correspondence files.... The lay leaders have money to spend—and you might be able to get some of it for some of your Univ. Penn. interests sometime."[62]

The growing involvement of voluntary health associations in medical research policy elicited criticism from other quarters. As the American Foundation report noted: "their annual 'drives' while useful in educating the public and in raising needed funds nevertheless distort the total public health picture by over-emphasizing one part of it, possibly focusing public attention sharply on a condition that may (in terms of mortality, morbidity, permanent disability) be less important medically and socially than some other condition not yet recognized by a specific organization or by specific drives."[63] The corporate-style public relations efforts of lay health organizations also bothered critics. In a 1945 report commissioned by the National Health Council, Selskar M. Gunn and Philip S. Platt noted that, unlike older benevolent societies, "voluntary health agencies are organized and operated in the manner of a corporation."[64] This had disturbing implications for their fundraising:

> Like a business organization, the typical voluntary health agency obtains its funds by processes that are akin to "selling." The ability of a national health agency to obtain public support seems to have little relation to the agency's age, the relative importance of its cause or its effectiveness in advancing the public's health. The money it gets depends rather upon the degree to which it can keep itself before the

public, its sponsors and leadership, and particularly upon
the use of special money-raising devices or techniques.[65]

These lay health groups effectively peddled sentimentality, particularly
in the reliance on images such as crippled children, in order to solicit
donations. As Gunn and Platt noted, "The picture of the suffering child
takes priority over any appeal concerning adults."[66] The NFIP honed their
skills at this kind of appeal, as seen in their yearly poster children.[67]

The Emerging Dominance of Federal Funding

In the immediate postwar years, the NFIP and the ACS patronized biomedical research on roughly the same scale as the extramural program of
the NIH, managing massive national public collection campaigns to raise
millions of dollars for research. While these organizations were private,
they were markedly different from interwar philanthropies (most notably the Rockefeller Foundation) in their support of research. The tens
of thousands of volunteers in the ranks of the health agencies and the
millions of donors held concrete expectations for medical breakthroughs
from laboratory research. A large portion of the funds collected by the
NFIP was spent on patient care ($94 million from 1938-1955), and
clinical research was also heavily supported, but research funds were
consistently committed to study "the physical, chemical and biological
nature of such minute objects as the cells in the body."[68] Because postwar
research on viruses, especially bacteriophage and TMV, contributed so
centrally to the formation of molecular biology, the NFIP served to
incubate this emerging field.[69]

By 1950, the growth of the NIH focused around several new categorical institutes, and the rapidly expanding extramural grant system available through these institutes, outstripped the funds available through the
voluntary health organizations. The National Cancer Institute had been
founded in 1937; to it were added the National Heart Institute (1948),
the National Institute of Dental Research (1948), the Microbiology
Institute (1948; this included the former intramural microbiologists and
was renamed the National Institute of Allergy and Infectious Diseases in
1955), the Experimental Biology and Medicine Institute (1948; renamed
the National Institute of Arthritis, Metabolism, and Digestive Diseases in

1950), a National Institute of Mental Health (1949), and a National Institute of Neurological Diseases and Blindness (1950).[70] Effectively, then, the organization of the NIH and its funding structures mirrored the disease-based voluntary health organizations that had been active for decades. The NIH was not the only source of support for experimental biologists: funding available through the Atomic Energy Commission and the NSF also expanded rapidly.[71] Nonetheless, the meanings and constraints of postwar "basic research" were indebted to these lay crusades against specific disease, linking university biologists and clinical researchers from diverse institutions in a coordinated effort.

Even once the NIH was supporting more biomedical researchers than any private agency, the efforts of voluntary health agencies continued to foster support for science. First, federal funding did not simply replace philanthropy; as the American Foundation noted in its 1955 report,

> The "remarkable correspondence" which the surgeon general's committee on medical school grants noted, [in] 1951, between increased collections of the American Cancer Society (from $285,000 in 1942 to $13,100,000 in 1948) and increased government appropriations to the National Cancer Institute (from $565,000 in 1942 to $14,000,000 in 1948) represents the progression from voluntary contributions to legislative appropriation of a public long educated by the American Cancer Society.[72]

In addition to the considerable efforts of Mary Lasker and other businessmen and philanthropists in lobbying Congress to allocate ever more funds to the NIH and the NCI, the American Cancer Society's advertising campaigns provided great media coverage for the value of research. For example, in one advertisement that depicted a stack of quarters under the phrase "The cure for cancer," the ACS articulated the assumption that also drove the popularity of federal funding for biomedical research: that more research money would generate medical breakthroughs. (Figure 1.) In 1960, the president of the NFIP, Basil O'Connor, asserted that "the national voluntary health agencies have caused the American people to become 'research minded,'" particularly in support of "basic research in the life sciences."[73]

Figure 1. American Cancer Society fundraising advertisement.

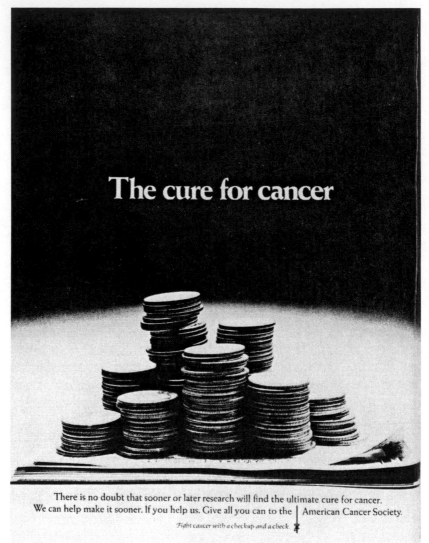

The cure for cancer

There is no doubt that sooner or later research will find the ultimate cure for cancer. We can help make it sooner. If you help us. Give all you can to the | American Cancer Society.

Fight cancer with a checkup and a check

Reprinted from *Cancer News*, 1970, *24*, no. 1: 1 by permission of the American Cancer Society, Inc.

The way in which such expectations for results were become part of funding systems for basic research troubled many scientists. One editorial writer in *Science* magazine expressed his opposition to the growing requirements for project reports for "design" research as opposed to "free research."[74] Nonetheless, a mode of accountability of research, to the scientific manager or peer review body of the granting agency, and more generally to the public, was being set in place by the 1950s. The degree of scientific freedom entailed by a "basic" research contract remained nebulous. One NSF official stated, "The concept 'basic research' may comprise the systematic endeavor, without preconception, to increase our knowledge and understanding of nature. It is the kind of research that some of our colleagues characterize as 'pure science.' If it is indeed pure, it derives that quality from uncompromising objectivity, unconcern over specific aims, and absence of intent to exploit results."[75] By contrast, the research director at Shell Oil Company differentiated pure from basic research:

> For my requirements, I suggest three categories. We have pure research, which I define as the inquiry after knowledge for its own sake, without consideration or hope of practical gain. We also have applied research, the investigation carried out in response to immediate, direct, and obvious needs. Basic research is in between.
>
> By basic research, then, I mean the scientific inquiry carried on, not under pressure of immediate needs or in hope of quick profit, but with reasonable hope of some eventual payout.[76]

He recognized that these usages were context-dependent: in the case of Shell-sponsored research grants to university chemists and chemical engineers: "These men are working on problems of their own selection; to us it is basic, to them it is pure."[77]

The NFIP's own investments in biomedical research enabled wide-ranging contributions to biological knowledge about viruses, proteins, and nucleic acids. Indeed, the philanthropy's understanding of the domain of basic polio research was remarkably broad, even contradictory, as assessed by its in-house historians of the late 1950s. For example, during the same year, 1949, the NFIP launched both its single most expensive project to date, Salk's virus typing program, which had highly specific objectives and applications, and also its large-scale grant to Wendell Stanley's laboratory "in support of the physical, chemical and biological studies of viruses with the *ultimate* aim of delineating the basic characteristics of polio virus." As one of the NFIP's historians noted, the second "was a long-term undertaking, broadly exploratory in nature, and of a kind that precluded any possibility of 'a yes or no answer.' We are forced to conclude that in this, as in other matters, the men who guided the Foundation's research program were supremely elastic in their practice."[78] In fact, it depended on the context whether the director of research boasted of or belittled these sorts of investments.[79]

Similarly, the NIH grants system was being presented to the Congress as fostering directed research towards specific diseases and organs even as it was simultaneously viewed as a mechanism for funding open-ended, basic research. As Kenneth Endicott and Ernest Allen summarized the development of NIH funding in 1953,

> Although the Public Health Service awarded a few grants for cancer research every year from 1937 on, the broad program began in 1946 with the transfer of 50 projects from the Office of Scientific Research and Development when that agency was dissolved. The new program had as its objective the improvement of the nation's health through the acquisition of new knowledge in all the sciences related to health. In the sense that new knowledge is sought for the purpose of improving health this program is one of applied research, but many of the grantees consider their projects basic. Those who established the program believed that maximum progress can be achieved only if the scientists enjoy freedom to experiment without direction or interference, and they drew up policies and procedures accordingly.... Congress imposes a degree of control and direction when it appropriates funds earmarked for research on a designated disease or a specific organ.... [I]n 1953 about 80 percent is earmarked. In actual practice, however, it has been possible to provide reasonably equal opportunity for scientists regardless of their specialty in the health field, since the earmarked areas are broad and overlap to a considerable degree, especially with regard to the basic medical sciences.[80]

Along similar lines, G. Burroughs Mider recalls that when "the NSF asked the NIH to identify its basic research projects..., [t]he NIH replied, 'none'; all of its awards were essential to its mission."[81]

In the 1950s, even as scientists appreciated the bountiful development of NIH extramural funding, they worried that public expectations of improved health, having justified phenomenal growth in biomedical research funds, would put unrealistic expectations on basic research. The report of an NSF Special Committee on Medical Research in 1955 criticized research funding that targeted specific diseases:

> This so-called "categorical approach" to the problems of certain diseases has been justified in some quarters (a) because it is believed that the support of Congress and the people is more easily obtained for research in diseases for which no cure is known and which all individuals in consequence fear, since they identify them in terms of themselves or their families; (b) the widely held belief, no doubt fostered by certain wartime successes, that the solution of pressing national needs is best met by drafting all available talent into the pursuit of the desired objective.

> The Committee believes that it must draw attention to the dangers inherent in accepting these reasons as justification for the "categorical approach" in medical research. In the first place, while the citizens of this country have been extraordinarily generous in their support of such programs, both through government and private agencies, they have been led to believe, consciously or unconsciously, that the donation of sufficient sums of money is all that is needed to eradicate diseases which have plagued mankind for centuries. Such a belief is contrary to experience... Mere numbers of investigators and countless dollars will not in themselves ensure success in a search where, in point of fact, the seeker does not know what to look for. *This is the essential difference between the production of a new weapon of war and a new weapon for the eradication of disease.*[82]

In effect, it was the very model of the successful wartime mobilization that the scientists fretted would lead to unrealistic public expectations. Yet however much these elite scientists objected to the framing of scientific research in terms of a war against disease, they were unable to dislodge this fundamental paradigm for the support of postwar biomedicine.

Concluding Reflections

Both Daniel Kevles and Saul Benison have argued for the significance of the NFIP in funding life science research in the mid-twentieth century.[83] Even so, the historical literature on scientific patronage, insofar as it attends to lay health organizations, tends to group them with the private philanthropies of industrial capitalists and in contrast to state funding.[84] This line of argument highlights the continuing relevance, even after World War II, of private funding of science. However, the targeting of basic biomedical research as part of a layperson-led fight against a specific disease was a marked departure from the interwar activities of large philanthropies such as the Rockefeller Foundation, with its undeniable impact on experimental biology.[85] If the Rockefeller Foundation was seeking to protect biological research from the encroachment of clinical concerns and build interdisciplinary connections between the life sciences and the physical sciences, then the NFIP and ACS were seeking to reopen the medical front of biological research, with expectations of therapeutic payoff.[86] The "scientific managers" of these organizations were well aware of the differences between their strategies.[87] The Rockefeller Foundation cited the experiences of the NFIP as well as the Department of Agriculture as examples of the dubious value of simply increasing research funds. For their part, leaders of the voluntary health organizations saw themselves, in contrast to the older robber-baron philanthropies, as trustees of public money.[88] As the NFIP's O'Connor scribbled in the margins of a 1944 report recommending a long study: "*No – No* – lets have a *new* philosophy of *doing* things in medicine. Let c [sic] how *quickly* we can do it (intelligently) and not how long we can *study* it. Remember we get money to spend–and from the people–(not like Rockefeller)–to spend intelligently–of course."[89]

Just as significantly, voluntary health agencies played a critical role in upholding the model of mobilized science after the war and adapting it to include support for basic laboratory research. Other contingent factors contributed to the channeling of public monies toward biomedical research. As Paul Starr argues, the demise of Truman's 1949 legislative proposal for universal health insurance gave the funding of medical research (and of hospital construction) a new political function; it served as the federal government's visible commitment to improving health.[90] By 1950, politicians realized that the "war against disease" was an almost invulnerable political formula, resulting in average yearly increases of almost 25 percent through that decade to the NIH's grants budget.[91] Scientists who had protested having their research priorities determined by laypeople and politicians found that they could live with the flexible terms of disease-relevant funding. The pattern of funding basic research through mission-oriented programs was more the rule than the exception in postwar American science. As Daniel Kevles has argued, much basic research in the physical sciences was similarly sponsored through federal programs whose ultimate aims were practical, particularly through the Atomic Energy Commission and the Department of Defense.[92]

At a more symbolic level, the NFIP and ACS solidified the perceived link between the mobilization of science for war and the postwar use of research to fight disease. The critical years for the establishment of the March of Dimes were during World War II: the organization was founded in 1938 and managed to raise increasing amounts of money throughout the war. In like manner, the lay activist takeover of the leadership of the ACS led to large public campaigns, raising millions of dollars (and more each year) through the 1940s. There is a sense in which the rhetoric of the NFIP *was* the rhetoric of war, with the obvious enemy of polio, which crippled American children at the same time as American soldiers were being maimed and killed in Europe and the Pacific.

Perhaps even more significant than any symbolic resemblance between the campaigns against the Axis forces and against polio was the fact that both efforts shared the same spokesperson, Roosevelt. In a public letter in 1944, O'Connor, president of the NFIP, wrote Roosevelt that only "unremitting research will provide the key which will unlock the door to victory over infantile paralysis." Roosevelt's response, written in the closing year of World War II and only four months before his death, called for the deployment of all-out research.

> We face formidable enemies at home and abroad.... Victory
> is achieved only at great cost—but victory is imperative on
> all fronts. Not until we have removed the shadow of the
> Crippler from the future of every child can we furl the flags
> of battle and still the trumpets of attack. The fight against
> infantile paralysis is a fight to the finish, and the terms are
> unconditional surrender.[93]

This exchange of letters provided the basis for an NFIP news release on
8 December 1944, building towards the collection of funds in January
1945. The military metaphor did not become obsolete in the postwar
period, in part because the outbreak of the Korean War gave it a renewed
pertinence. (Figure 2.) The transfer of the rhetoric and research organization of World War II to postwar disease research was made all the
more powerful because the biomedical war against polio was "won"
by scientists in the 1950s. The NFIP's strategic emphasis on the role
of laboratory research in the scientific war against polio was richly
vindicated in their development of the Salk and Sabin polio vaccines in
1955 and 1958.

Here the comparison of polio funding with the ongoing campaign
against cancer is revealing. The March of Dimes' fight against polio drew
strength from the perceptions that scientists had won World War II
and that basic research was critical to the victory over polio in the mid-
1950s. This was Roosevelt's final legacy against the crippler at home as
well as abroad. (And in 1946 the Roosevelt dime was introduced into
U.S. currency, commemorating his association with the March of
Dimes.) Throughout the 1950s and 1960s, the ACS fostered similar
expectations for novel research-based therapies or cancer vaccines and
contributed similarly to the new regime of public support for biomedical
research. However, the hopes for a cure for cancer were prolonged, and
ultimately disappointed, despite Nixon's great War on Cancer launched
in 1971.[94] Vigorous criticisms of the Cancer Establishment were part
of broader critiques of science and medicine in the 1960s and 1970s.[95]
Tellingly, one commentator declared in 1978, "By comparison with the
fight against polio, the war on cancer is a medical Vietnam."[96] This sentiment expresses the profound cultural shift since World War II in popular

Figure 2. March of Dimes fundraising poster from 1952, which juxtaposed polio victim Larry Jim Gross against a soldier during the Korean War.

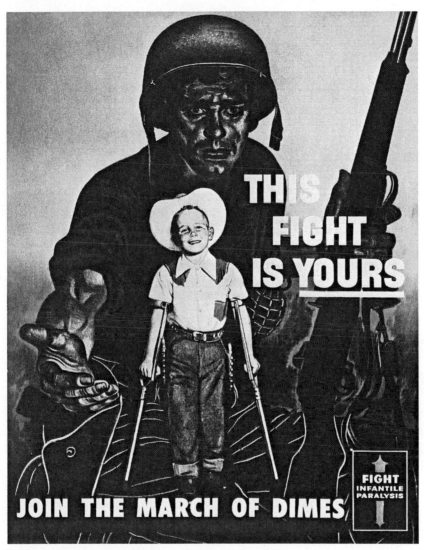

Reproduced by permission of the March of Dimes.

attitudes towards science as well as the unanticipated challenges biologists faced in understanding and controlling cancer.

James Patterson has compared "the popular support of voluntary health organizations in the 1940s and 1950s" to the environmentalism that emerged three decades later, both movements expressing American "demands for good health."[97] I have tried here to indicate how these health philanthropies contributed to the formation of new patterns of scientific research and patronage. More specifically, I have tried to indicate where the history of science policy in the United States must take into account not only party and presidential politics and the large capitalist philanthropies which have shaped the possibilities for research in this century, but also lay organizations which worked to equip biomedical researchers richly during the postwar decades. In the first part of the century, reverence for science and its methods did not mean that ordinary Americans gave their money, through donation or taxation, to pay for laboratory research. Voluntary health agencies, by cultivating a public demand for research, popularized government support of biomedical research in the name of fighting diseases.[98]

Notes

*   This essay includes material from my book, *The Life of a Virus: Tobacco Mosaic Virus as an Experimental Model, 1930-1965* (© 2002 by the University of Chicago Press). It is reprinted here with permission. I thank Jean-Paul Gaudillière and Daniel Kevles for sharing valuable research material, and for stimulating my interest in voluntary health organizations through their own work and our many conversations over the years. I acknowledge the National Academy of Sciences Archives, the March of Dimes, and the Bancroft Library for allowing me to quote from documents in their collections. An early version of this paper was presented at "Biology and Medicine– A Russian-American Overview," held at the American Philosophical Society, Philadelphia, in August 1998. Robert Kohler's perceptive comments at that meeting helped me refine the argument. In December 2005, I received valuable feedback from participants at the "Biomedicine in the Twentieth Century: Practices, Policies, and Politics" conference held at the National Institutes of Health; I especially thank Richard Lewontin, Harry Marks, Leo Slater, Warwick Anderson, and Keith Wailoo for their insightful responses and questions. Daniel Kevles and Buhm Soon Park provided astute suggestions on the written version, which was also improved by Michael Keevak's keen editing and kind encouragement.

1. Peter Keating and Alberto Cambrosio, *Biomedical Platforms: Realigning the Normal and the Pathological in Late-Twentieth Century Medicine* (Cambridge, Massachusetts: MIT Press, 2003), p. 25.
2. Daniel J. Kevles, "The National Science Foundation and the Debate over Postwar Research Policy, 1942-45: A Political Interpretation of *Science– The Endless Frontier*," *Isis*, 1977, *68*: 5-26; idem, "Principles and Politics in

Federal R&D Policy, 1945-1990: An Appreciation of the Bush Report," Preface to the 40th Anniversary Edition of Vannevar Bush, *Science, The Endless Frontier: A Report to the President on a Program for Postwar Scientific Research* (Washington, D.C.: National Science Foundation, 1990), pp. ix-xxv. For an account that stresses the role of business in these debates, see Daniel Lee Kleinman, "Layers of Interest, Layers of Influence: Business and the Genesis of the National Science Foundation," *Science, Technology, & Human Values*, 1994, *19*: 259-82.

3. Alice Kimball Smith, *A Peril and a Hope: The Scientists' Movement in America, 1945-47* (Chicago: University of Chicago Press, 1965); Jessica Wang, *American Science in an Age of Anxiety: Scientists, Anticommunism & the Cold War* (Chapel Hill: University of North Carolina Press, 1999).

4. In this respect I have been inspired by the late Nathan Reingold's call to historians to pay more attention to the relationship of postwar science patronage to mass, vernacular culture: see Nathan Reingold, "Science and Government in the United States since 1945," *History of Science*, 1994, *32*: 361-86, on p. 382.

5. American Foundation, *Medical Research: A Midcentury Survey*, 2 vols. (Boston: Little, Brown for the American Foundation, 1955), 1: 679.

6. James T. Patterson, *The Dread Disease: Cancer and Modern American Culture* (Cambridge, Massachusetts: Harvard University Press, 1987), p. 53.

7. Patterson, *Dread Disease*, p. 72.

8. Richard Harrison Shryock, *National Tuberculosis Association, 1904-1954: A Study of the Voluntary Health Movement in the United States* (New York: Arno Press, 1977; originally published in 1957 by the National Tuberculosis Association), p. 187. Only 5 percent of the gross sales went to the National Association's headquarters; most of the receipts were retained by local chapters to pay for community relief.

9. Shryock, *National Tuberculosis Association*, p. 188.

10. Despite the limited scale of their research grants, the National Tuberculosis Association is regarded by some as the first disease-oriented voluntary agency to support laboratory research as part of its mission; e.g., John R. Paul, *A History of Poliomyelitis* (New Haven, Connecticut: Yale University Press, 1971), p. 301.

11. Shryock, *National Tuberculosis Association*, p. 133.

12. Such as the American Bible Society and societies for crippled children. Shryock, *National Tuberculosis Association*, p. 133.

13. Shryock, *National Tuberculosis Association*, p. 182. Other health-related societies included the American Federation for Sex Hygiene, 1914, and the American Birth Control League, 1921. As Shryock comments elsewhere (p. 183), "The newer health movements emerged from much the same background which had earlier produced the tuberculosis societies. They all reflected the latest medical viewpoints, the American propensity for voluntary activities, and a growing concern about public health in general.

It seems probable that, even if the tuberculosis movement had not led the way in 1904, voluntary societies would have organized against other diseases during the decades which followed." Many, like the NTA, developed a "federal structure," with local, state, and national levels of organization.

14. Shryock, *National Tuberculosis Association*, p. 184, citing George E. Vincent, "Teamplay in Public Health," *American Journal of Public Health*, Jan. 1919, *9*: 14-20. According to Jane Smith, "In the first quarter of the century over seventy-five other groups were established to raise money for specific diseases. The National Tuberculosis Association had been founded in 1904, the American Cancer Society in 1913, the National Society for Crippled Children (now the Easter Seal Society) in 1919, and the American Heart Association in 1924. The Red Cross and the Salvation Army had become quasi-national causes during World War I, when they held rallies side-by-side with the sellers of government bonds and pledged themselves to care for the American soldiers overseas." Jane S. Smith, *Patenting the Sun: Polio and the Salk Vaccine* (New York: William Morrow, 1990), p. 69.

15. See Robert E. Kohler, *Partners in Science: Foundations and Natural Scientists, 1900-1945* (Chicago: University of Chicago Press, 1991), pp. 46-48.

16. Donald F. Shaughnessy, "The Story of the American Cancer Society" (Ph.D. dissertation, Columbia University, 1957), esp. chap. 8; Patterson, *Dread Disease*. The ASCC also created a Women's Field Army in their "War Against Cancer" in 1936, which distributed pamphlets and enlisted new supporters. But not until 1946 did the ASCC directly enroll researchers in their crusade against the disease. For more on Little's diverse activities, see Karen A. Rader, *Making Mice: Standardizing Animals for American Biomedical Research, 1900-1955* (Princeton, New Jersey: Princeton University Press, 2004).

17. "The American Foundation Proposals for Medical Care," *Journal of the American Medical Association*, 16 October 1937, *109*: 1280-81, quote on p. 1281.

18. Patterson, *Dread Disease*, p. 120. As Buhm Soon Park pointed out to me (personal communication, 17 April 2007), Roosevelt did use Social Security Title 6 appropriations to boost the research budget of the Public Health Service, with the enthusiastic cooperation of his Surgeon General, Thomas Parran, and the NIH Director, Lewis Thompson, who were both "ardent New Dealers." See Richard Mandel, *A Half Century of Peer Review, 1946-1996* (Bethesda, Maryland: Division of Research Grants, National Institutes of Health, 1996), p. 6. The title of the NIH was singular until 1948.

19. From the Certificate of Incorporation of the National Foundation for Infantile Paralysis Inc. Pursuant to Membership Corporation Files, as cited in Saul Benison, "The History of Polio Research in the United States: Appraisal and Lessons," in *The Twentieth-Century Sciences: Studies in the Biography of Ideas*, ed. Gerald J. Holton (New York: W. W. Norton, 1972), pp. 308-43, on p. 320.

20. National Foundation for Infantile Paralysis (hereafter NFIP), "Annual Report 1939," March of Dimes Archives, White Plains, New York (hereafter MDA), p. 11.

21. NFIP policy required that no grant be awarded without a vote of the relevant Committee, so these committees served as peer-review boards for the grants. This policy was not always adhered to; see Cornwell B. Rogers and George H. Jones, Chapter II, "Medical Administration, 1938-1943," Volume I of *The History of the National Foundation for Infantile Paralysis Through 1953*, Unpublished Historical Monographs, MDA.

22. As Rogers and Jones observe, "The General Statement of Plans of June 21, 1938, indicated that 'in the "after-effect" field' grants must 'redound to the medical benefit of all those afflicted with the disease.' In other words, the National Foundation should undertake, in technological and methodological ways, to raise the general level of care." To the degree that the awarding of grants followed these initial recommendations, the research funded by this committee was much more constrained to applied and clinical projects than was the research funded by the Committee on Scientific Research. Until 1940, all thirteen members of the Committee on Research for the Prevention and Treatment of After-Effects were orthopedic surgeons. Rogers and Jones, "Medical Administration, 1938-1943," pp. 70-73, quote from pp. 70-71.

23. That same year two additional advisory committees were formed: a Committee on Publications and a Committee on Nutrition. The second was short-lived. Rogers and Jones, "Medical Administration, 1938-1943," pp. 67, 81.

24. Paul de Kruif, author of *Microbe Hunters* (1926), is an interesting figure in his own right. On his research philosophy, his employment at and turbulent departure from the Rockefeller Institute, and his key role in supplying characterizations for Sinclair Lewis's *Arrowsmith*, see Paul de Kruif, *The Sweeping Wind: A Memoir* (New York: Harcourt, Brace & World, 1962); Benison, "History of Polio Research"; George W. Corner, *A History of the Rockefeller Institute, 1901-1953: Origins and Growth* (New York: Rockefeller Institute Press, 1964), p. 160; and William C. Summers, "On the Origins of the Science in *Arrowsmith*: Paul de Kruif, Félix d'Herelle, and Phage," *Journal of the History of Medicine and Allied Sciences*, 1991, 46: 315-32.

25. Rogers and Jones, "Medical Administration, 1938-1943," pp. 69-70.

26. The largest grant given by the President's Birthday Ball Commission went to Maurice Brodie of the New York City Health Department for development of a vaccine against polio. Spurred by the competition with John Kolmer of Temple University, who was developing a different vaccine against polio, Brodie tested his vaccine on a small group of children, and then extended the immunization to 3,000 children in 1935. Kolmer, too, administered his experimental vaccine widely that summer. As it turned out, the poliomyelitis virus in the Brodie-Park and Kolmer vaccines was only incompletely inactivated. The Brodie-Park vaccine was ineffective and could cause several

allergic reactions; the Kolmer vaccine was even more dangerous, having caused many cases of polio and several deaths. Although the President's Birthday Ball Commission had not supported Kolmer, its leaders realized that the public was not necessarily discriminating in its blame. Smith, *Patenting the Sun*, p. 72 and p. 132; Paul, *History of Poliomyelitis*, pp. 254-56.

27. Minutes, Meeting of the Committee on Scientific Research and the Committee on Public Health (Epidemics) and Committee on Education, 6 July 1938, p. 2. Bound Minutes, MDA. The committee assigned priority to the outstanding research questions the next spring; they were "(1) Pathology of poliomyelitis in human beings; (2) Portal of entry and exit of virus; (3) Purification and concentration of the virus; (4) What is to be called poliomyelitis?; (5) Mode of transmission of virus from man to man?; (6) Transmission of virus along nerves? (questions four, five and six received identical average ratings.); (7) Further attempts to establish poliomyelitis in small laboratory animals; (8) Settlement of question of chemical block-ade; (9) Chemotherapy of poliomyelitis; (10) Relation of conitution [sic] to susceptibility; (11) Production of good vaccine." Minutes, Meeting of the Committee on Scientific Research, 18 Apr 1939, Bound Minutes, MDA. On Stanley's crystallization of tobacco mosaic virus, see Lily E. Kay, "W. M. Stanley's Crystallization of the Tobacco Mosaic Virus, 1930-1940," *Isis*, 1986, *77*: 450-72; Angela N. H. Creager, *The Life of a Virus: Tobacco Mosaic Virus as an Experimental Model, 1930-1965* (Chicago: University of Chicago Press, 2002), chap. 3.

28. Milton Cantor, Chapter IV, "Medical Research Program, 1942-1945," Section A, Administration of the Medical Research Program, Volume 2 of *The History of the National Foundation for Infantile Paralysis Through 1953*, Unpublished Historical Monographs, MDA, pp. 352-53.

29. Edward L. Tatum, *The Contributions of the Basic Research Program of the National Foundation for Infantile Paralysis to Concepts of Modern Biology* (New York: National Foundation, 1963), p. 3.

30. A. Hunter Dupree, "The Great Instauration of 1940: The Organization of Scientific Research for War," in *Twentieth-Century Sciences*, ed. Holton, pp. 443-67.

31. Bush, *Science, The Endless Frontier*. On the significance of the mobilization for the physical sciences after the war, see Daniel J. Kevles, *The Physicists: The History of a Scientific Community in Modern America* (Cambridge, Massachusetts: Harvard University Press, 1995 [1971]); idem, "Scientists, the Military, and the Control of Postwar Defense Research: The Case of the Research Board for National Security, 1944-46," *Technology and Culture*, 1975, *16*: 20-47. Reingold argues that the Public Health Service (NIH) did not figure much in Bush's forecast of the relevant federal agencies. "That was a serious blind spot." Nathan Reingold, "Vannevar Bush's New Deal for Research: or The Triumph of the Old Order," *Historical Studies in the Physical and Biological Sciences*, 1987, *17*: 299-344, on 314.

32. Bush, *Science, The Endless Frontier*, p. 49. See also A. N. Richards, "The Impact of the War on Medicine," *Science*, 1946, *103*: 575-78.

33. Richard Harrison Shryock, *American Medical Research Past and Present* (New York: Commonwealth Fund, 1947), pp. 318-19.

34. See Stephen P. Strickland, *Politics, Science and Dread Disease: A Short History of United States Medical Research Policy* (Cambridge, Massachusetts: Harvard University Press, 1972).

35. Kevles, "National Science Foundation," p. 16. See also Reingold, "Vannevar Bush's New Deal" and the documentary selections in Part II, "Postwar Planning for Science, 1945-50," of *The Politics of American Science: 1939 to the Present*, ed. James L. Penick, Jr., Carroll W. Pursell, Jr., Morgan B. Sherwood, and Donald C. Swain (Chicago: Rand McNally, 1965).

36. For one example of this viewpoint, see Edwin J. Cohn, "History of the Development of the Scientific Policies of the University Laboratory of Physical Chemistry Related to Medicine and Public Health: A Memorandum of the Unwisdom of Projects and Reports," pamphlet in series *University Laboratory of Physical Chemistry Related to Medicine and Public Health* (Cambridge, Massachusetts: Harvard Printing Office, 1952).

37. Strickland, *Politics, Science and Dread Disease*; Harry Marks, "Leviathan and the Clinic," unpublished paper prepared for the History of Science Society Meeting, 27-30 December 1992.

38. U.S. Congress, P.L. 410, 78th Congress, 2nd session, 1944, as quoted in Strickland, *Politics, Science and Dread Disease*, p. 19.

39. Marks, "Leviathan and the Clinic."

40. Daniel M. Fox, "The Politics of the NIH Extramural Program, 1937-1950," *Journal of the History of Medicine and Allied Sciences*, 1987, *42*: 447-66, on p. 460. For the history of the NIH, see Victoria A. Harden, *Inventing the NIH: Federal Biomedical Research Policy, 1887-1937* (Baltimore, Maryland: Johns Hopkins University Press, 1986); Mandel, *Half Century of Peer Review*; Buhm Soon Park, "The Development of the Intramural Research Program at the National Institutes of Health after World War II," *Perspectives in Biology and Medicine*, 2003, *46*: 383-402; and idem, "Disease Categories and Scientific Disciplines: Reorganizing the NIH Intramural Program, 1945-1960," this volume. On the significance of private funding between the end of the war and 1948, see Clarence A. Mills, "Distribution of American Research Funds," *Science*, 1948, *107*: 127-34.

41. Here I follow Strickland (*Politics, Science and Dread Disease*) in calling into question Swain's influential interpretation that the Public Health Service had deliberately planned its pattern of postwar expansion based on the success of the Office for Scientific Research and Development; Donald C. Swain, "The Rise of a Research Empire: NIH, 1930 to 1950," *Science*, 1962, *138*: 1233-37.

42. See Patterson, *Dread Disease*, pp. 170-71. On the postwar involvement of voluntary health organizations in the medical research scene (and some of the resulting conflicts), see Harry M. Marks, "Cortisone, 1949: A Year in

the Political Life of a Drug," *Bulletin of the History of Medicine*, 1992, *66*: 419-39.

43. Benison, "History of Polio Research."

44. Both laboratories were extending epidemiological studies of poliomyelitis to include use of the physical and chemical tools. Minutes, Meeting of the Committee on Virus Research, 12 March 1946, Bound Committee Minutes, MDA. Max Lauffer, who had just left Stanley's laboratory to direct a Laboratory of Biophysics at the University of Pittsburgh, also received NFIP funding to isolate and study poliomyelitis.

45. I have rounded these numbers from those listed in Schedule 1 of the Annual Reports of the NFIP, 1945 and 1946, MDA.

46. Joseph H. Mori, Chapter V, "Medical Research Program, 1946-1949," Volume 3 of *The History of the National Foundation for Infantile Paralysis Through 1953*, p. 653. Unpublished Historical Monographs, MDA.

47. John Storck, Chapter V, "Consolidating the Early Achievements, 1942-44," Volume 1 of *The History of the National Foundation for Infantile Paralysis Through 1953*, p. 170. Unpublished Historical Monographs, MDA.

48. NFIP Campaign Handbook 1945, MDA.

49. NFIP, Tenth Annual Report, 1947, p. 36, MDA.

50. Jean-Paul Gaudillière, "The Molecularization of Cancer Etiology in the Postwar United States: Instruments, Politics and Management," in *Molecularizing Biology and Medicine: New Practices and Alliances, 1910s-1970s*, ed. Soraya de Chadarevian and Harmke Kamminga (Amsterdam: Harwood Academic Publishers, 1998), pp. 139-70.

51. National Research Council, Committee on Growth, *The Research Attack on Cancer, 1946, A Report on the American Cancer Society Research Program* (Washington, D.C.: National Research Council, 1946), Foreword.

52. On the activities of the National Research Council during the interwar period, see Glenn E. Bugos, "Managing Cooperative Research and Borderland Science in the National Research Council, 1922-1942," *Historical Studies in the Physical and Biological Sciences*, 1989, *20*: 1-32.

53. Frank B. Jewett to Karl T. Compton, 28 July 1946, in National Academy of Sciences-National Research Council Archives, Washington, D.C.: Central File: DNRC: MED: Committee on Growth: 1946.

54. National Research Council, Committee on Growth, *Research Attack on Cancer, 1946*, pp. 3-4.

55. By 1947, this panel was folded into the Panel on Experimental Genetics and the Panel on Viruses. See "Committee on Growth of the Division of Medical Sciences, National Research Council, 1947-1948," 1 September 1947, National Academy of Sciences-National Research Council Archives: Central File: DNRC: MED: Committee on Growth: 1947. On the milk agent, see Jean-Paul Gaudillière, "Circulating Mice and Viruses: The Jackson Memorial Laboratory, the National Cancer Institute, and the Genetics of Breast Cancer, 1930-1965," in *The Practices of Human Genetics*, ed. Michael Fortun and Everett Mendelsohn, Sociology of the Sciences Yearbook

Vol. 21 (Dordrecht, The Netherlands: Kluwer Academic Publishers, 1999), pp. 89-124.

56. Reginald G. Coombe to Frank B. Jewett, 2 Aug 1946, National Academy of Sciences-National Research Council Archives: Central File: DNRC: MED: Committee on Growth: 1946. At the same time Alfred P. Sloan, Jr., made a gift of $4 million to establish the Sloan-Kettering Institute for cancer research. Thus, the full amount received by Memorial Hospital was between $7 and $8 million. On the Sloan-Kettering Institute, see Robert F. Bud, "Strategy in American Cancer Research after World War II: A Case Study," *Social Studies of Science*, 1978, *8*: 425-59.

57. National Research Council, Committee on Growth, *Research Attack on Cancer, 1946*, Foreword. The same language can be found in a report the following year: "Members of the Committee on Growth Acting for the American Cancer Society through the National Research Council, Including a List of Research Grants and Fellowships, 1947-1948," copy in National Academy of Sciences-National Research Council Archives: Central File: DNRC: MED: Committee on Growth: 1947.

58. James S. Adams to Lewis H. Weed (Chairman, Division of Medical Sciences, NRC), National Academy of Sciences-National Research Council Archives: Central File: DNRC: MED: Committee on Growth: 1947.

59. James S. Adams to Frank Jewett, 11 February 1947, National Academy of Sciences-National Research Council Archives: Central File: DNRC: MED: Committee on Growth: 1947. There were also disagreements over how to handle an additional $1 million set aside by the ACS for "fluid research grants," money they wished to direct to institutions of their choosing. The leadership of the ACS overruled the recommendations of the Committee on Growth in deciding to give $250,000 to Memorial Hospital; this decision had been opposed by C. P. Rhoads of Memorial Hospital, also Chairman of the Committee on Growth, on account of the obvious and embarrassing conflict of interest in which he found himself.

60. Kevles, "National Science Foundation."

61. Douglass Poteat to A. N. Richards, 17 September 1947, National Academy of Sciences-National Research Council Archives: Central File: DNRC: MED: Committee on Growth: 1947.

62. E. B. Wilson to A. N. Richards, 12 September 1947, National Academy of Sciences-National Research Council Archives: Central File: DNRC: MED: Committee on Growth: 1947.

63. American Foundation, *Medical Research: A Midcentury Survey*, 1: 685.

64. Selskar M. Gunn and Philip S. Platt, *Voluntary Health Agencies: An Interpretive Study* (New York: Ronald Press, 1945), p. 206.

65. Gunn and Platt, *Voluntary Health Agencies*, p. 206.

66. Gunn and Platt, *Voluntary Health Agencies*, p. 219.

67. For some examples, see Tony Gould, *A Summer Plague: Polio and its Survivors* (New Haven, Connecticut: Yale University Press, 1995).

68. American Foundation, *Medical Research*, 1: 681.

69. See Daniel J. Kevles, "Renato Dulbeco and the New Animal Virology: Medicine, Methods, and Molecules," *Journal of the History of Biology*, 1993, *26*: 409-42; see esp. footnotes on pp. 420-21, and Creager, *Life of a Virus*.

70. Five more categorical institutes were added between 1962 and 1974. See G. Burroughs Mider, "The Federal Impact on Biomedical Research," in *Advances in American Medicine: Essays at the Bicentennial*, ed. John Z. Bowers and Elizabeth F. Purcell, 2 vols. (New York: Josiah Macy, Jr., Foundation and the National Library of Medicine, 1976), 2: 806-71, list on 854. I am indebted to Buhm Soon Park for helping me recover the original names of the institutes created before 1950.

71. See Toby A. Appel, *Shaping Biology: The National Science Foundation and American Biological Research, 1945-1975* (Baltimore, Maryland: Johns Hopkins University Press, 2000).

72. American Foundation, *Medical Research*, 1: 687.

73. Basil O'Connor, "A Special Message," National Foundation Annual Report 1960, MDA.

74. On the pre-World War II history of scientists' derogatory comments about "design" research and "project" science, see Michael Aaron Dennis, "Accounting for Research: New Histories of Corporate Laboratories and the Social History of American Science," *Social Studies of Science*, 1987, *17*: 479-518; David A. Hollinger, "Free Enterprise and Free Inquiry: The Emergence of Laissez-Faire Communitarianism in the Ideology of Science in the United States," *New Literary History*, 1990, *21*: 897-919. Marks discusses these debates as they played out for biomedical researchers situated in private medical schools in "Leviathan and the Clinic."

75. Paul E. Klopsteg, "Role of Government in Basic Research," *Science*, 1955, *121*: 781-84, on 781.

76. Monroe E. Spaght, "Basic Research in Industry," *Science*, 1955, *121*: 784-92, on 785.

77. Ibid. For another historical perspective on "basic" as a value system, see Reingold, "Science and Government."

78. Joseph H. Mori, Chapter V, "Medical Research Program, 1946-1949," Volume 3 of *The History of the National Foundation for Infantile Paralysis Through 1953*, p. 657. Unpublished Historical Monographs, MDA.

79. Ibid.

80. Kenneth M. Endicott and Ernest M. Allen, "The Growth of Medical Research 1941-1953 and the Role of Public Health Service Research Grants," *Science*, 1953, *118*: 337-43, on p. 341.

81. Mider, "Federal Impact on Biomedical Research," p. 848.

82. "NSF Special Committee on Medical Research Report," December 1955, pp. 28-30, Wendell M. Stanley papers, Bancroft Library, University of California Berkeley, 78/18c, carton 17, folder National Science Foundation, Special Committee on Medical Research. Emphases added. On the political origins of this committee, see Marks, "Leviathan and the Clinic" and Strickland, *Story of the NIH Grants Program*, chap. 7.

83. Daniel J. Kevles, "Foundations, Universities, and Trends in Support for the Physical and Biological Sciences, 1900-1992," *Daedalus*, 1992, *121*: 195-235; Benison, "History of Polio Research."

84. See Kohler, *Partners in Science*; Kevles, "Foundations, Universities, and Trends"; and, for a broader view, Barry D. Karl and Stanley M. Katz, "The American Private Philanthropic Foundation and the Public Sphere, 1890-1930," *Minerva*, 1981, *19*: 236-70.

85. Benison claims that even among the voluntary health agencies, the NIFP was the "first to open the field of philanthropy to the so-called 'common man.' Before the organization of the Foundation, philanthropy was generally an attribute and activity of the wealthy." Benison, "History of Polio Research," p. 323.

86. On the Rockefeller Foundation, see Kohler, *Partners in Science*.

87. Robert E. Kohler, "The Management of Science: The Experience of Warren Weaver and the Rockefeller Foundation Program in Molecular Biology," *Minerva*, 1976, *14*: 279-306.

88. Reingold, "Science and Government," p. 372.

89. As excerpted in John Storck, Chapter VII, "Administrative Problems and Changes, 1944-1953," Volume I of *The History of the National Foundation for Infantile Paralysis Through 1953*, p. 210. Unpublished Historical Monographs, MDA.

90. Paul Starr, *The Social Transformation of American Medicine* (New York: Basic Books, 1982).

91. "NIH Obligations and Amounts Obligated for Grants and Direct Operations," *NIH Almanac*, http://www.nih.gov/about/almanac/obligations/nih.html.

92. Daniel J. Kevles, "Cold War and Hot Physics: Science, Security, and the American State, 1945-56," *Historical Studies in the Physical and Biological Sciences*, 1990, *20*: 239-64. I am indebted to Daniel Kevles for drawing this connection to my attention.

93. Paul, *History of Poliomyelitis*, p. 319.

94. See Richard A. Rettig, *Cancer Crusade: The Story of the National Cancer Act of 1971* (Princeton, New Jersey: Princeton University Press, 1977).

95. For example, see Elizabeth Brenner Drew, "The Health Syndicate: Washington's Noble Conspirators," *Atlantic Monthly*, December 1967, *220*: 75-82.

96. Donald Kennedy, "What Animal Research Says About Cancer," *Human Nature*, May 1978, *1*: 84-89, on p. 84; also quoted in Patterson, *Dread Disease*, 252.

97. Patterson, *Dread Disease*, p. 138.

98. Benison, "Polio Research in the United States," p. 323.

Genes, Disease, and Patents: Cash and Community in Biomedicine

Daniel J. Kevles

In 1988, in a report on the emerging Human Genome Project, the National Research Council called for keeping open the data the project would generate, declaring that ". . . access to all sequences and material generated by these publicly funded projects should and even must be made freely available." Shortly thereafter, the National Institutes of Health (NIH), the lead agency in the project, chimed in, holding that the data should be "in the public domain, and redistribution of the data should remain free of royalties."[1] The admonitions to openness of course expressed the scientific community's longstanding communitarian norm, part ethical and part practical, that knowledge of nature is to be publicly shared.

But the project had hardly gotten under way before it felt a counter-communitarian jolt toward privatization. The blow came in 1991 from J. Craig Venter, a biologist at the NIH, in Bethesda, Maryland, who proposed the wholesale patenting of human gene fragments called "expressed sequence tags," or ESTs. Although just 150 to 400 base pairs long, each served to identify the gene of which it was a part. Venter claimed that ESTs would have utility as diagnostic probes for genes, but he also seemed bent on using the fragments to gain control of the intellectual property in the entire gene that the EST identified even though the EST revealed nothing about the gene's function. Within a year, the number of ESTs covered by the Venter/NIH patent application had multiplied to almost 7,000. A lawyer for the leading biotechnology firm Genentech noted, "If these things are patentable, there's going to be an enormous cDNA arms race."[2]

Much to the relief of most academic scientists and a sizable fraction of the biotechnology industry, the U.S. Patents and Trademarks Office (USPTO) rejected the Venter/NIH application, holding that ESTs were not patentable proxies for entire genes.[3] But the episode reveals that, from the beginning, human genomics has been torn between a commitment to communitarianism and an impulse to privatization and cash. Communitarians disparaged the cash impulse as a major and unwelcome departure from a longstanding commitment to cooperativeness in seeking to understand the workings of nature. There is a good deal of truth in the assumption of communitarianism in science, but the assumption is also suffused with a good deal of mythology, a romanticization of scientific practices in the past.

First, then, a few words about past scientific norms and practices in the interest of throwing into perspective the issue of cash and community in contemporary genomics.

******

Cooperativeness is a cultural value of ancient lineage in science. It was and remains undergirded by the standard of humility before the mysteries of nature to which so many scientists have adhered. The reasoning has gone that nature is infinitely complex, no one scientist can untangle its intricacies, and so all scientists must cooperate in the joint pursuit of understanding. The search for truth thus transcends the individual scientist, the local scientific group, even the national scientific community. Cooperation across national boundaries is one of the fundamental ethics of science. Scientists have often repeated the remark of the British chemist Humphrey Davy, who in 1807 accepted a prize for his research from Napoleon: "If the two countries or governments are at war, the men of science are not–that would indeed be a civil war of the worst sort."[4]

Through the long nineteenth century, scientific internationalism was reinforced by the increasing integration of the globe that technology was accomplishing via steamships, railroads, telegraphs, telephones. A number of cooperative scientific endeavors emerged in fields such as astronomy, geology, and geodesy. Scientists in these fields were concerned with global tasks–e.g., mapping the heavens and the earth–tasks that could be efficiently pursued by melding the results of local effort into a cooperative global network.

But competitiveness has also characterized fields that lent themselves to cooperative effort, and it has been perhaps even more manifest in fields that have not–for example, the branches of physics and chemistry that are grounded in the small, individualistic endeavor. More than fifty years ago, the pioneering sociologist of science Robert K. Merton pointed out that at least since the seventeenth century science has been marked by rivalries, some of them ferocious. For example, Galileo attacked competitors for stealing credit for his invention of the military compass and the telescope; and Newton, who was periodically obsessed with getting proper credit, battled with Robert Hooke over priority in optics and celestial mechanics, and waged a sustained war with Leibniz over the invention of the calculus. Merton wrote that priority disputes have not been the exception in science. On the contrary, they "have long been frequent, harsh, and ugly."[5]

One has to think back only to James D. Watson's memoir, *The Double Helix,* to be reminded that even without commercial incentives the practice of science could be marked by aggressive secretiveness, competitiveness, and even ruthlessness. In a review of the book the biologist Richard Lewontin wrote, "What every scientist knows, but few will admit, is that the requirement for great success is great ambition. Moreover, the ambition is for personal triumph over other men, not merely over nature. Science is a form of competitive and aggressive activity, a contest of man against man that provides knowledge as a side product."[6] Natural competitiveness has also been exacerbated by the exponentially increasing number of players in the game.

Since the late nineteenth century, the longstanding propensity to personal competitiveness was compounded by the increasing utilitarian payoffs of laboratory science. Physics and chemistry fueled what is known as the second industrial revolution that has continued through our own day. In branches of these fields, commercial competition penetrated academic science far more widely than it had hitherto. World War I, World War II, and the Cold War introduced national policies that fostered international rivalry in areas of science related to the technologies of national defense. The close interweaving of science and national security put many laboratories under the wraps of national security, and it brought many of those that remained open into sharp competition with the West's principal antagonist.[7]

Even so, cooperation continued in high-energy particle physics, the most prestigious and expensive area of that science. Openness in the development of the technologies themselves had helped speed development of accelerators before World War II, and so did a similar policy pursued by the Atomic Energy Commission (AEC) after it.[8] Unlike participants in human genomics, the early accelerator scientists and engineers thus worked in an environment largely free from patent constraints that greatly speeded accelerator development. Both law and policy have tended to vest in the AEC ownership of patentable inventions made in its laboratories or under its contracts and to make freely available the technologies of particle physics to scientists engaged in basic research.[9]

During the Cold War and since, a similar freedom characterized the exchange of basic data among high-energy physicists. They have achieved a formidable level of integration, now via the Internet, in respect of creating, evaluating, and banking data about the properties of elementary particles. Whence this exemplary cooperation and consensus? The answer, according to a member of a British group: "Particle physics data have no economic or strategic worth."[10]

In the life sciences, circumstances contributed to a strong anti-commercial orientation. With some exceptions—for example, hybrid corn—most university research, especially in the basic life sciences, yielded little that was commercializable or patentable, and of that, less that commanded significant, if any, market value. For example, the workhorse of classical genetics was, of course, *Drosophila*. Although fruit fly geneticists developed these creatures into standardized strains at the cost of much time and painstaking effort, no one attempted to profit from them; indeed, fruit fly stocks were freely exchanged among genetics laboratories on an international basis.[11] Similarly with bacteriophage in the middle third of the twentieth century, which were also standardized and made widely available among geneticists. Cooperation worked because there was little reason not to cooperate, and many reasons to cooperate, including the prospect of professional rewards. Besides, most living organisms and their parts were held not to be patentable as a matter of law.[12]

Academic culture's resistance to commercialization was particularly strong in the life sciences related to health and medicine. The University of Toronto scientists who were responsible for the isolation of insulin excluded themselves from shares in revenue from the insulin patent, assigning their rights to the University of Toronto for one dollar each. Ditto for Harry Steenbock, at the University of Wisconsin, who ceded his patent on a process for producing Vitamin D to the institution, which made millions on it until it was declared invalid. In the mid-1930s, Harvard promulgated the explicit policy that innovations in medical research arising from its laboratories must not be patented or, if they were, should be given freely to the public.[13]

******

Harvard's policy now seems quaint. Molecular biology has been demonstrating for some thirty years that it is highly practical, capable of generating both products and profits. Academic institutions and entrepreneurial faculty, with strong support from the federal government, have used the technologies of recombinant DNA, gene sequencers, and research tools to establish an astonishing fund of new biomedical knowledge. They have also joined with entrepreneurs to establish the modern biotechnology industry and the intellectual property protection on which it is built, including the commercialization of human genes. And they have been assisted by the courts and the USPTO, which have together expanded the scope of patentability to include living organisms and their parts.[14]

Commercialization sharply challenged communitarian access to genomic data. If Craig Venter failed at the wholesale patenting of human genes, he sought, successfully, to capitalize on human genomics ultimately through the creation of Celera and fast, shotgun sequencing. Celera's original business plan called for its data to be held as proprietary by the company and released at first only to paying subscribers, while patents would be sought on genes of interest.[15] After the human sequence was completed in 2001 jointly by Celera and the National Human Genome Research Institute at the National Institutes of Health, Celera

allowed academic scientists to download data only on a restricted basis–
e.g., requiring that they not be given to anyone else.[16]

Other firms in the United States and Europe have managed to achieve
exclusive control over genomic databases. Perhaps the best known is the
arrangement of DeCode with the Icelandic government: The company
enjoys exclusive access for commercial purposes to the national medical
database; an agreement it entered into with the government in 1998,
for twelve years. The drug firm LaRoche, which financed DeCode, got
exclusive rights to develop pharmaceuticals for twelve diseases, in
exchange for which it contracted to provide the Icelandic population
with any such drugs free of charge.[17]

A number of critics both in and out of science have objected strongly
to such proprietary arrangements, especially where it involves human
genomic sequence data. Many have advanced an ethical argument–
that the human genome is humanity's birthright, that it belongs to the
human community and ought not to be privatized in any way.[18] That
ethical argument has been largely ineffective against the commercial drive,
but consequentialist claims arising from the mutual self-interest of most
genomic researchers have kept genomic databases largely public.

Several models demonstrated how this could be done. Among them
was the *Centre d'études du polymorphisme humain* (CEPH), established in
1984 in France with genetic material from French and American families
that was made freely available to scientists constructing a human genetic
map.[19] There was also the *Worm Breeder's Gazette,* a record of the worldwide effort to map and sequence and characterize the *C. elegans* genes,
including their multiple mutations. The worm breeders shared data,
methods, instruments, and stocks, including mutants. Within this
community John Sulston began construction of a physical map of the
worm's genome, and the community at large linked this map to the
genetic map it had been developing collectively.[20] The enterprise was
characterized by the award of credit within communitarian norms.

The worm model influenced representatives of the multinational
human genome enterprise when they met in Bermuda in 1996 to strategize
the project scientifically and draw up rules for the treatment of data.
Clearly a response to the growing commercialization of the genome,
the rules stated that: "all human genomic DNA sequence information,

generated by centers funded for large-scale human sequencing, should be freely available in the public domain in order to encourage research and development and to maximize its benefit to society."[21] They urged that all primary genomic sequence data should be in the public domain.

The publicly funded human genome effort, which since the early 1990s has operated on an international scale, has of course undercut privatization by retaining its commitment to openness in its databases. Since the beginning of the sequencing phase of the Human Genome Project, all data generated by participants have been deposited in publicly available databases every twenty-four hours. By 2003, the human genome sequence, essentially complete, was posted on the Internet with no barriers to use, no subscription fees, no obstacles.[22] A growing number of journals will not publish genomic articles without proof that the authors have submitted their data electronically to GenBank, in Los Alamos, the central genomic database in the United States. The National Center for Biological Information, which runs GenBank, places no restrictions on reasonable use and distribution of its data.[23]

Large, well-established pharmaceutical firms have recognized the value of publicly available databases. Ten of them were instrumental in the establishment of the SNP (for single nucleotide polymorphisms) consortium, in 1999. Far more interested in using genomic data than in generating it, they saw in the consortium a means of reducing costs for the employment of such data and recognized that making it freely available to all would accelerate the growth in the knowledge base and benefit the public good.[24]

In all, the communitarian commitment in modern life science remains strong and has kept genomic databases widely available.

******

But despite the ubiquitousness of open genomic data, communitarianism and cash competitiveness remain in conflict in human genomics. The key reason is patents. The Bermuda rules, like CEPH, recommend against patenting human gene sequences. But there is nothing inconsistent with disclosing data and patenting the data if the disclosure occurs after a patent has been filed. And even if academic and biotech scientists submit genomic data to the public databases, they are free to file patents on it first.

What is wrong with patenting human genes? Nothing, many say, adding that much is right with it because it encourages investment and innovation in genomics. But one might counter that patenting human genes is at the least problematic because the practice entails costs to both the enterprise of research and the delivery of medical services.[25] In contemporary academic research, the expectation of patentability discourages open discussion of technical detail during the critical R&D phase before patent filing. Then, too, patented genes are research tools, and such tools, according to a decision by a federal court in 2002, are controlled by the patent holder, who may restrict and charge for their use because research even in its most abstract form is part of the "legitimate business" of the university and is not exempt from threats of patent infringement suits.[26]

A human gene patent establishes what has been called "a chain of dependency" in biomedical research. The chain reaches to efforts to characterize the gene and its functions more fully and to develop diagnostic tests based on it. It thus has a chilling effect on all research that involves the gene.[27] One firm patented a gene encoding the CCR5 lymphocyte receptor without any knowledge of its link to HIV infection. When the latter was established by another laboratory, the patent holder declared that it would enforce its patent against anyone making use of the discovery in the development of any pharmaceutical to combat HIV. In 1999, a survey of 74 clinical laboratories revealed that a quarter of them had abandoned a clinical test they had developed because of pending patents and almost half had decided not to develop a clinical test because of the patent.[28]

In the medical service area, gene patent holders have tended to insist that only they can conduct diagnostic tests using their gene. The practice threatens, among other consequences, to concentrate expertise in only a few centers; to fragment molecular medical services; to elevate the prices consumers pay for diagnostic tests; and to make doctors vulnerable for infringement suits. It also flies in the face of sound medical practice in that it can deny patients access to second and independent diagnostic opinions.

Such threats are not merely hypothetical, as is evident from Myriad Genetics' management of BRCA1 and BRAC2, the two genes known to dispose women to breast cancer. Myriad's BRCA1 patent covers the sequence not only as a descriptor of the gene but as the substance in and of itself and its mutant forms; also the uses of the gene as a probe or a primer; and its protein. Myriad's patent claims cover all and any diagnostic method that uses the gene, including those developed by others.[29]

For various reasons, by the end of the 1990s Myriad held monopoly control through patents and exclusive licenses over the DNA sequence of BRCA1 and BRCA2.[30] Myriad demands that all commercial testing for the two genes be done in its laboratory. It will not license the test to anyone, with the result that a woman diagnosed positively by Myriad cannot obtain a second opinion from an independent laboratory.[31]

Myriad has enforced its patent rights against various universities, a hitherto exceptional practice. In 1999, for example, it notified Arupa Ganguly, of the University of Pennsylvania clinical genetics laboratory, that she was infringing the Myriad patents because she had independently developed a test to screen for mutations in the BRCA genes and was charging her patients a fee to undergo the test. Myriad advised the university to halt Ganguly's activities or risk suit. To meet criticism from academic researchers, Myriad negotiated an agreement with the NIH in 2000 whereby NIH-funded researchers would be charged $1,200 per test instead of the usual $2,580 so long as the purpose was research. In exchange, Myriad would have access to resulting research data.[32]

******

How should we now think about the evolving conflict between cash and community in human genomics? BRCA1 was identified by Mark Skolnick, of the University of Utah. He had founded Myriad Genetics, and the university granted the fledgling firm an exclusive license on the sequence. Skolnick, contesting the idea that DNA is information, insists that it is a chemical and must be treated as such for patent purposes. He has said, "If you discover a new molecule, whether its's a pharmaceutical or a paint or a dye or a gene, it's a new molecule, you should be protected; . . . genetic patents really follow the model that's been set up in organic chemistry." The USPTO has affirmed that view, saying that if genes are treated as are "other chemicals, progress is promoted because the original inventor has the possibility to recoup research costs, because others are motivated to invent around the original patent, and because a new chemical is made available as a basis for future research."[33]

The fact of the matter, however, is that no one can invent around a human gene, including the mutated form that causes a disease. Human genes are the only ones we have got and, as such, they are natural monopolies. As a society, we exclude private property rights in some natural monopolies–say, Yellowstone National Park or the Cape Cod Seashore. We allow private property rights in others–say, railroads or the radio spectrum–but we do not permit the property holders to use their rights of ownership absolutely. We regulate the property right.

The time has arguably come to regulate the kind of property right–the intellectual property right–that is represented by a patent in human genes and possibly in human proteins, too. There is ample foundation in the structure of American law for the regulation of patented innovations that are essential to public interests, including health. Congress may grant the federal government "march-in" authority to license a patent to third parties if the patent holder has not made the invention available within a reasonable time or does not reasonably satisfy needs of health or safety.[34]

The regulation of human-gene patents might take the form of compulsory or voluntary licensing, or patent pools. It might even take the form of denying patentabilty to human gene sequences, which would then make them available to anyone for research into the gene, the development of diagnostic tests for it, and discovery of its functions and malfunctions, and the creation of pharmaceuticals based on it. This is a position advocated by many scientists, patient groups, and medical practitioners, including the American College of Medical Genetics. The strategy would allow for the patenting of the tests and the drugs while leaving the gene freely available for research.[35]

Few places are better situated to advance this analysis and suggestion for a modified patent policy on human genes than the National Institutes of Health, the nation's principal patron and safeguard of biomedical research in the public interest.

Notes

1. Committee on Intellectual Property Rights in Genomic and Protein Research and Innovation, Board on Science, Technology, and Economic Policy, Committtee on Science, Technology, and Law, Policy, and Global Affairs, National Research Council, *Reaping the Benefits of Genomic and Proteomic Research: Intellectual Property Rights, Innovation, and Public Health* (Washington, D.C.: National Academies Press, 2005), p. 22. Hereafter, NRC, *Reaping the Benefits*. I am indebted to Bruno Strasser for comments, criticisms, and suggestions.

2. Daniel J. Kevles and Ari Berkowitz, "Patenting Human Genes: The Advent of Ethics in the Political Economy of Patent Law," *Brooklyn Law Review*, Fall 2001, *67*: 237.

3. Ibid., p. 239.

4. Daniel J. Kevles, *The Physicists: The History of a Scientific Community in Modern America* (Cambridge, Massachusetts: Harvard University Press, 1995), p. 141.

5. Robert K. Merton, ""Priorities in Scientific Discovery" [1957] ," in *Sociology of Science: Theoretical and Empirical Investigations; Robert K. Merton*, ed. Norman W. Storer (Chicago: University of Chicago Press, 1973), p. 289; Mario Biagioli, "Instruments and Intellectual Property: Galilei vs. Capra," 2005, unpublished paper, cited with permission.

6. Richard C. Lewontin, "'Honest Jim' Watson's Big Thriller About DNA," *Chicago Sunday Sun-Times*, 25 February 1968, pp. 1-2, reprinted in Gunther S. Stent, *James D. Watson, The Double Helix: A Personal Account of the Discovery of the Structure of DNA: Text, Commentary, Reviews, Original Papers* (New York: W. W. Norton, 1980), p. 186.

7. Kevles, *The Physicists*, pp. 141, 378-81.

8. Government Accounting Office, *DOE's Physics Accelerators: Their Costs and Benefits* (GAO: RCED-85-96, 1 April 1985), p. 45. A not-for-profit organization, the Research Corporation, obtained rights to the cyclotron from its inventor, the Berkeley physicist Ernest O. Lawrence, on the understanding that his Berkeley Laboratory would continue to be a beneficiary of the Corporation's policy of investing proceeds from its patents in university research. The Corporation hoped that these proceeds would include royalties from licenses to commercial firms using cyclotrons to make radioisotopes for biological and medical applications. No radio-pharmaceutical industry developed before World War II, however, and after the war, owing to inventions made to exploit atomic energy, the cyclotron appeared to have little commercial value. The Research Corporation then wrote all cyclotron laboratories to grant royalty-free use of the machine. J. L. Heilbron and Robert W. Seidel, *Lawrence and His Laboratory* (Berkeley: University of California Press, 1989), pp. 192-93, 196-99.

9. Atomic Energy Act of 1946, Secs. 4, 6; Atomic Energy Act of 1954, Sec. 152. Executive Order 10096, 23 January 1950, gave the government rights to all inventions made by government employees during working hours or while using government facilities. Case law originating in implementation of the Order is reviewed by John O. Tresansky, "Patent Rights in Federal Employee Relations," Patent and Trademark Society, *Journal*, 1985, *67*: 451-88.

10. F. D. Gault, "Physics Databases and Their Use," *Computer Physics Communications*, 1981, *22*: 125-32.

11. Robert Kohler, *Lords of the Fly: Drosophila Genetics and the Experimental Life* (Chicago: University of Chicago Press, 1994), chaps. 2, 3, 5; Ernst Peter Fischer and Carol Lipson, *Thinking About Science: Max Delbruck and the Origins of Molecular Biology* (New York: W. W. Norton, 1988), pp. 153-54.

12. Daniel J. Kevles, "Ananda Chakrabarty Wins a Patent: Biotechnology, Law, and Society, 1972-1980," *HSPS: Historical Studies in the Physical and Biological Sciences*, 1, 1994, *25*: 111-12.

13. Daniel J. Kevles, "Principles, Property Rights, and Profits: Historical Reflections on University/Industry Tensions," *Accountability in Research*, 2001, *8*: 12-26.

14. "Of Mice and Money: The Story of the World's First Animal Patent," *Daedalus*, Spring, 2002, *78*: 81-88; Daniel J. Kevles and Glen Bugos, "Plants as Intellectual Property: American Law, Policy, and Practice in World Context," *Osiris*, 2nd series, 1992, *7*: 88-104; Kevles and Berkowitz, "Patenting Human Genes," pp. 233-48.

15. Kevin Davies, *Cracking the Genome: Inside the Race to Unlock Human DNA* (New York: Free Press, 2002), p. 208; NRC, *Reaping the Benefits,* p. 29.

16. Maurice Cassier, "Private Property, Collective Property, and Public Property in the Age of Genomics," *International Social Science Journal*, 2002, *171*: 87.

17. Ibid., p. 85.

18. Lori Andrews, "Genes and Patent Policy: Rethinking Intellectual Property Rights," *Nature Reviews Genetics,* October 2002, *3*: 803.

19. Cassier, "Private Property," p. 84.

20. John Sulston and Georgina Ferry, *The Common Thread: A Story of Science, Politics, Ethics and the Human Genome* (New York: Bantam, 2002), pp. 38-55; NRC, *Reaping the Benefits,* pp. 45-46.

21. NRC, *Reaping the Benefits,* p. 46.

22. Ibid.

23. Ibid., p. 27. See the statements of policy on sequencing and other data on the National Human Genome Research Institute website: http://www.genome.gov/

24. Cassier, "Private Property," pp. 84, 94.

25. Andrews, "Genes and Patent Policy," pp. 803-6.

26. *Madey v. Duke University,* 307 F3d 1351 (Fed. Circuit 2002); NRC, *Reaping the Benefits,"* p. 23.

27. Cassier, "Private Property," p. 90.
28. Ibid.; NRC, *Reaping the Benefits*, p. 44.
29. Cassier, "Private Property," pp. 89-90.
30. NRC, *Reaping the Benefits*, p. 52.
31. Cassier, "Private Property," p. 88.
32. NRC, *Reaping the Benefits*, p. 52.
33. Cassier, "Private Property," p. 88.
34. Andrews, "Genes and Patent Policy," p. 806. Andrews notes that "under the Clean Air Act, courts can, when necessary, order compulsory licensing of patents on equipment or technology used in air pollution control on reasonable terms to ensure competition." Ibid.
35. Cassier, "Private Property," pp. 84, 95.

The Critical Role of Laboratory Instruments at the Rockefeller: Biomedicine as Biotechnology

Darwin H. Stapleton

This examination of the importance of scientific instruments in the history of biomedicine begins with the premise that the role of instrumentation in the history of medicine and the history of science, or more specifically the history of biomedicine in the twentieth century, has been underreported. Instead, the published record of biomedical research has overplayed the conceptualization of research projects and the pursuit of theoretical confirmation, while underplaying the central role of instrumentation.[1] As two historians of instrumentation have suggested, "the philosophical debate over whether theory drives experiment or experiment drives theory has tended to obscure the independent role of instruments in science."[2] More broadly, the eminent historian of science Derek de Solla Price stated that "the scientific revolution…was largely the invention and improvement and use of a series of instruments of revelation that expanded the reach of science in innumerable directions."[3] Indeed, new and powerful scientific instruments of the twentieth century–such as the ultracentrifuge, the Tiselius apparatus, and the peptide synthesizer–were "instruments of revelation" that opened up new vistas of research and discovery in biomedical science.

To explore the key role of instrumentation in twentieth-century science, this paper will examine several significant episodes in the history of the Rockefeller University, the current name for the biomedical research institution in New York City that for most of the twentieth century was the Rockefeller Institute for Medical Research. The relevance of this framework for considering the importance of instrumentation in modern biomedicine is supported by historian and sociologist J. Rogers Hollingsworth, who in a recent essay titled "Institutionalizing Excellence in Biomedical Research," noted that "more major discoveries occurred in biomedical science at Rockefeller University than at any other research organization during the twentieth century."[4]

This study will begin by reviewing briefly several Rockefeller researchers (four of whom were winners of Nobel Prizes) for whom instruments of science were central to their accomplishments. It will then examine at greater length the critical function of instrumentation in perhaps the most important series of experiments of the twentieth century–the identification of DNA as the genetic material in cells.

Lindbergh-Carrel Perfusion Pump

Alexis Carrel won his Nobel for inventing remarkable surgical techniques, but he is equally important for his work in tissue culture.[5] Carrel came to the Rockefeller Institute in 1906 after demonstrating both in his native France and at the University of Chicago (1904-1906) an amazing dexterity and skill in laboratory and surgical techniques. In the 1930s he carried on an ingenious series of experiments with aviator Charles Lindbergh to test the possibilities of maintaining animal tissues and even organs outside of the body. These experiments were based on ingenious blown-glass devices and mechanical pumps. While Carrel's many years of experience with tissue culture were crucial to the research project, Lindbergh's practical knowledge of valves, pumps, and fluids made him a true partner in the project. Also a collaborator with Carrel and Lindbergh was Rockefeller's glassblower, Otto Hopf, a full-time contributor to laboratory work throughout the institute, who made a series of increasingly intricate pieces of glassware for the perfusion pump.

The Lindbergh-Carrel experiments failed to show conclusively that an organ could be kept alive outside of the body for experimental purposes, let alone for the purpose of repairing it or transplanting it. That was years in the future. But the work of the two men did show that modern engineering and biomedicine could easily join in the laboratory.[6] One of the Lindbergh-Carrel laboratory notebooks documents the beginning of an experiment with a chicken thyroid, in March 1935, the moment of their greatest success. The continued functioning of the thyroid for several days gave Lindbergh and Carrel the subject for a joint publication three months later in *Science*.[7] Their work was deemed important enough for the Rockefeller Foundation to pay for the training of a Danish researcher in the functions of the Carrel-Lindbergh apparatus, with the expectation that he would train other European researchers in the associated techniques.[8]

Neurophysiology: Cathodes and Computers

Another field of biomedicine at the Rockefeller Institute, neurophysiology, from the beginning depended upon instruments originally developed for physics. When Herbert Gasser came to the Rockefeller in 1935 to assume the directorship, he brought along his well-developed research program "that focused on the fundamental properties of nerve cells, dendrites, and the primary synaptic endings of nerve fibers."[9] His research was based on the development in 1920 or 1921, by Western Electric, of a suitable "low vacuum Braun tube [i.e., an oscilloscope] with a hot cathode which operated at a low voltage," and which Gasser judged to be "the most important factor in aid of [his] work on the electro-physiology of nerves."[10] Gasser began research with this oscilloscope, combined with an amplifier, at Washington University in St. Louis, in collaboration with Joseph Erlanger. He then spent the years 1923 to 1925 in the laboratory of A.V. Hill at University College, London, and later moved to Cornell University Medical College in New York City, before coming to the Rockefeller.

Although a small instrument shop had been created at the institute in 1920, Gasser greatly expanded it to support his research program. In his first annual report to the Rockefeller Institute's Board of Scientific Directors in 1936, he told board members that "The first step toward the establishment of a physiological laboratory…is the establishment of an instrument shop."[11] By 1937, with the aid of newly hired skilled workers, Gasser had created a sophisticated electronic apparatus that combined six of the latest model of oscilloscopes with a powerful vacuum tube, the thyratron. His apparatus could take either still or moving pictures of the oscilloscopes, which were measuring the electrical impulses carried by nerve fibers excised from several laboratory species.[12] Gasser's Nobel Prize was based on the effective use of this technology.[13]

Although not a student of Gasser, in the 1950s and 1960s, Haldan Keffer Hartline continued the strong Rockefeller tradition in neurophysiology. Hartline came to Rockefeller in 1953 from the Johns Hopkins University when his close colleague Detlev Bronk left Hopkins's presidency to become the head of the Rockefeller. Hartline already had a considerable record of research on the neurophysiology of vision, using oscilliscopy to study "the long optic nerves" of the horseshoe crab, which could be "frayed into thin bundles which are easy to split until just one active fiber remains."[14] He later extended his studies to vertebrates, particularly the frog. At Johns Hopkins he already was known for working closely with an instrument-maker and an electronics engineer.[15]

In 1960 or 1961, Hartline's technical inclination led him to begin exploring the capabilities of a computer owned by a colleague at Johns Hopkins.[16] In 1962, Hartline purchased the Rockefeller Institute's first computer, a Control Data Corporation 160-A, to improve his ability to analyze his data from "the experimental stimulation of nerve fibers."[17] This computer, priced at $90,000, was described in a Control Data Corporation press release as having "a magnetic core memory of 8,192 12-bit computer words [expandable to 32,768 words]….and an unusually large and powerful list of 91 instructions." Possible peripherals included "a magnetic tape system, high-speed line printer, card reader/[card] punch, and [an] electric typewriter."[18] After installation, the Rockefeller electronics laboratory created an interface that "translate[d] the information coming from the experiment into data which [could] be handled by the computer."[19]

A contemporary article described the value of the computer to the Hartline laboratory:

> An advantage of…the computer is, of course, that experiments can be modified or rerun at the moment on the basis of the information received. Another advantage of such "on-line" work, in addition to the time-saving feature, is the effect on the investigator–the stimulation of being able to monitor his own experiment as it is going on.[20]

Hartline received the Nobel Prize in 1967 for his accomplishments in understanding vision.

Counter-current Apparatus

Lyman C. Craig, regarded as a "gifted experimentalist," came to the Rockefeller in 1933. He held a Ph.D. from Iowa State University, and had spent the previous two years at Johns Hopkins. During war work in the early 1940s he developed the counter-current apparatus for separating constituents of mixtures otherwise thought to be compounds. Craig continued to improve his apparatus through the 1950s. The counter-current device was particularly important in work on proteins and antibiotics, and its use spread widely in the biomedical research community.[21] For example, Nobel Prize winner Sune Bergström noted that his early work on prostaglandins was aided significantly by a Craig counter-current device that Bergström had brought to Sweden after a fellowship in the United States in the 1940s.[22] Craig himself received the Albert Lasker Award in 1963 for the apparatus and associated methodology "which [according to the award citation] has made possible the isolation and identification of countless substances that occur in nature and that [as a result] can be synthesized in the laboratory for therapeutic purposes."[23]

Peptide Synthesizer

Bruce Merrifield won a Nobel Prize in 1984 for creating the peptide synthesizer. He had graduated from UCLA, where he also received his Ph.D. (1949). He joined Wayne Woolley's laboratory at the Rockefeller immediately, and a decade later began work on a device that would assemble amino acids into peptide chains.[24] A successful result held the promise of making proteins to order in the laboratory. Merrifield took three years to create a device that would synthesize a nine-amino-acid-long hormone. Then, "Merrifield and his colleagues from his laboratory and Rockefeller's instrument shop began automating the process.... By 1965 they had a working model and in 1969 they synthesized ribonuclease.... Merrifield's invention...revolutionized protein chemistry."[25]

The Centrifuge and DNA

The final and most substantial case of instrumentation at the Rockefeller Institute to be considered relates to what may be the most significant series of experiments in twentieth-century biomedicine–the work of Avery, MacLeod and McCarty on DNA. Oswald T. Avery carried out this work for more than a decade, culminating in the famous publication of 1944 with his two collaborators, Colin MacLeod and Maclyn McCarty. Avery was on the staff at the Rockefeller Institute for Medical Research's hospital, a hospital dedicated to research on infectious diseases.[26]

Soon after he joined the hospital staff in 1913 Avery focused his studies on pneumococci, a subject that occupied his succeeding 30 years of research. Avery was fascinated, therefore, in 1928 when Frederick Griffith published an article demonstrating that in the laboratory one type of the pneumonia bacterium could be changed into another type. Griffith had injected a non-virulent pneumonia type into mice, and then followed with an injection of killed pneumonia of the virulent type: to his surprise the non-virulent type was "transformed" into the virulent type, and the mice died. This unexpected result was of great interest to disease researchers primarily because better understanding of the characteristics of pneumonia might provide clues for the development of vaccines; but Avery gradually came to recognize the Griffith experiment's significance for genetics.

Avery's laboratory was known for its modest equipment and its reliance on well-known chemical procedures.[27] It was only in his intensifying hunt for the key to the "transforming principle," as it was known in his laboratory, that Avery began to take advantage of recent developments in research instrumentation. Not until 1938 did he have "centrifuges and other electrical laboratory equipment" installed in his laboratory.[28]

The appearance of centrifuges, in particular, should be understood in the context of what had gone on at the Rockefeller in recent years.[29] On the campus of the Rockefeller Institute was a laboratory of the International Health Division (IHD) of the Rockefeller Foundation. This laboratory was pursuing the development of vaccines for various diseases, including yellow fever, typhus, and influenza. In 1934 the IHD laboratory instituted a program of ultracentrifuge development, temporarily borrowing from the University of Virginia Edward Pickels, a promising graduate student of J. W. Beams, who was developing the air-driven centrifuge.[30] Pickels joined the IHD staff on a full-time basis in 1937, and with officer Johannes Bauer developed "an ultracentrifuge with which they were able to sediment the virus of yellow fever and with which they [studied] a number of other viruses."[31] In this work the IHD laboratory had the support of the inventor of the ultracentrifuge, The Svedberg of Sweden, whose work was being supported by the Rockefeller Foundation, and the collaboration with the Rockefeller Institute staff.[32] Variations of the ultracentrifuge were built at the institute by Ralph Wycoff and Alexandre Rothen.[33] It was Rothen's version which proved to be useful to Avery's investigations.

There was also another device available to Avery, a less-sophisticated centrifuge derived from the cream separators in use by the dairy industry since the late 1800s. The Sharples Company of West Chester, Pennsylvania, a major manufacturer of cream separators, moved into the manufacture of laboratory centrifuges by the mid-1930s.[34] Edward Pickels served as a consultant and "designed for them [an] air-driven centrifuge," that they manufactured in at least two models.[35] One or more of the Sharples models was installed in Avery's updated laboratory as early as 1938.[36]

We can now return to Avery's pursuit of the "transforming principle." According to the account of his collaborator Maclyn McCarty, the Sharples centrifuge was modified in 1940 to handle large quantities of pneumococcal cultures. In his words

> ...this cream separator-centrifuge was just the thing for dealing with mass cultures of bacteria, but it had one serious flaw.... In the course of its operation at high speed, it emitted an invisible aerosol laden with bacteria...this may have been tolerable when dealing with various nonpathogenic bacteria, [but] was totally unacceptable when one was centrifuging living, virulent type III pneumococci. Some-time before the fall of 1940...Colin MacLeod set about a way to overcome this defect.... With the assistance of a mechanically talented technician he designed an airtight,

sealed housing…which was fixed tightly by a series of bolts like those used on automobile tires. In fact, an ordinary tire wrench was used to remove and tighten them.[37]

According to McCarty, "thousands of liters of pneumococcal culture were passed through this machine" over the next three years, and "the increased yields of starting material had a major impact on progress of the work; one could now try a variety of fractionation and purification procedures without being limited by the amount of crude active extract."[38]

Another important step in Avery's project was the use of Rothen's modified ultracentrifuge in the spring of 1942. This device was in a separate laboratory and, according to McCarty, filled "most of the space in a medium-sized room." Unlike the Sharples centrifuge, which was designed and used to concentrate substantial quantities of fluid, Rothen's ultracentrifuge was analytical.[39] It held "only about one-half [a] cubic centimeter of extract."[40]

McCarty recalled the results of the analytical work as follows:

> Very quickly we learned that the active substance must be an exceptionally large molecule and that it was not present in very high concentration, since it was sedimented more rapidly than the material that gave the fastest-moving visible boundary. Even at the relatively moderate speed of 30,000 rpm, only 1 hour of centrifugation was required to concentrate 99 percent of the activity in the lower third of the chamber. The only other known component of the extract that was similarly concentrated under these conditions was DNA. Here, then, was totally independent evidence to suggest that transforming activity and DNA were somehow associated.[41]

Although some additional research was carried out, the studies done with the aid of the Sharples centrifuge and the Rothen ultracentrifuge had by the summer of 1942 convinced the Avery laboratory that the "transforming principle" was DNA.[42] They worked during the next year to refine their laboratory techniques so as to have a clearly reportable procedure, and carried out further tests with the Rothen ultracentrifuge. Rothen, in his unpublished report on the experiments, was unambiguous in his description of the result. He stated that "the [transforming] activity is a property of the nucleic acid."[43]

It is useful to note here that Avery's team took the further step of utilizing electrophoresis as another means of confirming that the transforming principle was inherent in DNA. As with Svedberg and the ultracentrifuge, the Rockefeller Foundation had been a supporter of Arne Tiselius's development of the apparatus, and researchers at the Rockefeller Institute were early adopters of the technique.[44] In 1939 it was reported that five of the fourteen Tiselius electrophoresis devices in the United States were either at the Rockefeller or in the IHD laboratory on the Rockefeller campus.[45] Thus, although Avery was himself not a very technology-oriented researcher, to confirm the results of his work he had utilized two of the most advanced laboratory techniques of his time—ultracentrifuging and electrophoresis.[46]

In February 1944 Avery, MacLeod, and McCarty published their landmark paper, "Studies on the chemical nature of the substance inducing transformation of pneumococcal types. Induction of transformation by a desoxyribonucleic acid fraction isolated from pneumococcus type III."[47] Interestingly, major historical works have not focused nearly as much on the role of instrumentation in their accomplishment as did McCarty in his later memoir, *The Transforming Principle*, from which I have quoted above. René Dubos, for example, who had worked in Avery's laboratory, wrote a volume on Avery and the DNA work. He gave only a brief mention each to the Sharples centrifuge and Rothen's ultracentrifuge, although he recognized the importance of advanced techniques in Avery's laboratory's research, and noted that "these technical advances were not published at the time."[48] Robert Olby devoted an early chapter to the history and use of the ultracentrifuge in his classic *The Path to the Double Helix*, but made no mention at all of its role—or of the role of any instrumentation—in his account of Avery's research.[49] Horace Judson, in *The Eighth Day of Creation*, did mention the role of instrumentation in Avery's project, but without highlighting its significance. In another context, however, Judson quotes Nobelist Sidney Brenner as stating that the availability of a "tremendous technological armamentarium" was one of the critical preconditions for the development of molecular biology.[50]

******

All together, I come back to my original points: whether looking at the discovery of DNA as the genetic material, or at some of the other leading discoveries over the last century at Rockefeller University, instruments have played a very important, yet seldom-appreciated, role. I will leave the last word to Rockefeller professors Stanford Moore and William H. Stein, who received a shared Nobel Prize in 1972 "for their contribution to the understanding of the connection between chemical structure and catalytic activity of the active center of the ribonuclease molecule." In their Nobel address, after reviewing the experimental procedures that led to their accomplishment, they concluded: "The sharing of knowledge among academic scientists and industrial designers of instruments... has played an important role in [the] progress of biomedical research."[51]

Notes

1. However, a recent brief essay provides a counterpoint: Guiliano Pancaldi, "Instruments, Biological," in *The Oxford Companion to the History of Modern Science,* ed. J. L. Heilbron, et al. (Oxford: Oxford University Press, 2003), pp. 411-13.
2. Albert Van Helden and Thomas L. Hankins, "Introduction: Instruments in the History of Science," *Osiris,* 1994, *9*: 6.
3. Quoted in William J. Broad, "Is Technology the Hero of the Scientific Revolution?" *Plain Dealer* (Cleveland, Ohio), 21 August 1984, p. 1-B. See Derek de Solla Price, "The Science/Technology Relationship, the Craft of Experimental Science, and Policy for the Improvement of High Technology Innovation," *Research Policy,* February 1984, *12*: 1-20.
4. J. Rogers Hollingsworth, "Institutionalizing Excellence in Biomedical Research: The Case of the Rockefeller University," in *Creating a Tradition of Biomedical Research: Contributions to the History of the Rockefeller University,* ed. Darwin H. Stapleton (New York: Rockefeller University Press, 2004), p. 17.
5. Shelley McKellar, "Innovation in Modern Surgery: Alexis Carrel and Blood Vessel Repair," in Stapleton, ed., *Creating a Tradition,* pp. 142, 146; Hannah Landecker, "Building 'A new type of body in which to grow a cell': Tissue Culture at the Rockefeller Institute, 1910-1914," in Stapleton, ed., *Creating a Tradition,* pp. 151-74.

6. McKellar, "Innovation in Modern Surgery," p. 146; George W. Corner, *A History of the Rockefeller Institute, 1901-1953: Origins and Growth* (New York: Rockefeller Institute Press, 1965), pp. 232-37.

7. Alexis Carrel and Charles A. Lindbergh, "The Culture of Whole Organs," *Science*, 21 June 1935, *81(2112)*: 621-23.

8. See documentation of a 1936 grant to the Carlsberg Biological Laboratory in Copenhagen in folder 26, box 2, series 713, Record Group (RG) 1.1, Rockefeller Foundation Archives (RFA), Rockefeller Archive Center (RAC), Sleepy Hollow, New York.

9. Hollingsworth, "Institutionalizing Excellence in Biomedical Research," in Stapleton, ed., *Creating a Tradition*, p. 36.

10. Herbert S. Gasser to William W. Stanhope, 10 January 1962, folder 5, box 4, RG 302.2, Herbert S. Gasser Papers, Rockefeller University Archives (RUA), RAC. This letter gives a date of December 1920 for the date when Gasser heard about the development of this type of oscilloscope; another document gives the date of December 1921: J. Erlanger and H. S. Gasser, "The Beginning of Nerve Oscillography," n.d., folder 1, box 6, RG 302.6, Herbert S. Gasser Papers, RUA.

11. "Report of Dr. Gasser (assisted by Drs. Toennies, Grundfest, and Lehmann)," Reports to the Board of Scientific Directors, October 1935–October 1936, vol. XXIV, RG 105, RUA, RAC.

12. Laboratory Scrapbook, 1935-1945, RG 302.6, RUA, RAC; "Report of Dr. Gasser (assisted by Drs. Grundfest, Lehmann, Lorente de Nó, Odoriz, and Toennies)," Reports to the Board of Scientific Directors, 17 April 1937, RG 105, RUA, RAC.

13. Abigail Tierney, "Gasser, Bronk, and the International Network of Physiologists," in Stapleton, ed., *Creating a Tradition*, pp. 241-44; Corner, *History of the Rockefeller Institute*, pp. 333-35.

14. H. Keffer Hartline, "Visual Receptors and Retinal Interaction," *The Rockefeller University Review*, November-December 1967, 5: 2. This is a reprint of Hartline's Nobel Prize speech.

15. Robert L. Schoenfeld, *Explorers of the Nervous System: With Electronics, An Institutional Base, A Network of Scientists* (Boca Raton, Florida: Universal Publishers, 2006), p. 195.

16. Schoenfeld, *Explorers of the Nervous System*, p. 197.

17. Robert L. Raney to R. L. Schoenfeld, 19 December 1962, "Control Data Corp." folder, box 9, H. Keffer Hartline Papers, RUA; "New Computer," *The Rockefeller University Review*, March-April 1966, 4: 23.

18. "Control Data Corporation Announces its New 160-A Computer, Broadening its Computer Line," 24 April 1961, press release, copy courtesy of archivist Karen Spilman, Charles Babbage Institute, Minneapolis, Minnesota.

19. "New Computer," p. 23; C. L. Ricker to E.[sic] Hartline, 25 January 1963, "Control Data Corp." folder, box 9, H. Keffer Hartline Papers, RUA.

20. "New Computer," p. 23.

21. Nicole Kresge, Robert D. Simoni and Robert L. Hill, "Lyman Creighton Craig: Developer of the Counter-Current Distribution Method," *Journal of Biological Chemistry*, 18 February 2005, *280*, at jbc ONLINE, site visited 7 November 2005; E. H. Ahrens, Jr., "After 40 Years of Cholesterol-Watching," *Cardiovascular Drug Reviews*, 2002, *20*: 245; Corner, *History of the Rockefeller Institute*, pp. 350-52.

22. Sune Bergström, "The Prostaglandins: From the Laboratory to the Clinic," Nobel Lecture, 8 December 1982, at www.nobel.se.

23. "1963 Albert Lasker Award for Basic Medical Research: Lyman C. Craig," at http://www.laskerfoundation.org/awards/library/1963b_cit.shtml. Site visited 7 November 2005.

24. Corner, *History of Rockefeller Institute*, pp. 378, 592; Bruce Merrifield, "Solid State Synthesis," Nobel Lecture, 8 December 1984, at www.nobel.se.

25. Elizabeth Hanson, *The Rockefeller University Achievements: A Century of Science for the Benefit of Humankind, 1901-2001* (New York: Rockefeller University Press, 2000), p. 111.

26. Saul Benison, "The Development of Clinical Research at the Rockefeller Institute before 1939," in *Trends in Biomedical Research, 1901-1976,* Proceedings of the Second Rockefeller Archive Center Conference, 10 December 1976 (North Tarrytown, NewYork: Rockefeller Archive Center, 1977), pp. 39, 44; E. H. Ahrens, Jr., "Changing Patterns in Clinical Investigation," in *Trends in Biomedical Research*, p. 59.

27. René J. Dubos, *The Professor, the Institute, and DNA* (New York: Rockefeller University Press, 1976), pp. 70-71.

28. Bernard Lupinell to E. B. Smith, 13 June 1938, folder 1, box 1, Oswald T. Avery Papers, RG 450 Av37, RUA.

29. An excellent exploration of the role of the ultracentrifuge in biological research may be found in Angela N. H. Creager, *The Life of a Virus: Tobacco Mosaic Virus as an Experimental Model, 1930-1965* (Chicago: University of Chicago Press, 2002), chap. 4, "That 'Whirligig of Science': The Ultracentrifuge in Virus Research," pp. 79–140. However, this work does not note the role of the ultracentrifuge in Avery's DNA research.

30. W. A. Sawyer, memorandum to Dr. Russell, 1 August 1935, folder 260, box 22, series 4, RG 5, RFA, RAC.

31. Proposed appointment action, 19 September 1936, folder 260, box 22, series 4, RG 5, RFA, RAC; "The Ultracentrifuge," January 1938, an article in the *International Health Division Newsletter* (January 1938), copy in folder 723, box 60, series 200, RG 1.1, RFA, RAC. See Christopher S. W. Koehler, "Developing the Ultracentrifuge," *Today's Chemist at Work*, February 2003: 63-66, at www.tcawonline.org; and "Centrifuge and Ultracentrifuge," in Heilbron, et al., eds., *Oxford Companion to the History of Modern Science*, pp. 135-36.

32. Warren Weaver diary, 28 August 1936, 22 September 1936 RG 12.1, RFA, RAC. See also Darwin H. Stapleton, "With the Best Intentions: Rockefeller Philanthropy and the Development of Atomic Bomb Technology," paper read at the annual meeting of the Society for the History of Technology, August 1-4, 1996, London, United Kingdom.

33. Warren Weaver diary, 28 August 1936, 22 September 1936, 5 November 1937, RG 12.1, RFA, RAC.

34. Elements of the history of the Sharples Cream Separator Company are found in: Creager, *Life of a Virus*, pp. 95-96; Martha Carson-Gentry and Paul Rodebaugh, *Images of America: West Chester [Pennsylvania]* (Charleston, South Carolina: Arcadia Publishing, 1997), pp. 62-63; Chester County Historical Society with the Chester County Camera Club, *Chester County [Pennsylvania]: Then and Now* (Charleston, South Carolina: Arcadia Publishing, 2004), p. 11; Sam Stephens, Mike Fournier, and Robert Benoit, *Cream Separator Memorabilia: De Laval, Sharples and Others* (Pierrefonds, Quebec: Benoit Publications, 2000), p. 169. A useful summary of the operation of contemporary cream separators is in W. E. Petersen, *Dairy Science: Its Principles, and Practice in Production, Management, and Processing* (Chicago: J. B. Lippincott, 1939), pp. 550-58.

35. Warren Weaver diary, 24 February 1938, RG 12.1, RFA, RAC.

36. The industrially produced Sharples centrifuges were much less expensive than ultracentrifuges, each of which was built to order. In 1938 it was estimated that an air-driven ultracentrifuge would cost $3,000-5,000, while about two years later a Sharples centrifuge was purchased for $312. Warren Weaver to C. Sidney Burwell, 18 February 1938, folder 1742, box 141, series 200, RG 1.1, RFA, RAC; and "Rockefeller Foundation Gift for Special Equipment, 1939-1940," 22 August 1940, folder 1743, box 141, series 200, RG 1.1, RFA, RAC.

37. Maclyn McCarty, *The Transforming Principle: Discovering That Genes are Made of DNA* (New York: W. W. Norton, 1985), p. 104.

38. McCarty, *Transforming Principle*, p. 104.

39. "Report of Dr. Rothen," in *Reports to the Scientific Directors*, vol. 27, October 1938-October 1939, p. 131, RUA, RAC; "Report of Dr. Rothen," in *Reports to the Scientific Directors*, vol. 28, October 1939-October 1940, p. 36, RUA, RAC.

40. McCarty, *Transforming Principle*, p. 138.

41. McCarty, *Transforming Principle*, pp. 138-39.

42. McCarty, *Transforming Principle*, p. 142.

43. "Report of Dr. MacInnes (assisted by Drs. Belcher, Longsworth, Rothen and Shedlovsky)," in *Reports to the Scientific Directors*, vol. 32, October 1943-October 1944, p. 27, RUA, RAC. The quoted section of the report is attributed in the text to Rothen.

44. Warren Weaver diary, 5 November 1937, 22 September 1939, RG 12.1, RFA, RAC; Lily E. Kay, "Laboratory Technology and Biological Knowledge: The Tiselius Electrophoresis Apparatus, 1930-1945," *History and Philosophy of the Life Sciences*, 1988, *10*: 51-72.

45. Warren Weaver diary, 22 September 1939, RG 12.1, RFA, RAC.

46. It is worth noting here that the close relationship between the Rockefeller Foundation and the Rockefeller Institute for Medical Research undoubtedly contributed to the early adoption of advanced instrumentation by institute researchers. While the Foundation and the Institute were separate organizations, the first two directors of the Institute, Simon Flexner (1901-1934) and Herbert Gasser (1935-1952) also served as trustees of the Foundation, and the Institute was regularly visited by Foundation officers, in part because of the Foundation's International Health Division laboratory on campus. As Angela Creager has noted, "the effects" of the Foundation's promotion of the use of instrumentation "on scientific practices have only begun to be appreciated." Creager, *Life of a Virus*, p. 10. For a brief commentary on the relationship between the Foundation and the Institute, see Darwin H. Stapleton, "The Rockefeller (University) Effect: A Phenomenon in Biomedical Science," in Stapleton, ed., *Creating a Tradition*, pp. 7-10.

47. O. T. Avery, C. M. MacLeod, and M. McCarty, "Studies on the chemical nature of the substance inducing transformation of pneumococcal types. Induction of transformation by a desoxyribonucleic acid fraction isolated from pneumococcus type III." *Journal of Experimental Medicine*, 1944, *79*: 137-58.

48. Dubos, *The Professor, the Institute, and DNA*, pp. 140-41, quote on p. 141. Dubos also stated that "surprising as it may seem, the Avery group never published a complete detailed account of the steps that led them to this remarkable and unexpected conclusion (p. 142)." McCarty's volume, *Transforming Principle*, substantially remedied the situation.

49. Robert Olby, *The Path to the Double Helix: The Discovery of DNA*, rev. ed. (New York: Dover, 1994), pp. 11-21, 181-89.

50. Horace Freeland Judson, *The Eighth Day of Creation: Makers of the Revolution in Biology*, expanded ed. (Plainview, New York: Cold Spring Harbor Laboratory Press, 1996), p. 183.

51. Stanford Moore and William H. Stein, "The Chemical Structures of Pancreatic Ribonuclease and Deoxyribonuclease," Nobel lecture, 11 December 1972, at www.nobel.se.

Clinical Research in Postwar Britain: The Role of the Medical Research Council

Carsten Timmermann

Introduction

In this essay I deal with probably the closest relative of the National Institutes of Health (NIH) in the United Kingdom, the Medical Research Council (MRC). The MRC oversaw and actively promoted the rise of biomedical ideals and the proliferation of institutions devoted to bio-medical research in Britain. In my work in recent years, developments in medical research in the post-World War II period have been my main concern. I have looked at high blood pressure, both debates over the etiology of hypertension and the introduction of new therapies, and at lung cancer, the search for its causes and, again, for effective therapies.[1] When I looked at these issues I was struck by how much postwar practices in clinical research in Britain were informed by a specific MRC ethos and informal MRC networks constituted in the interwar period, and by research traditions that representatives of the Council saw as embodying its ethos. In the first part of this paper, I will discuss the emergence of these traditions and the people who shaped them.[2] In the second part, I will discuss how these traditions left their imprint on postwar clinical research on high blood pressure and lung cancer. This paper is about continuity more than change. Some of the post-war administrative changes, however, especially those linked to the introduction of the British National Health Service (NHS), allowed the MRC to broaden its influence on British clinical research by vigorously promoting the traditions invented in the interwar period. While older research traditions permeated and shaped the policies of the postwar period, the new NHS provided the MRC with an opportunity to reflect on what to them constituted good clinical science. I will describe the reorganization of clinical research later, but at this point let me briefly introduce the definition of clinical science the Council espoused at this time.

Clinical research, according to the MRC's 1952 Annual Report, had to go "beyond the stage of observation and description of syndromes."[3] It was to engage with "planned investigations of illness."[4] The author of the article in the 1952 report clearly valued the experimental more than the observational, when he stated that "a branch of research which is debarred from using the experimental method is heavily handicapped in the general advance of science."[5] Experimentation in clinical medicine, however, was "limited to investigations which involve no risk to the patient and enlist his willing co-operation," and such practical limitations explained "the relatively slow development in the direct application of the investigational method to the study of illness."[6] But clinical research also included objects of study not susceptible to the experimental method: "clinical research covers not only work on patients in hospital but also field studies in epidemiology and social medicine, and observations in general practice."[7] The aim was to build on knowledge gained in the pre-clinical fields and to devise "accurate techniques for the investigation of illness in human patients."[8]

> It is the devising of such techniques in adequate variety and with increasing speed over the last two or three decades that is putting new opportunities within our grasp. Chemical and instrumental methods are now available for accurate investigation in many types of illness, without risk to the patient. The development of statistical techniques has refined the methods of planned observation and controlled clinical trials.... Progress in clinical knowledge need, therefore, no longer depend entirely upon the chance observation of naturally occurring events. The clinical observer can now become, in addition, a clinical investigator.[9]

In other words, the time was ripe for a new type of clinical research in Britain, based on the foundations laid and the traditions established by the MRC in the interwar period and during the war, and on the new opportunities provided by the reorganization of healthcare. Before I return to the post–World War II period, in the first part of the chapter I will discuss the origins of the MRC traditions and the context of academic medicine in Britain in the early twentieth century. A brief word of warning: this essay is by no means a comprehensive account. Rather, I am attempting to highlight some of the trends that are most relevant for a broad comparison with contemporary developments in the United States.

The Origins of the MRC Traditions

The Medical Research Committee, which in 1919 became the Medical Research Council, was set up in 1913 with funds provided by the British government in the 1911 National Insurance Act. Initially intended for research on tuberculosis, as Linda Bryder has shown, the Council's research agenda got much broader very quickly.[10] The MRC agenda was shaped to a considerable extent by a small group of men, some of them close friends, most with ties to Cambridge physiology, who seized this opportunity to create a new platform for their brand of medical research.[11] A key figure was Sir Walter Morley Fletcher, MRC secretary from 1914 until his death in 1933, a medically qualified physiologist and Fellow of the Royal Society.[12] His background and continued interest in physiology secured basic science an important place in the MRC research agenda, and the Cambridge tradition with its emphasis on neurophysiology, pharmacology, and nutritional research was strongly represented in the research projects supported by the Council. According to his obituary, Fletcher "loved Cambridge first and foremost," and Cambridge played a special role in the policies of the Council, as home for many of its institutions and also of the intellectual traditions the Council embraced.[13] Joan Austoker argues that "Fletcher believed that all medical research should be influenced by the MRC" and ultimately come under some form of MRC control, and many of the MRC policies from the beginnings until well into the postwar period, under Fletcher as well as his successors, were designed to extend this influence to areas of medicine which they perceived as following different agendas, incompatible with MRC ethos.[14] One example was cancer research, which initially was dominated by the Imperial Cancer Research Fund (ICRF), an organization that had close ties with the Royal College of Physicians.[15]

While there was considerable emphasis on fundamental research, clinical research was part of the MRC program almost from the beginning. Fletcher's obituary for the Royal Society, for example, was written by his friend, Thomas Renton Elliott, the first full-time Professor of Medicine at University College Hospital (UCH) London, himself a Cambridge man and one of the central players when it came to importing Cambridge research traditions and MRC ethos into the clinic. It was Elliott who proposed Fletcher for the post of MRC secretary in 1913. Theirs was an approach to the clinic that was new for Britain, modeled on continental European examples refracted through the prism of United States institutional reform. The men who shaped the policies of the council in the early years believed that investigations in the physiology laboratory provided the best model for good clinical research and practice. As long as only a few "rational" remedies were available, foundations had to be laid in the laboratory, which explains the initial emphasis on fundamental research. Medical education at the clinical level also was to be reorganized, following the model of the basic sciences, and students were to be taught by full-time clinicians who were also researchers.

This may sound banal for us now, as most medical research and teaching is organized along these lines today, but it was not banal in interwar Britain, where most medical schools, in the words of Donald Fisher, "remained essentially 'trade schools,'" with clinical teachers holding part-time appointments and living on income generated by private practice.[16] Most of London's medical schools were associated with voluntary hospitals, and they maintained a considerable degree of independence from the University of London until well into the twentieth century, despite joining the university as "schools" in 1900. The promoters of the MRC disapproved of the prevailing attitude at these schools which viewed research as a "private hobby."[17] There was also, as Christopher Lawrence has argued, more fundamental opposition to the approaches promoted by the MRC from members of the medical elite who objected to the extension of experimental practices to the clinic and insisted that clinical knowledge was different from the knowledge generated in the laboratory. It was incommunicable, they argued, and could only be acquired by way of bedside practice.[18]

The conflicts between the MRC and the Royal Colleges, the traditional representatives of all things medical in Britain, as David Cantor has shown, found their expression in controversies over the uses of radium for research and in treatment of cancer in the interwar period.[19] In 1919, the Medical Research Committee had acquired five grams of hydrated radium bromide, an extremely valuable and scarce resource that provided the basis for the MRC's program of radiological research. This program was initially predominantly clinical rather than biological, as it proved difficult for Fletcher to promote an experimentalist agenda in the face of the increasing visibility of cancer and the growing belief that radium might provide a solution to the problem of therapy, as an alternative or in combination with surgery. Surgeons, initially extremely critical towards radium, became interested in the new therapeutic modality towards the late 1920s. In the 1930s, the creation of a National Radium Commission and a division in the control of radium allowed the MRC to expand experimental research. This was not defeat, however: the Commission, while controlled by the Colleges, allocated radium to the various centers under similar conditions concerning record keeping and data evaluation to those the MRC had imposed. The British Empire Cancer Campaign (BECC) was another example of an organization colonized by the Council. Initially founded by a group of London doctors, Fletcher managed to secure the MRC control over the Campaign's Scientific Advisory Committee. The controversies between the Council and the Colleges continued well into the postwar period, when the reorganization of the British healthcare system allowed the MRC significantly to expand its influence and the Colleges, too, changed their outlook.[20] Before I turn to these postwar developments, however, let me take a closer look at the traditions that prepared the ground for the postwar clinical research that I will discuss later, above all in two institutions, UCH and the MRC's own National Institute for Medical Research (NIMR).

Clinical Science at University College Hospital and the Role of the Rockefeller Foundation

The two major pioneers of the clinical science tradition in the MRC were Thomas Lewis and Thomas Renton Elliott.[21] Both had their institutional home at UCH, then the flagship for those who worked to develop British medical studies according to the German-American model. After World War I, University College Medical School and its hospital received substantial amounts of funding from the Rockefeller Foundation in order to enable its transformation into a university medical center modeled on the Johns Hopkins University.[22] The UCL center was to serve as a model for other medical schools in Britain and in the Empire. Much of the funding went into the pre-clinical departments on one side of Gower Street, but the Foundation also funded two clinical "units" in the hospital across the road, staffed with full-time researchers and teachers and with direct access to laboratories. The MRC provided additional funding, as its statutes prevented it from making capital grants. Its architects intended the unit system as a model for clinical research in Britain. The Rockefeller Foundation subsequently also supported the establishment of units elsewhere in London and in the country and funded the transformation of the School of Tropical Medicine into the new London School of Hygiene and Tropical Medicine (LSHTM), a postgraduate school for hygiene and public health within the University of London, which would become the institutional home of Major Greenwood and Austin Bradford Hill and the influential MRC Statistical Unit, to which I will return later. [23]

T. R. Elliott's medical unit and Thomas Lewis's MRC-funded department of clinical research and experimental medicine turned into important staging posts in the careers of many clinical researchers in Britain. Lewis, unlike Elliott and Fletcher, was not a Cambridge graduate. He studied at Cardiff before he went to UCH in 1902, where he met Elliott and Henry Dale, another member of the "club" that was going to shape MRC research traditions.[24] An important influence on Lewis, besides his work in E. H. Starling's physiology laboratory, was a friendship with James Mackenzie. In his research Lewis focused on the heart, its functions and diseases. An active, hands-on researcher, he pioneered the routine clinical use of the electrocardiogram and of many other laboratory techniques. Elliott's early research at Cambridge followed the traditions established by Michael Foster and John Langley, his director of research, and dealt with the physiology of the autonomic nervous system. Later, as professor of medicine, his publications became infrequent, and Elliott's more important roles were those of an administrator and teacher. Elliott and Lewis were close friends and even shared lodgings for a period of time. Lewis self-consciously and repeatedly described his work as "clinical science," as though he was laying claim to the term. He changed the title of the journal he founded and edited from *Heart* to *Clinical Science*.

Lewis's approach to and understanding of clinical science was immensely important for the directions subsequently taken by the MRC. Many young medical graduates who were interested in research spent a year or more in either Lewis' department or Elliott's unit, often supported by Beit Memorial Fellowships, where they were exposed to approaches to the clinic that integrated technologies and practices from the physiology laboratory. [25] These disciples shaped medical research in Britain and the Empire in the decades to come. They included George Pickering and Frederick Smirk, about whom more will be said later, as well as Harold Himsworth, secretary of the MRC from 1949 to 1968, and John McMichael, later director of the new Postgraduate Medical School in Hammersmith. [26]

The National Institute of Medical Research

The other important birth place of MRC traditions included under "clinical research" in the postwar definition was the Council's National Institute of Medical Research (NIMR). The institute was set up originally for the Medical Research Committee just before the outbreak of World War I in 1914, in the buildings of the North London Hospital for Consumption, Mount Vernon. [27] During the war the buildings were used by the Army Medical Service, and Thomas Lewis did his research work on "soldier's heart" at what was then Hampstead Military Hospital. [28] The institute had four departments: Bacteriology, initially under the directorship of the eminent Sir Almroth Wright; Biochemistry and

Physiology with Henry Dale as director; Applied Physiology under Leonard Hill, and Medical Statistics under John Brownlee. I will focus here on Dale's and Brownlee's departments, as these are important for the postwar case studies I want to look at. The four directors initially had equal standing and the institute was run by a staff committee and a general secretary, but de facto Dale gained more and more control over both day-to-day and strategic decisions. This arrangement was formalized in 1928 when Dale was appointed overall director of the institute.[29]

Dale, like Elliott was a Cambridge man and a product of the Foster School. Another major professional experience that shaped his approach to research and, more important, the ways in which Dale and the Council dealt with the pharmaceutical industry, was his time as director of the Wellcome Physiological Laboratories.[30] Dale had joined Wellcome's new research center in 1902 and, contrary to what some of his colleagues assumed, this excursion out of the university and into the expanding corporate world of the pharmaceutical industry did not ruin his academic career. Wellcome left Dale plenty of freedom to pursue his own research. The Wellcome laboratories were the first corporate research establishment of this kind in Britain and Dale's appointment may have provided a model for other companies. As Tilly Tansey has shown, Dale managed to combine productive research in the Cambridge physiology tradition with commercial exploration.[31] He also valued the experiences he gained with routine tasks and in his later career at the NIMR used what he learned about the everyday work in a corporate laboratory, for example, on the bread and butter issue of standardizing biological compounds. Dale managed to turn the NIMR into not only a national, but an international center for the standardization of therapeutic substances. The institute under Dale also actively promoted therapeutic substances that were products of laboratory research and thus embodied the new ethos of scientific medicine as embraced by the MRC, such as insulin or penicillin.[32]

The NIMR's Department of Medical Statistics, and later the London School of Hygiene and Tropical Medicine (LSHTM), were home to another tradition that shaped the self understanding of the MRC in the postwar world and, with its work on the health effects of smoking, also the public image of the Council.[33] The first director of the Department,

John Brownlee in this regard was far less effective than a Ministry of Health employee transferred to the NIMR in 1920, Major Greenwood.[34] Both were disciples of the eugenicist Karl Pearson.[35] Greenwood was a personal friend of Walter Fletcher. By then chair of the MRC Statistical Committee, he accepted an appointment to the London School of Hygiene and Tropical Medicine and when Brownlee died in 1927, the Council decided to bring all statistical work under Greenwood's direction. In 1945 Greenwood was succeeded by Austin Bradford Hill and the LSHTM group became the MRC Statistical Research Unit.[36] As we will see, this unit left its mark on many of the MRC's postwar activities, not least through its crucial involvement in the iconic streptomycin trials and work on smoking and health.[37]

Postwar Reorganization

Rockefeller money and MRC initiatives turned the UCH center into a moderate success (researchers there complained about the heavy teaching load), but such activities initially were mainly centered on London, and the status of medical academics remained precarious, in relation to other consultants or compared, for example, to professors in the United States or Germany. From three in 1939, the number of MRC clinical research units rose to eighteen by 1948.[38] However, organized clinical research struggled, as Helen Valier has shown, until the massive influx of funds to British medicine in the years following World War II provided a new basis for its organization.[39] In 1948 the National Health Act came into operation. Centrally funded through general taxation and national insurance contributions, the new National Health Service, encompassing general practice, hospital medicine, and public health, was designed to provide care from cradle to grave and be free at the point of use.[40] This provided the MRC with an opportunity to broaden its remit. Britain's hospitals were now owned by the state. The MRC, since the interwar period the body on which the government drew in most questions of medical research, was the ideal partner for new negotiations over access for researchers. Harold Himsworth, secretary of the Council from 1949, along with other members of the influential "42 Club" of medical academics (many of them with MRC links) had liaised with Ministry of Health officials and Members of Parliament about provisions for teaching and research even before the National Health Act was passed.[41] There was by now also a sufficient supply of trained researchers to staff new positions. The reorganization provided an opportunity to secure their career paths and "export" MRC ethos to provincial hospitals.

One important vehicle through which the Council broadened its control over clinical research was the Clinical Research Board (CRB), set up following the report of a Joint Committee chaired by Sir Henry Cohen, published in 1953 as a government White Paper.[42] The remit of the CRB, whose members were appointed by the MRC after consultation with the Health Departments, was to advise on the placement of new research units and the running and staffing of existing ones, as well as on decentralized research (i.e., research not organized and funded by the MRC), research grants and training awards. MRC spending on investigations directly concerned with patients rose from circa £400,000 in 1951-52, before the Cohen Report to circa £700,000 in 1955-56. [43] Much clinical research in Britain, if not funded by the MRC, responded to MRC advice, was performed by researchers trained in the clinical units, or drew on extensive, formal and informal MRC networks. In the following sections I will look at two complexes of postwar research that exemplified the role that these networks played in disseminating the traditions established in the interwar period, on the etiology and treatment of high blood pressure and on bronchial carcinoma. [44]

Hypertension

Much attention in medical research in the postwar era turned from infectious to non-infectious and chronic conditions such as cancer or cardiovascular disease. British researchers left their marks in both these fields, and MRC networks had a role in this research. In hypertension, two major shifts could be observed, one in the understanding of its etiology and the other therapeutic.[45] First, high blood pressure turned into a disorder where the boundary between normal and pathological was blurred, defined by statistics and notions of risk. Second, while the origins of essential hypertension remained obscure and contested, new therapies, including drugs, became available for the treatment of high blood pressure. The early medicines had quite drastic side effects, and their use was only justifiable for malignant hypertension, cases where the high blood pressure had led to clearly diagnosable and often life threatening pathological changes. These drugs demonstrated that it was possible to use drugs for the management of blood pressure over long periods of time, and new drugs with less drastic side effects made it acceptable to treat ever lower blood pressures.[46] Both in controversies over the etiology of high blood pressure and in the development of new drugs, formal and informal MRC networks played major parts.

At the node of one of these networks was George White Pickering, member of the second generation of full-time professors and director of one of the new clinical units in London, at St. Mary's Hospital Medical School. Pickering was a Cambridge graduate and a Lewis disciple who had joined the UCH department with a Beit fellowship.[47] At UCH he had taken up research on blood pressure. Before World War II, this research was mostly physiological, concerned with mechanisms and particularly with the hormonal regulation of blood pressure.[48] After the war, triggered by a publication by Robert Platt, Manchester's first full-time professor of medicine, Pickering turned to the etiology of high blood pressure and the role of inheritance.[49] With colleagues at St. Mary's he sought to organize an epidemiological study to test Platt's assumption that hypertension was a single-gene trait whose inheritance followed a simple Mendelian pattern. While Platt had studied the relatives of patients treated for high blood pressure in his Manchester clinic, Pickering and his colleagues surveyed the blood pressures of surgical outpatients at the hospital, a sample that they hoped to be representative of the wider British population.[50]

Initially unsure about the best way of dealing with the data, Pickering turned to an expert within the MRC network, the geneticist and statistician John Alexander Fraser Roberts at the London School of Hygiene and Tropical Medicine, who devised a score method that allowed for correction by age and sex.[51] As a consequence of the study, Pickering and his colleagues came to challenge the predominant view of hypertension as a distinct disease entity, contributing to its conceptual transformation into a quantitative rather than a qualitative phenomenon.[52] Guided by Fraser Roberts, Pickering looked to Galton and Pearson, the founding fathers of the biometric tradition for examples, comparing blood pressure to body height. Hypertensive patients, according to Pickering, did not suffer from a specific disorder. Rather, just as for very tall or very short people, the difference was quantitative. The distribution of blood pressure in the population could be described by a normal distribution, and patients with high blood pressure found themselves on one extreme of the bell curve. Blood pressure rose with age and close relatives resembled one another in blood pressure as in other characteristics. According to the MRC Annual Report, these "observations suggested that what is called essential hypertension is not an entity but a convenient label given to those with arterial pressures above a level selected on arbitrary grounds."[53] Pickering disseminated his thinking about high blood pressure as author of some of the most important textbooks on the subject.[54] He continued to collaborate with epidemiologists at the MRC's pneumoconiosis research unit in South Wales.[55] Moving from St. Mary's to Oxford, where he was appointed as Regius Professor of Medicine in 1956, he played an important role in the reorganization of medical research and medical teaching in Britain for years to come.

The transformation of high blood pressure was associated not only with changing views about its etiology but also with new treatment methods, and here, too, MRC networks were important. One of the first drugs for the treatment of hypertension, hexamethonium, was the product of such a network.[56] Pickering's work on the etiology of high blood pressure gained its decisive innovative impetus from contacts between the clinical science and statistical traditions. In the development of hexamethonium, pharmacology in the Dale tradition met clinical science, with the MRC assuming the role of a booster. The node of the network in this case was William Paton, a physiologist and pharmacologist in Henry Dale's former laboratory at the NIMR.[57] Paton stumbled on the methonium drugs while testing a antibiotic compound for a colleague in the institute in 1947. As became clear fairly quickly, the methonium compounds, depending on the length of the carbon chain, had a variety of effects on the autonomic nervous system—a subject of much research in Cambridge physiology. They were characterized as ganglion blockers, a label that had been used by pharmacologists at Harvard to describe the effects of Tetraethylammonium (TEA), a drug with a related structure. [58] While in previous decades such experimental compounds rarely made it into the clinic, this was different for the methonium compounds in the postwar period. Curare and its active principle had long been subjects of research at the NIMR. [59] As Paton and colleagues established in animal tests and heroic self experiments, decamethonium (C10) had clinical potential for use in surgery as a synthetic curare analogue, while pentamethonium and hexamethonium (C5 and C6) promised to be useful in the treatment of high blood pressure and stomach ulcers. [60]

The search for clinical applications was actively promoted by the MRC, and Paton was put in charge of an ad-hoc committee for evaluating the drug in further clinical experiments. [61] Clinicians in a number of centers in the United Kingdom were contacted, and a number of small-scale clinical trials organized whose results were published between 1948 and 1950, when the Council hosted a conference on these clinical tests. [62] The responses for blood pressure treatment were optimistic, but very cautious, due to difficulties with dosage and considerable side effects.

The decisive breakthrough came from Frederick Horace Smirk, a clinician who, supported by a Beit Fellowship, had trained with Elliott at UCH in the 1930s. [63] In 1940 he found himself in the dominions, as the first full-time professor of medicine at the Otago Medical School in Dunedin, New Zealand, where he attempted to construct a center modeled on UCH. In 1949, during a sabbatical spent at the Postgraduate Medical School in Hammersmith on the invitation of John McMichael, another former Beit fellow at UCH, Smirk was introduced to the effects of hexamethonium on blood pressure. He had long been screening compounds for their antihypertensive effects and, on his return to New Zealand, took a supply of hexamethonium, provided by the drug house May and Baker at the initiative of the MRC, with him.

Smirk was a therapeutic enthusiast, believing (like Edward Freis in the United States) that clinicians were justified in treating patients with high blood pressure even without much knowledge about its causes. [64] With his colleagues, Smirk developed a regime that overcame the problems of dosage by administering the drug subcutaneously with a tuberculin syringe and training the patients how to do this themselves (like the way diabetics injected their insulin). They also developed a number of simple fixes for the most common side effects. [65] Partly thanks to Smirk's advocacy–like Pickering he wrote a textbook[66]–it became acceptable to treat hypertensive patients, initially those with malignant hypertension, over long periods of time, with the intention not to cure the disorder but to manage the blood pressure.[67]

Lung Cancer

Hypertension research was one example of the MRC extending its influence by promoting approaches from a combination of traditions established in the interwar period. Clinical cancer research was another case, and in this section I want to look particularly at lung cancer.[68] The MRC had sought to incorporate the prestigious field of cancer research into its activities from early on in its history.[69] The restructuring of the British health system with the introduction of the NHS in 1948 enabled the Council to assume the central role long aspired to by its officers and advocates. However, the territory of cancer research that the Council attempted to colonize in the 1950s and 1960s was contested. Clinicians and scientists interested in cancer research already had the resources of the ICRF, the BECC, and cancer centers such as the Marsden and Christie hospitals to draw on.[70] However, as has been indicated, the MRC already played a central role in the organization of radiotherapy. Below I will take a brief look at two further inroads into cancer research, based on traditions established in the interwar period. The first of these is lung cancer epidemiology, especially the work by Richard Doll and Austin Bradford Hill on the effects of smoking, and the second is the attempt to organize therapeutic trials for cancer on the back of the successful trials of streptomycin in the treatment of tuberculosis.

Lung cancer emerged after World War II as the major cause of cancer deaths and a particular public health problem. A rare disease at the turn of the century, incidence and mortality had been increasing noticeably and exponentially since the 1920s. Initially, it was controversial if this was a real increase or just coincidental as changes in the health system and insurance coverage led to more men dying in hospital and subsequently being autopsied, the only way of conclusively diagnosing the disease. After the war, the increase was generally accepted as real and controversy turned to its causes. Cigarette smoking was one of the chief suspects, along with air pollution, industrial exposure or tarring of the roads.[71] The controversy over "Tobacco Smoking and Cancer of the Lung" was one of the few occasions on which the MRC, in 1957, issued a public statement.[72] The statement drew on the innovative epidemiological work on the subject by Hill and Doll at the Statistical Research Unit at LSHTM.[73]

Doll and Hill first undertook a retrospective investigation, in the course of which they collated interview data relating to nearly 5,000 hospital patients, including circa 1,500 suffering from lung cancer, revealing only one significant difference between patients with and without lung cancer: lung cancer patients were much more likely to be cigarette smokers and to smoke heavily.[74] Still, many in politics and the wider public remained unconvinced, especially as experimental research on the effects of tobacco smoking yielded inconclusive results.[75] In response to such doubts, Doll and Hill devised a prospective study, sending out a questionnaire to all registered members of the medical profession. More than 40,000 doctors replied, were classified according to their smoking habits, and followed up.[76] This study produced results that led to the 1957 MRC Statement and a Report of the Royal College of Physicians in 1962, and to a broad consensus in the United Kingdom that cigarette smoke was the main cause of lung cancer.[77]

Lung cancer was not only a subject of epidemiological research, but also part of the MRC's strategy to develop therapeutic cancer research, and here the statistical tradition was combined with clinical research in a narrower sense. In the early 1950s, before the link with smoking became general consensus, carcinoma of the bronchus was not yet framed as a disease that had to be prevented rather than cured. While the expectations of survival were bleak for lung cancer patients, they were not significantly worse than those for other malignant diseases. In 1957 the MRC held a Conference on the Evaluation of Different Methods of Cancer Therapy. The conference, under the chairmanship of the renowned Professor of Radiotherapy at Middlesex Hospital Medical School, Brian W. Windeyer, recommended that the Council "should consider undertaking an investigation into the treatment of certain tumours which appeared particularly suitable for short-term study."[78] The purpose of the meeting was to prepare a series of therapeutic studies for cancer along the lines of the Council's preferred, biomedical model of controlled intervention. Lung cancer was included in the list of cancers that were thought suitable explicitly because much was known about its etiology and because of its short natural history after diagnosis.[79]

The agenda set by the recommendations of the 1957 conference was heavily geared towards the evaluation of new approaches in radiotherapy. Radiotherapy was the form of therapy from which British cancer specialists most expected innovative impulses. [80] The studies were motivated, as much by the urge to tackle a major public health problem, as by the desire to extend the MRC's remit by applying and combining a set of promising new technologies in which the Council had invested. Besides radiotherapy, there was the randomized controlled trial (RCT), a set of methods that had gained public attention and professional acclaim through use in the evaluation of the effects of streptomycin in the treatment of tuberculosis.[81] The central role assigned to statistics was reflected by the fact that Bradford Hill, credited with some of the more innovative aspects of the RCT approach, was a member of most of the working parties set up for the different cancers. He was joined by radiotherapists and by specialists who traditionally treated the respective organs, in the case of lung cancer, chest physicians and surgeons. The chairman of the lung cancer working party, J. G. Scadding, and its secretary, J. R. Bignall, both based at the Brompton Hospital for Diseases of the Chest in London, were also veterans of the streptomycin trials.

The organization of the lung cancer trials proved difficult, not least, as I have argued elsewhere, because with surgical resection of the affected lung (or parts of it) there was a mature, generally accepted therapy in place.[82] The working party was confronted with long and frustrating debates over the ethics and the feasibility of trials, focusing especially on randomization and the withholding of surgery. Was it acceptable to treat operable patients with radiotherapy? How reliable were the results of experimental radiotherapy if only "surgical rejects" were treated?[83] Trials that were practically feasible and addressed questions of interest could not be justified ethically, and ethically justifiable trials addressed problems that were comparably marginal. Radiotherapists and chest surgeons, when invited for consultations, were distinctly unenthusiastic (in many ways continuing some of the controversies of the interwar period).

The working party finally, in 1961, decided on a trial that compared surgery and radiotherapy for small cell lung cancer, a cell type that metastasized particularly quickly and for which the use of surgery was controversial, and a second trial looking at two different forms of adjuvant chemotherapy. The studies were organized by the MRC Tuberculosis Research Unit under Philip d'Arcy Hart, the unit that had also been in charge of the streptomycin trials. However, while the latter assumed iconic status, the results of the lung cancer trials were disappointing, and along with the problems that had emerged during their preparation left their organizers frustrated.[84] And this had nothing to do with bad organization: a note in the administrative file dealing with the study states: "It seems to me that there is nothing at all controversial about this report, which is a straightforward account of a difficult but well organized clinical trial, the outcome of which has been as depressing as it was predictable."[85] Along with the increasing recognition of the link with smoking, this frustration about the results of therapeutic trials contributed to a shift of focus from therapy to prevention and the prevailing notion that lung cancer was a particularly hopeless cancer.

Conclusion

Lung cancer therapy, in contrast with hypertension research, was a case where the Council's strategy of combining MRC networks, traditions, and methods developed with MRC investment to facilitate the desired extension of the Council's influence and ethos, ultimately to all areas of medical research in Britain, did not work particularly well. Radiotherapists, especially those in well established regional centers like, for example, Manchester's Christie Hospital, had developed their own statistical methods and their interest in an RCT comparing radiotherapy with surgery was limited. They felt, with some justification, that their work was already sufficiently scientific. The surgeons proved difficult to convince, too. And these were not the most conservative of surgeons. Thoracic surgery at the time was an innovative field, and lung resection had only very recently become a routine operation.[86] Such a failure to convince crucial specialists was unfortunate, as the RCT, probably like few other methods, embodied the ethos that the MRC wanted to see applied to clinical research. It represented the successful use in the clinic of experimental methods: a carefully planned investigation and more than just observation, this was what the MRC Annual Reports meant when they called for use of "the scientific method" in clinical research. However, other working parties were more successful, and by the 1970s the MRC organized whole series of randomized controlled trials for different forms of malignant disease, working alongside with the ICRF and the CRC (the successor organization to the BECC).[87] This may have less to do with the MRC's activities, however, and more with contemporary developments in the United States, especially the successes with experimental chemotherapy in the treatment of leukemia and lymphomas, leading to the notion in the 1970s that these diseases were curable.[88] For leukemia and lymphomas, it seems, the trial organizers managed to create and maintain the sense of hope that activists are now keen to bring to lung cancer research.

Notes

Acknowledgment: I am grateful to the Wellcome Trust for funding the research for this essay.

1. Carsten Timmermann, "Lung Cancer, Clinical Trials, and the Medical Research Council in Post-War Britain," *Bulletin of the History of Medicine*, 2007, *81*: 312-34; Carsten Timmermann, "Hexamethonium, Hypertension and Pharmaceutical Innovation: The Transformation of an Experimental Drug in Post-War Britain," in *Devices and Designs: Medical Technologies in Historical Perspective*, ed. Carsten Timmermann and Julie Anderson (Basingstoke: Palgrave Macmillan, 2007), pp.156-74; Carsten Timmermann, "A Matter of Degree: The Normalisation of Hypertension, circa 1940-2000," in *Histories of the Normal and the Abnormal*, ed. Waltraud Ernst (London: Routledge, 2006), pp. 245-61; Carsten Timmermann, "To Treat or Not to Treat: Drug Research and the Changing Nature of Essential Hypertension," in *The Risks of Medical Innovation: Risk Perception and Assessment in Historical Context*, ed. Thomas Schlich and Ulrich Tröhler (London: Routledge, 2006), pp. 133-47.

2. The main works on the history of the MRC are a two-volume history by a senior administrator of the Council, A. Landsborough Thomson, *Half a Century of Medical Research* (London: HMSO, 1973, 1975) and a collection of essays edited by Joan Austoker and Linda Bryder, *Historical Perspectives on the Role of the MRC* (Oxford: Oxford University Press, 1989). Especially relevant for this paper is Christopher C. Booth, "Clinical Research," in Austoker and Bryder, eds., *Historical* Perspectives, pp. 205-41. See also

Christopher C. Booth, "From Art to Science: The Story of Clinical Research," in his *A Physician Reflects: Herman Boerhaave and Other Essays* (London: Wellcome Trust Centre for the History of Medicine at UCL, 2003), pp. 79-101; Christopher C. Booth, "Clinical Research," in *Companion Encyclopedia of the History of Medicine*, ed. William F. Bynum and Roy Porter (London and New York: Routledge, 1993), pp. 205-29. Many of the important figures in the early history of the Council were fellows of the Royal Society, and their biographies have been published in the *Obituary Notices*, later *Biographical Memoirs of Fellows of the Royal Society*. I will cite these where I draw on them.

3. MRC Annual Report 1951-1952, p. 3.
4. Ibid.
5. Ibid., p. 4.
6. Ibid.
7. MRC Annual Report 1955-1956, p. 5. This passage is a quote from the 1953 Cohen Report.
8. MRC Annual Report 1951-1952, p. 4.
9. Ibid.
10. Linda Bryder, "Tuberculosis and the MRC," in Austoker and Bryder, eds., *Historical Perspectives*, pp. 1-21.
11. On the Foster school, see Gerald L. Geison, *Michael Foster and the Cambridge School of Physiology: The Scientific Enterprise in Late Victorian Society* (Princeton, New Jersey: Princeton University Press, 1978). On networks that had their roots in the Cambridge school, see also Abigail O'Sullivan, "Networks of Creativity: A Study on Scientific Achievement in British Physiology, c. 1881-1945" (D.Phil. dissertation: University of Oxford, 2002).
12. Joan Austoker, "Walter Morley Fletcher and the Origins of a Basic Biomedical Research Policy," in Austoker and Bryder, eds., *Historical Perspectives*, pp. 23-33. See also Thomas R. Elliott, "Sir Walter Morley Fletcher," *Obituary Notices of Fellows of the Royal Society*, 1935, *1*: 153-63.
13. Ibid., p. 163.
14. Austoker, "Walter Morley Fletcher," p. 24.
15. On the history of the ICRF, see Joan Austoker, *A History of the Imperial Cancer Research Fund, 1902-1986* (Oxford: Oxford University Press, 1988).
16. Donald Fisher, "The Rockefeller Foundation and the Development of Scientific Medicine in Great Britain," *Minerva*, 1978, *16*: 20-41, p. 23.
17. Ibid., p. 25.
18. Christopher Lawrence, "Still Incommunicable: Clinical Holists and Medical Knowledge in Interwar Britain," in *Greater than the Parts: Holism in Biomedicine, 1920-1950*, ed. Christopher Lawrence and George Weisz (New York and Oxford: Oxford University Press, 1998), pp. 94-111.
19. David Cantor, "The MRC's Support for Experimental Radiology During the Inter-War Years," in Austoker and Bryder, eds., *Historical Perspectives*, pp.181-204.

20. See Christopher C. Booth, "Smoking and the Gold-Headed Cane: The Royal College of Physicians Enters the Modern World," in Booth, *A Physician Reflects*, pp. 155-60.
21. Henry H. Dale, "Thomas Renton Elliott," *Biographical Memoirs of Fellows of the Royal Society*, 1961, *7*: 53-74; A. N. Drury, R. T. Grant, "Thomas Lewis," *Obituary Notices of Fellows of the Royal Society*, 1945, *5*: 179-202.
22. Fisher, "Rockefeller Foundation."
23. Ibid. See also Helen K. Valier, "The Politics of Scientific Medicine in Manchester" (Ph.D. dissertation: University of Manchester, 2002).
24. On Dale, see W. S. Feldberg, "Henry Hallet Dale," *Biographical Memoirs of Fellows of the Royal Society*, 1970, *16*: 77-174; E. M. Tansey, "What's in a Name? Henry Dale and Adrenaline, 1906," *Medical History*, 1995, *39*: 459-76; E. M. Tansey, "Sir Henry Dale and Autopharmacology: The Role of Acetylcholine in Neurotransmission," *Clio Medica*, 1995, *33*: 179-93.
25. The Beit Memorial Trust was founded in 1909. Both Lewis and Elliott received Beit Memorial Fellowships. Lewis was the first Beit Fellow in 1909. See Dale, "Thomas Renton Elliott," p. 68.
26. See Booth, "Clinical Research." See also Booth, *A Physician Reflects*; Douglas Black and John Gray, "Sir Harold Percival Himsworth, K.C.B.," *Biographical Memoirs of Fellows of the Royal Society*, 1995, *41*: 200-18; Colin Dollery, "Sir John McMichael," *Biographical Memoirs of Fellows of the Royal Society*, 1995, *41*: 282-96.
27. Joan Austoker and Linda Bryder, "The National Institute for Medical Research and Related Activities of the MRC," in Austoker and Bryder, eds., *Historical Perspectives*, pp. 35-57.
28. Joel D. Howell, "'Soldier's Heart': The Redefinition of Heart Disease and Speciality Formation in Early Twentieth-Century Great Britain," *Medical History*, 1985, *Supplement No 5*: 34-52.
29. Austoker and Bryder, "National Institute for Medical Research."
30. See references in note 24.
31. Tansey, "What's in a Name?"
32. See Jonathan Liebenau, "The MRC and the Pharmaceutical Industry: The Model Insulin," in Austoker and Bryder, eds., *Historical Perspectives*, pp.163-180; Jonathan Liebenau, "The British Success with Penicillin," *Social Studies of Science*, 1987, *17*: 69-86.
33. Edward Higgs, "Medical Statistics, Patronage and the State: The Development of the MRC Statistical Unit, 1911-1948," *Medical History*, 2000, *44*: 323-40.
34. Lancelot Hogben, "Major Greenwood," *Obituary Notices of Fellows of the Royal Society*, 1950, *19*: 139-54.
35. Eileen Magnello, "The Introduction of Mathematical Statistics into Medical Research: The Roles of Karl Pearson, Major Greenwood and Austin Bradford Hill," *Clio Medica*, 2002, *67*: 95-123.
36. Richard Doll, "Austin Bradford Hill," *Biographical Memoirs of Fellows of the Royal Society*, 1994, *40*: 128-40.

37. J. Rosser Matthews, *Quantification and the Quest for Medical Certainty* (Princeton, New Jersey: Princeton University Press, 1995). On streptomycin, see Alan Yoshioka, "Streptomycin in Postwar Britain: A Cultural History of a Miracle Drug," *Clio Medica*, 2002, *66*: 203-27; Alan Yoshioka, "Use of Randomisation in the Medical Research Council's Clinical Trial of Streptomycin in Pulmonary Tuberculosis in the 1940s," *British Medical Journal*, 1998, *317*: 1220-3. On smoking, see S. A. Lock, L. A. Reynolds, and E. M. Tansey, eds., *Ashes to Ashes: The History of Smoking and Health* (Amsterdam & Atlanta: Rodopi, 1998).
38. MRC Annual Report 1951-1952, p. 5.
39. Valier, "Politics of Scientific Medicine."
40. For an overview of the origins and development of the NHS, see Charles Webster, *The National Health Service: A Political History* (Oxford: Oxford University Press, 1998); Rudolf Klein, *The New Politics of the NHS*, 3rd ed. (London: Longman, 1995); Geoffrey Rivett, *From Cradle to Grave: Fifty Years of the NHS* (London: The King's Fund, 1998).
41. See L. A. Reynolds and E. M. Tansey, eds., *Clinical Research in Britain, 1950-1980: A Witness Seminar held at the Wellcome Institute for the History of Medicine, London, on 9 June 1998* (London: Wellcome Centre, 2000), pp. 12, 16; Christopher C. Booth, "Pioneers in the World of Academe: History of the '42 Club,'" in Booth, *A Physician Reflects*, pp. 103-15.
42. Medical Research Council, Ministry of Health, Department of Health for Scotland, Central Health Services Council, Advisory Committee on Medical Research in Scotland, *Clinical Research in Relation to the National Health Service* (London: HSMO, 1953).
43. MRC Annual Report 1951-1952; MRC Annual Report 1955-1956.
44. For the official MRC take on these episodes, see MRC Annual Reports 1948-1950, pp. 20-21; 1952-1953, pp. 30-33; 1953-1954, pp. 4-8; 1955-1956, pp. 10-14.
45. For reflections on these changes, see Colin T. Dollery, "A Clinician Looks at the Future," *British Journal of Clinical Pharmacology*, 1982, *13*: 127-32.
46. See Timmermann references in note 1; Jeremy Greene, "Releasing the Flood Waters: Diuril and the Reshaping of Hypertension," *Bulletin of the History of Medicine*, 2005, *79*: 749-94.
47. On Pickering, see John McMichael and W. S. Peart, "George White Pickering," *Biographical Memoirs of Fellows of the Royal Society*, 1982, *28*: 431-49.
48. MRC Annual Report 1952-1953, pp. 30-33.
49. Robert Platt, "Heredity in Hypertension," *Quarterly Journal of Medicine*, 1947, *16*: 111-33. The debate is documented in J. D. Swales, *Platt Versus Pickering: An Episode in Recent Medical History* (London: Keynes Press, 1985).
50. M. Hamilton, G. W. Pickering, J. A. Fraser Roberts, G. S. C. Sowry, "The Aetiology of Essential Hypertension. 1. The Arterial Pressure in the General Population," *Clinical Science*, 1954, *13*: 11-35.

51. On Fraser Roberts, see P. E. Polani, "John Alexander Fraser Roberts," *Biographical Memoirs of Fellows of the Royal Society*, 1992, *38*: 306-22.

52. I have discussed this study in greater detail elsewhere. See Timmermann, "A Matter of Degree."

53. MRC Annual Report 1952-1953, p. 32.

54. For example, George W. Pickering, *High Blood Pressure* (London: Churchill, 1955); George W. Pickering, *The Nature of Essential Hypertension* (London: Churchill, 1961); George W. Pickering, I. W. Cranston, and M. A. Pears, *The Treatment of Hypertension* (Springfield, Illinois: Charles C. Thomas, 1961).

55. Pickering Papers, PP/GWP/C.6/51, Wellcome Library, London.

56. I have analyzed the development of this drug in detail in Timmermann, "Hexamethonium."

57. For Paton's account of the story, see William D. M. Paton, "Hexamethonium," *British Journal of Clinical Pharmacology*, 1982, *13*: 7-14. See also H. P. Rang and P. Walton, "Sir William Drummond MacDonald Paton, CBE," *Biographical Memoirs of Fellows of the Royal Society*, 1996, *42*: 290-314.

58. George H. Acheson, "Tetraethylammonium, Ganglionic Blocking Agents, and the Development of Antihypertensive Therapy," *Perspectives in Biology and Medicine*, 1975, *19*: 136-48; Gordon K. Moe, Walter A. Freyburger, "Ganglionic Blocking Agents," *Pharmacological Reviews*, 1950, *2*: 61-95.

59. MRC Annual Report 1948-1950, pp. 20-21.

60. Ibid. See also "The Methonium Compounds" [editorial], *British Medical Journal*, 1950, *i*: 474-5.

61. Green to William Paton, 18 July 1950, FD1/1172, U.K. National Archives, London.

62. Conference on Clinical Tests of Methonium Drugs, 22 June 1950, Minutes of the Meeting, UK National Archives, FD1/1172.

63. Austin E. Doyle, "Sir Horace Smirk: Pioneer in Drug Treatment of Hypertension," *Hypertension*, 1991, *17*: 247-50.

64. For Freis's views, see Edward D. Freis, "Recent Developments in the Treatment of Hypertension," *Medical Clinics of North America*, 1954, *38*: 363-74.

65. F. Horace Smirk, *Instructions for Patients on C6 Injections*, and *Organisation of a Hypertensive Clinic, more particularly for patients on methonium treatment*, typescripts, October 1951, FD1/1172, U.K. National Archives.

66. F. Horace Smirk, *High Arterial Pressure* (Oxford: Blackwell, 1957); F. N. Fastier, "Biography: Sir Horace Smirk: Professor Emeritus," *New Zealand Medical Journal*, 1968, *67*: 258-65.

67. "Methonium and Hypertension" [editorial], *Lancet*, 1951, *257*: 395-96. See also MRC Annual Report 1952-1953, p. 33.

68. For a more detailed analysis, see Timmermann, "Lung Cancer."

69. An early, successful chapter in the history of the Council was, for example, its role in the distribution of radium in the interwar period. See Cantor, " The MRC's Support for Experimental Radiology."

70. On the ICRF, see Austoker, *A History of the Imperial Cancer Research Fund*.

71. On the debates over smoking and health, see Lock, Reynolds, and Tansey, eds. *Ashes to Ashes*. For the United States, see also Allan M. Brandt, *The Cigarette Century: The Rise, Fall, and Deadly Persistence of the Product That Defined America* (New York: Basic Books, 2007).

72. Medical Research Council, "Medical Research Council's Statement on Tobacco Smoking and Cancer of the Lung," *Lancet*, 1957, *272*: 1345-7. See Thomson, *Half a Century*, vol. 1, p. 185.

73. On smoking and epidemiological innovation, see Luc Berlivet, "'Association or Causation?' The Debate on the Scientific Status of Risk Factor Epidemiology, 1947-c.1965," *Clio Medica*, 2005, *75*: 39-74.; Colin Talley, Howard I. Kushner, and Claire Sterk, "Lung Cancer, Chronic Disease Epidemiology, and Medicine, 1948-1964," *Journal of the History of Medicine and Allied Sciences*, 2004, *59*: 329-74; Gerry Hill, Wayne Millar, and James Connelly, "'The Great Debate': Smoking, Lung Cancer, and Cancer Epidemiology," *Canadian Bulletin of Medical History*, 2003, *20*: 367-86.

74. Richard Doll and Austin Bradford Hill, "A Study of the Aetiology of Carcinoma of the Lung," *British Medical Journal*, 1952, *ii*: 1271-86.

75. See Virginia Berridge, "Science and Policy: The Case of Postwar British Smoking Policy," *Clio Medica*, 1998, *46*: 143-62.

76. Richard Doll and Austin Bradford Hill, "Lung Cancer and Other Causes of Death in Relation to Smoking: A Second Report on the Mortality of British Doctors," *British Medical Journal*, 1956, *ii*: 1071-81.

77. Royal College of Physicians, *Smoking and Health: A Report of the Royal College of Physicians on Smoking in Relation to Cancer of the Lung and Other Diseases* (London: Pitman Medical Publishing, 1962). See also Booth, "Smoking and the Gold-headed Cane."

78. Evaluation of Different Methods of Cancer Therapy, Recommendations of the Council's Steering Committee, NA, FD7/327.

79. Ibid.; Working Party for the Evaluation of Different Methods of Therapy in Carcinoma of the Bronchus, Minutes of the meeting held on 24 June 1958, FD7/327, U.K. National Archives.

80. On radiotherapy, see Caroline C. S. Murphy, "A History of Radiotherapy to 1950: Cancer and Radiotherapy in Britain, 1850-1950" (Ph.D. dissertation: University of Manchester, 1986), and Cantor, "The MRC's Support for Experimental Radiology."

81. See Yoshioka references in note 37.

82. Timmermann, "Lung Cancer."

83. Minutes of a Special Meeting with Consultant Surgeons and Radiotherapists, 25 July 1961, FD 7/327, U.K. National Archives.

84. J. G. Scadding, et al., "Comparative Trial of Surgery and Radiotherapy for the Primary Treatment of Small-Celled or Oat-Celled Carcinoma of the Bronchus: First Report to the Medical Research Council by the Working-Party on the Evaluation of Different Methods of Therapy in Carcinoma of the Bronchus," *Lancet* 1966, *288*: 979-86; J. G. Scadding, "Treatment of

Bronchial Carcinoma" [letter], *Lancet*, 1967, *289*: 157; Medical Research Council Working Party, "Study of Cytotoxic Chemotherapy as an Adjuvant to Surgery in Carcinoma of the Bronchus," *British Medical Journal*, 1971, *ii*: 421-8.

85. Note by J. R. H. [Herrald?], 22 August 1966, FD 7/1151 U.K. National Archives.

86. See Roger Abbey Smith, "Development of Lung Surgery in the United Kingdom," *Thorax*, 1982, *37*: 161-68.

87. See Helen C. Tate, Janet B. Rawlinson, and Laurence S. Freedman, "Randomised Comparative Studies in the Treatment of Cancer in the United Kingdom: Room for Improvement?" *Lancet*, 1979, *314*: 623-25.

88. See Gretchen M. Krueger, "'A Cure is Near': Children, Families, and Cancer in America, 1945-1980" (Ph.D. dissertation: Yale University, 2003).

Towards a History of "The Vaccine Innovation System," 1950-2000

Stuart Blume

Introduction

The most familiar histories of vaccines and vaccination are variants on a narrative of progress. Written by practitioners in the field, scattered through the professional literature, they recount the contributions that vaccination has made to reductions in mortality and morbidity from one infectious disease after another: polio, diphtheria, measles, and whooping cough among others. The eradication of smallpox is, rightly, hailed as one of the greatest of vaccination's successes. Senior vaccine scientists are frequently inclined to remind us of the remarkable advances in vaccine science and technology that have made all this possible. To be sure, progress has not always been at the same pace. In the early 1960s an optimistic view of the future seemed particularly appropriate. Control of viral diseases seemed within reach, despite continuing and heated debate concerning the relative merits of live and killed virus vaccines. Jonas Salk's inactivated (killed) polio vaccine and then Albert Sabin's rival live vaccine had, together, vastly reduced the ravages of this terrible disease. Jonas Salk, in particular, had achieved world renown. Soon afterwards, successes in developing vaccines against other diseases of childhood, less feared than polio but in much of the world still killers, followed. Measles was the first, with a vaccine introduced in the United States in 1963. In the 1950s only two vaccines had been given to all children in the United States: against smallpox, and a compound DTP (diphtheria, tetanus and pertussis) vaccine. By the late 1980s, smallpox vaccination was no longer needed, and children were given four vaccines by the time they entered school: DTP, oral polio, MMR (measles, mumps, and rubella) and Hib (*Haemophilus influenzae type b*). By 2005, American children received nine vaccines, offering protection against twelve diseases.[1]

Past successes and recent discoveries seem to imply that we can continue to look forward with optimism. Such extrapolations are common. For example, in his foreword to a 1996 government report, the British Chief Medical Officer of Health, Sir Kenneth Calman, uses characteristic language:

> Two hundred years after Jenner's first observations, we are seeing a new era beginning for vaccines. With the application of genetic manipulation techniques, better understanding of processes of infection and immunity, and a widespread recognition that investment in disease prevention is one of the best uses of resources, we can expect ever more vaccines, and ever more diseases eradicated.[2]

The history that I want to try to sketch out in this paper is a less familiar and a less comforting one. It will not be an account of progress in vaccine technology, or of the scientific breakthroughs on which progress has been built. Rather, my focus will be on the institutional changes, and the changes in rhetoric, associated with successes and failures in developing and producing vaccines. An apology is required at the very start, for what I will have to say is more an agenda for future research than an account of what we know. Most of the work still has to be done, and for two reasons. One has to do with the power of the familiar narrative of progress: a narrative that speaks to the professional and institutional interests that helped shape it, and that at the same time provides reassurance in a world beset by risks and by doubts. It is difficult to escape its influence. The second reason has to do with the kind of scholarly enterprise entailed. Writing the history of the institutions involved in developing and supplying the tools of public health, and their interrelations, is a much more formidable task than writing a history that takes a vaccine or group of vaccines as its focus.

The history of what I am calling the "vaccine innovation system" must draw its materials from around the globe, for some of the institutions that comprise it are located far from the scientific metropolis. We know a little of how they came to be there: of the important roles played by colonial relations, by the Rockefeller Foundation[3] and by the Institut Pasteur[4] a century ago. We know much less of what happened thereafter, or of their evolution–let alone interrelations–in an era marked by decolonization, the Cold War, and free trade ideologies. Underlying what I shall have to say, therefore, is not so much a set of convictions regarding the (unquestionable) benefits of vaccines and vaccination, as it is a set of questions regarding the changing roles of states, supranational organizations, and private corporations in this vaccine innovation system. I hope that in this paper I can at least hint at the fruitfulness and the significance of this alternative agenda for future historical research.

The Social Organization of Vaccine Innovation

The middle decades of the twentieth century were a turbulent time in the vaccines field. At the end of World War II, interest on the part of the pharmaceutical industry, that in the 1930s had been substantial, had now turned elsewhere. This was partly a consequence of the emergence of new and powerful, and potentially profitable, antibiotics. For example, a pneumonia vaccine developed in the 1940s was virtually ignored because treatment with the new penicillin and sulfonamide drugs was much the more attractive option. The pharmaceutical industry was expanding the scope of its research and production into several therapeutic areas, all of which appeared more profitable than vaccines. Elsewhere, however, research was going on that was to change matters dramatically. Notably, at Harvard University, John Enders, Thomas Weller, and Frederick Robbins were developing new and far safer methods of culturing live viruses: work for which they were later to receive a Nobel Prize.[5] This work was to lead to the development of a range of new viral vaccines (attenuated polio vaccine, measles, rubella, mumps...), but, most important for the argument here, the prospects of breakthroughs in this area catalyzed new attention for vaccine development.

The career of Maurice R. Hilleman, possibly the twentieth century's most renowned and successful developer of new vaccines, shows the changes taking place in the vaccine world.[6] Having completed graduate work at the University of Chicago, he joined the virus laboratories of E. R. Squibb and Sons of New Jersey in 1944. There he worked on development of a vaccine against Japanese encephalitis B, needed by troops fighting in the Pacific. In 1948 he left Squibb to join the Walter Reed Army Institute of Research, where he worked principally on influenza: the "drift and shift" in antigens, and how a future flu pandemic could be averted. In 1957, by which time the implications of the Harvard research were clear, Vannevar Bush, then chairman of the newly merged Merck, Sharp & Dohme, decided that the company needed a new push in the virus field. Hilleman was recruited to establish and run a virus vaccine research initiative that would encompass basic research, development, and (through a collaboration with the University of Pennsylvania School of Medicine) clinical research. Hilleman was provided with ample support, and launched a major and ambitious program of work directed at the major diseases of childhood, starting with measles.[7]

There was little or no patent protection for vaccines in those days, and knowledge of vaccine production techniques was either exchanged or leaked out as discoveries were disclosed to government regulatory bodies. However, lack of patent protection—which was to continue as the norm in the vaccines field until the 1980s—was not a barrier. Spurred by the new scientific possibilities, and by the more active role being taken by the federal government in promoting the use of selected vaccines (starting with Salk's polio vaccine), by the late 1950s the number of manufacturers licensed to produce vaccines in the United States was growing. Industrial commitment, however, was to remain uncertain and unreliable.

By the 1970s, the vaccine market was once more losing its appeal for pharmaceutical companies: a situation to which the swine flu fiasco of 1976 certainly contributed.[8] And now, in the United States in particular, this was becoming a matter of political concern. Like the majority of Western industrialized countries, the United States was wholly dependent on private pharmaceutical companies for its supplies of vaccines. In the United States it was noted that from the mid-1960s to the end of the 1970s (a twelve-year period) the number of licensed vaccine manufacturers had dropped from thirty-seven to eighteen, whilst the number of licensed vaccine products was also falling.[9]

The Office of Technology Assessment (OTA) of the United States Congress, investigating the matter, felt that "The apparently diminishing commitment–and possibly capacity–of the American pharmaceutical industry to research, develop, and produce vaccines…may be reaching levels of real concern."[10] As far as nineteen vaccines, including the polio vaccine, were concerned, the United States was dependent on only a single American pharmaceutical company. What if that producer decided to exit the vaccine field? There were precedents enough. For example, in the mid-1970s, Eli Lilly was working on an experimental pneumococcal vaccine with support from the National Institutes of Health (NIH). Then the company decided to terminate almost all its vaccine research and development (R&D) and production activities. Company executives told the OTA that this reflected the costs and difficulties of developing vaccines, market considerations, and carrying out the testing of each batch of vaccine as required by federal regulations.[11] Vaccines were more difficult to develop, test, and license than pharmaceutical products. They were also less profitable, and there were much greater risks of liability actions and huge damages if anything went wrong. After all, vaccines were typically administered to millions of healthy children.

Influential vaccine spokesmen, including D. A. Henderson, who had spearheaded the World Health Organization's smallpox eradication program, were now arguing for a more active federal government role in stimulating and coordinating vaccine R&D. In the United States, these concerns, and the desirability of government policies aimed at facilitating vaccine development and stimulating industrial commitment, remained an issue.[12] William Jordan, director of the Microbiology and Infectious Diseases Division of the National Institute of Allergy and Infectious Diseases (NIAID), estimated that all federal agencies (NIH, Center for Disease Control, Food and Drug Administration, Army, Navy, and USAID) had together spent only $23 million on vaccines R&D addressing eleven domestic and seven tropical diseases in 1978. "Clearly the vaccine effort needed to be expanded."[13] In 1986 the U.S. Congress established a National Vaccine Program (NVP), with the task of coordinating the vaccine-related activities of federal agencies and private industry, and of determining what vaccines are needed. But the NVP led an uncertain existence, with "little money and less clout" as a *Science* reporter put it in 1994.[14] By that time leading vaccine scientists were arguing for the creation of a more powerful National Vaccine Authority.[15] The proper role of the federal government continued to be a matter of political debate. Some argued, for example, that the 1993 Vaccines for Children Act, providing an entitlement to free vaccines for uninsured and certain other groups of children, acted as a serious disincentive to vaccine manufacturers[16]

Whilst political discussion continued, in the 1980s more American pharmaceutical companies left the vaccine business. By the mid-1990s, only four private wholly owned United States firms were active, of which only two (Lederle-Praxis Biologicals and Merck) were active developers of new pediatric vaccines. However, the picture is more complex than this suggests, and other elements have to be added. One is the influx of small biotechnology companies into the field, the result of the emergence of new biotechnology-based ways of making vaccines. A second is 1986 legislation that provided important encouragement to vaccine manufacturers. In that year, driven largely by widespread popular concern at side effects of the pertussis vaccine, and the concomitant surge in damage actions against manufacturers, the U.S. Congress passed legislation establishing the National Childhood Vaccine Injury Compensation Program. This limited the liability of manufacturers and established a public fund from which possible compensation claims could be paid. Reassured by the protection this act afforded, pharmaceutical firms began to reconsider their commitment to vaccines.

Changes in the vaccine field in the 1980s and 1990s did not affect the United States alone. Far from it. In 1998 Seung-il Shin, of the International Vaccine Institute (IVI), then recently established in Korea, characterized these changes as follows:

> The most important thing driving the transformation of the vaccine enterprise (which encompasses the development, clinical testing, production, licensure and distribution of vaccine) is the increasingly complex scientific and technological base that is required....

The second factor…is the changing nature of technology ownership…vaccine development has become primarily the purview of large industrial laboratories…. In Pasteur's day, and even as recently as forty years ago when the polio vaccines were first developed, most of the new technologies needed to manufacture vaccines were owned by the public. The scientists and organizations that developed them often assisted and funded the technology transfer to institutions in developing countries….

The third factor is the globalization of international commerce…. The global vaccine industry in 1998 is thus dominated by a small number of large multinational companies, instead of the smaller, publicly owned and public-spirited national vaccine production centers that were until recently the norm. Consequently, some of the key decisions regarding which vaccines to develop and how to distribute (market) them are no longer made by scientists and public health officials but by business executives….

Finally, the increasingly stringent international product safety standards required of vaccines.[17]

What consequences have these changes, and in particular the growing role of business executives, had for institutions involved in developing and producing vaccines? A comprehensive answer to this question must await a good deal of further research, for consequences certainly differed from country to country, and between the public and private sectors. One of the few detailed studies we have is Louis Galambos's comprehensive history of vaccine development at Merck: one company that has maintained its commitment throughout.[18] This is a success story, attesting to the crucial role that the company has played in vaccine development and production. The study shows how Merck was able successfully to adapt to new scientific opportunity. As the focus in vaccine development shifted from bacteriology to virology (starting in the 1940s and lasting through the 1980s), and then to recombinant DNA technology, so Merck (and the companies it absorbed) modified their organizational structures and–crucially–their scientific capabilities and networks.

To be successful, however, Merck had to respond not only to changes in vaccine science, but changes in the vaccine market also. This is a market that is particularly sensitive to changing government policies. From a business point of view government policies, in the United States, had two sorts of effect: one negative and one positive. On the negative side, Galambos refers to the growth of the public sector market, both nationally and internationally. The Vaccines for Children Program had been just one in a series of measures through which public sector agencies negotiated rock-bottom prices for their bulk vaccine purchases, and so drove down the profits available for investment in R&D. The share of this public market was growing, to the extent that, according to Galambos, economic motives for remaining in the vaccine business were continuously eroding. On the positive side, Galambos refers to relaxation in antitrust laws in the 1980s and 1990s. These changes had made it possible for large companies like Merck to establish strategic alliances "that broadened the front across which it innovates and enabled it to strengthen its position in global markets."[19] And this is what it did.

As David Mowery and Violaine Mitchell wrote in 1995, "the extent of acquisitions and alliance formations among vaccine manufacturers during the past decade, especially from 1990 to 1993, is staggering."[20] The diagram that they provide to illustrate their argument links Merck with a number of other major manufacturers (notably Pasteur-Mérieux in France), with a number of smaller biotech companies (including Biogen and MedImmune), and with a few public sector institutes, RIVM [National Institute for Public Health and the Environment] in the Netherlands and the Commonwealth Serum Laboratory in Australia).

Reflecting the developments listed by Shin, the vaccine system was changing in shape and size. But the implications of these changes varied greatly from country to country. Consider, for example, the implications for what Shin refers to as the "publicly owned and public-spirited national vaccine production centers," that had previously been the mainstay of vaccine production. In both China and India private vaccine manufacturers emerged and flourished alongside the older public sector ones. In some countries, including Sweden and Australia, the public sector institutes (the Swedish State Bacteriological Laboratories and the Australian Commonwealth Serum Laboratory), were privatized (in

1993 and 1994, respectively). There were other countries, including Colombia, where public sector production was gradually phased out.[21] In the Netherlands, by contrast, private sector attempts at acquiring the public sector vaccine facility (then part of the Dutch Institute of Public Health, RIV, later renamed RIVM) continued to be resisted. Though vaccine production remained in the public sector, the institute was not immune to developments taking place in the vaccine field at large. In order to understand how it was affected, however, we have to focus down to consider the vaccine development work being conducted there.

With responsibilities for vaccine supply (including development, manufacture and/or purchase) of vaccines located in a single public sector institution, the Netherlands[22] was not faced with the concerns regarding security of supply that were arising in the United States in the late 1970s. But the point to be made here concerns not security of supply but incentives to innovate. Since their foundation early in the twentieth century, state vaccine institutes like the Dutch Institute of Public Health were concerned with meeting the vaccine requirements of national public health systems. The incentives to innovate were not principally commercial but could be public health needs. Innovation could indeed fly in the face of commercial reasoning. This is shown clearly by RIV's collaboration with Jonas Salk in developing an improved inactivated polio vaccine (IPV).[23]

Disputes regarding the relative merits of live and killed vaccines, compounded by personal animosity between the principal investigators, had marked the search for a polio vaccine since the early 1950s. Though Salk's killed (IPV) vaccine was first to be licensed, in the course of the 1960s most major manufacturers abandoned it and switched to production of the rival Sabin oral polio vaccine (OPV). In doing this they responded to majority scientific and medical opinion. There seemed reason to believe that the OPV would be quicker acting and would control the disease more effectively. Thus, whilst in the mid 1960s, some 4 to 5 million doses of IPV were being distributed annually in the United States, by 1967 this had fallen to 2.7 million and a year later to zero. By contrast, distribution of OPV had reached some 25 million doses annually. With the exception of a few small West European countries with very high rates of vaccination coverage, the whole world switched to OPV.

By the 1970s, as evidence that, in a small number of cases, the weak-ened virus used in the OPV reverted to virulence and led to vaccine-induced disease, matters became more complex. By then, choice for one vaccine or the other should have entailed weighing the presumed benefits of OPV (greater acceptability, community protection and so on) against what were now known to be small, but definite risks associated with its use. The evidence was ambiguous and could be read as showing the superiority of the OPV, or of the IPV, or as suggesting the need for some intermediate strategy using both vaccines. In the event, the virtually complete consensus around the OPV was not threatened. Few experts were willing to take the risk of recommending a switch back to the Salk vaccine.

Tracing the process by which the IPV was reconstituted as a credible option leads us to an innovation process driven, in its beginnings at least, by a logic that did not derive from economic incentives. In the Netherlands, children were (and still are) vaccinated using a combina-tion diphtheria tetanus pertussis polio (DTPP) vaccine, of which the inactivated polio vaccine was one component. The Sabin vaccine, which is taken orally, could not replace IPV in the Dutch cocktail. Introducing it would necessitate major changes in immunization practice, and given the success of the existing program there was no reason to make these changes. But there were problems with the IPV being produced by the institute. One was the enormous supply of monkeys needed for cultur-ing the polio virus and in testing the vaccine. Ways were thus found of using cultured kidney cells for growing the virus, in place of tissue taken directly from live monkeys. In this way the need for live monkeys was reduced from 5000 per annum in 1970 to just 50 by 1975. In other ways, too, the production process was improved and the strength of the vaccine enhanced. Crucial here is that these developments were motivated in part by perceived inadequacies in the production process, and in part by the attempt to provide the Netherlands with a more powerful weapon in the fight against infectious disease, given existing vaccination practices.

In the 1970s, the RIV succeeded in developing a technology for effi-ciently producing a high potency, standardized IPV, on a scale sufficient for domestic needs. There was little interest in exploring the possibilities of (re)developing an international market for IPV. Both Jonas Salk and the (French) Institut Mérieux, with which they were also collaborating, *were* interested in demonstrating that the enhanced IPV was as effective in tropical countries as the OPV that was by now in virtually universal use. Field trials were organized in Africa, though not without difficulty and even opposition. According to Philippe Stœckel, (then with the Institut Mérieux, now of the Fondation Mérieux) the improved IPV threatened political and economic interests: "we were bothering the WHO. We were an alternative, we were another solution. We were, they said, distracting people. With one goal, the use of OPV. We were sort of challenging them and they didn't like that." [24] As Stœckel sees it, it was protection of their home market by pharmaceutical companies with no IPV production facilities that was principally at stake here.

In his review of "the ten most important discoveries in vaccinology during the last two decades"[25] Stanley Plotkin places the acellular pertussis vaccine first on his list. Although it had been widely used for decades, the older "whole cell" pertussis (or whooping cough) vaccine was long acknowledged to have nasty side effects: mostly not serious but worrying to parents. Far more worrying were reports in the 1970s linking the vaccine with possibly permanent brain damage in a small number of cases. In the light of these suggestions, and of the declining incidence of the disease in the industrialized world, widespread resistance to pertussis vaccination emerged in a number of countries. Japan and Sweden stopped vaccinating children against pertussis in the late 1970s, whilst in some other countries vaccination levels fell precipitously (e.g., in the United Kingdom from 70/80 percent to 40 percent).[26] In the United States a spate of law suits against vaccine manufacturers, demanding compensation for damage, led all but two manufacturers to abandon production of pertussis vaccine. This was a major stimulus to introduction of the National Childhood Vaccine Injury Compensation Program, designed to protect manufacturers against crippling claims, in 1986.

By the mid-1980s several research groups were working on the development of alternative "acellular" pertussis vaccines from which reactogenic and non-protective components had been removed.[27] By the early 1990s the global pharmaceutical industry had made a clear commitment to the new acellular pertussis vaccine. Indeed, it has been suggested that the market prospects of acellular pertussis vaccine (costing approximately three times as much as the older vaccine) were an important factor in the expansion of the global vaccine market since 1992.[28] Clinical trials were initiated in a number of countries, with the NIAID playing a major role.

The results of the trials were complex. Just as in the case of the polio vaccines earlier, data did not lend themselves to unambiguous interpretation. Some of the older whole cell vaccines were clearly very good (for example, those used in Britain and France), whilst others (including that used in Canada) seemed to be poor. Some acellular vaccines seemed to be as effective as good whole cell vaccines, others less so. Side effects, however, were generally less with the new vaccines. "Health authorities are thus faced with a difficult choice. Should the better efficacy of certain whole cell vaccines be traded for the better tolerance of acellular vaccines?"[29] Recognizing that this trade-off is not only political but also depends upon the particular whole cell vaccine in use, there is no simple and unambiguous answer. "The answer may vary in different parts of the world. In the U.S. the greater safety afforded by acellular vaccines, as well as the recent demonstration of the lower efficacy of one of the whole cell vaccines used in a three-dose regimen, will elicit recommendations to favor acellular over whole cell vaccines. The same will be true of those countries of Europe where pertussis vaccine has not been accepted for fear of reactions."[30]

Today the majority of industrialized countries, including the United States, Canada, and most West European countries, have switched to one or other commercially available acellular vaccine. In the Netherlands, the Health Council has repeatedly advised that the country should switch to acellular vaccine. Disease incidence suggests that the whole cell vaccine being used, and produced by the Dutch institute, is not effective enough (or, not as effective as it used to be). However, Dutch scientists were not convinced that, in the long term, the acellular vaccine would prove the optimal solution for the Netherlands.

The answer to the pertussis problem in the Netherlands, these scientists agree, is a whole cell vaccine–but a better one than the one they had been producing. Though instructed by the Dutch Minister of Health to develop a combination vaccine incorporating a (commercial) acelullar component, the Dutch vaccine institute (by now called NVI)[31] was also trying to produce a combination vaccine incorporating a good whole cell pertussis component. Though they had failed to produce the vaccine they wanted themselves within the time they had, good whole cell vaccines do still exist. They are used, officially, in both France and the United Kingdom. The next best thing would be to import one of these. However, it appeared that import of the British or the French vaccines was not possible, since their manufacturers appeared unwilling to expand production: perhaps a consequence of the fact that they were also producing the new (and more profitable) acellular alternative. In the meantime, the Minister of Health, responding to yet a further recommendation of the Health Council, and a growing public furore over side effects, decided that the country would switch to the acellular vaccine. This it recently did.

This example shows two views of the relative merits of the distinct kinds of vaccine locked in uneasy equilibrium. Grounded in epidemiology and appeal to the (positive) experience of other countries, the view of the Health Council reflects what has become the orthodoxy in the industrial world. The view of the NVI is rather different. Bacteriologists and immunologists interpret the current state of knowledge differently than do epidemiologists. Dutch vaccine scientists have doubts regarding the long-term advantages of acellular vaccines. The current "uneasy equilibrium" contrasts with the situation in the 1970s and 1980s. It is more difficult than it was then to diverge from majority opinion and practice. As one microbiologist put it:

> I think that the variation in vaccines between different countries will get less and less. This is of course on the one hand dangerous, but I see it as a factor that makes it more and more difficult for individual countries to escape from international advice or international consensus regarding what a vaccination scheme should or can be. [...] You see how experts have tried to get consensus, at the level of South America, North America, at the European and Australian levels, regarding how it should be.... I think more and more synchronization is taking place, as the world becomes increasingly global.[32]

Neither with respect to polio nor to pertussis did Dutch "vaccinologists" accept that the vaccine that had achieved, or seems set to achieve, global dominance was best for the Netherlands. In the case of polio, reasoning from the health needs of the population as well as from their technical mastery of the production process, the scientists decided that the Netherlands needed a better version of the IPV already being used, and that a more efficient production process was necessary. There was no good reason, in their view, to follow most of the world in introducing the alternative vaccine. Expertise needed to solve the technical problems was available. An improved IPV was developed not because of commercial considerations, which initially played no role. Crucial was the institute's responsibility for producing and providing the vaccines the country's vaccination program needed. Twenty years later, in the face of the controversy over pertussis, scientists at the Dutch Vaccine Institute were again convinced that the Netherlands needed a vaccine like the one they had, but better. Again, they reached this conclusion on the basis of scientific arguments and analysis of the epidemiology of the disease in the Netherlands itself. The preferred pertussis vaccine is not the one in which the pharmaceutical industry, sensitive to the growing political weight of public concern, had invested so much. Again the scientists tried to act on their convictions, but this time they faced difficulties of a kind that had not arisen twenty years earlier.

Global preference for the OPV had only become problematic for the RIVM when attempts were made to test their enhanced IPV in developing countries. Trials in Africa, and any demonstration of the efficacy of the enhanced IPV there, were a potential threat to investments (financial and symbolic) in the OPV, and to the strategy the WHO had built around it. Today, by contrast, the fact that acellular pertussis vaccine has become the preferred solution to disease control in the industrialized world inhibits producing the improved DTP-P even for domestic needs. Technical problems are greater, and the pharmaceutical industry, possibly looking to abandon the older and less profitable vaccine, may be less willing to collaborate. It has become more difficult to go against the grain of global consensus or, in more sociological language, the force of "institutional isomorphism"[33] has become far greater.

Underlying this "force" is a change in the structure of the vaccine field: one marked by changing relationships both between individual scientists and between institutions. Prior to the mid-1980s, vaccine researchers were a relatively homogeneous and relatively small group, mostly microbiologists and virologists. Knowledge was freely available and freely exchanged irrespective of place of work. That changed. Vaccines-related research is now pursued not only by microbiologists and virologists but also by molecular biologists, geneticists, immunologists, and organic chemists; working in competing networks jealously guarding their findings.

Scientists who have been in the field long enough are well aware of the changes in the vaccine field that have taken place:

> In terms of the way in which the whole vaccine community talks to each other, my experience in going to meetings in the last two or three years is that in the vaccines field the number of commercial companies involved is really quite large. In the old days, you'd go to a conference and it would be mainly your colleagues, people from universities throughout the world. Now you see a lot of representation from companies, who are certainly willing to talk about their data, often talking about their data far more freely than academics would. Probably knowing that their basic technologies, or basic ideas, have been covered by patenting anyway. I'm sure that that's a key issue in the whole thing. [34]

Institutional relationships have changed in a similar way. Decades ago they were rooted in a common commitment to public health. Hans Cohen, who was for many years director general of the Dutch Institute of Public Health responsible for producing/supplying the country's vaccine needs, tells of his earlier relationships with industry, specifically with Pasteur Mérieux

> They [Mérieux] got all our know-how, and we weren't always happy about that, but on the other hand we got a great deal of know how back in return. For example, I got a rabies vaccine. We exchanged. It took three minutes. A matter of

"what do you want from me?" then the boss says "I'll have some polio, and what do you want?" And I'd say "Give me a measles strain, and some of that and some of that…" It was good. Really a free exchange [35]

The knowledge generated in the new networks is no longer freely available or freely exchanged. A 1983 survey of United States vaccine manufacturers had revealed only two patents for twenty-seven vaccine products. A decade later, SmithKline Beecham had to assemble fourteen patents to produce and market its recombinant hepatitis-B vaccine.[36] Vaccine development and production had become "privatized." Despite the important role of governments in funding basic research and in subsidizing vaccine distribution, it was the private sector that had acquired "the pivotal intermediate role in deciding whether research gets translated into products available for public use."[37] That this "privatization" had been accompanied by remarkable scientific progress is in no doubt. Between the 1950s and the 1980s, vaccines offered to children in the United States (and through the WHO Expanded Program of Immunization in much of the world) had multiplied. By 2005, at least in the United States, they had multiplied again, with the IPV having replaced the OPV, acellelular pertussis having replaced whole cell vaccine, and new hepatitis B, varicella, influenza, and pneumococcal conjugate vaccines having been added to the schedule. But progress had come at a price. The new vaccines were expensive. Whereas vaccines provided through the public sector in 1987 had cost $33.70 per child, by 2005 this figure had risen to $517.12.[38]

Discursive Change: From *Scientific Discipline* to *Global Enterprise*

With changing structures comes a changing discourse. Historians and sociologists of science have long been intrigued by the kinds of disciplinary histories that practitioners write: their functions, and their publics. Most of these practitioner histories have some kind of a legitimating function. Not infrequently, they are directed towards the public, governments, and foundations that provide financial support for science.

"Legitimations of this sort typically assume the format of popularised accounts of heroic achievements and adventures at the frontiers of knowledge."[39] So it is here. The vaccine literature is studded with references to past heroes (Edward Jenner, Louis Pasteur, Jonas Salk...); to the extension of vaccination programs into the world's poorest regions; and to the dramatic decline in infant mortality that has been achieved. Despite the recalcitrance of HIV/AIDS and of malaria, the range of diseases against which effective vaccines are available is constantly growing. The significance of these references to the past, typically and commonly to be found in prefaces and in personal memoirs, is not only a matter of their reasonableness or veracity. Their significance, evident in the fact of their constant reiteration, derives from their function as a source of confidence for the public and of motivation and inspiration for the professionals involved. They attest to what has been possible in the past and by implication, but crucially, to what will be possible in the future.

Confronting the prospect of an apparently imminent and devastating epidemic of SARS a few years ago, or of bird flu more recently, we are routinely consoled by the idea that soon there will be a vaccine to protect us. Scientists are already hard at work and they are making rapid progress. Industry is ready, and will be in a position rapidly to produce millions of doses of the vaccine, just as soon as the last hurdles have been cleared. We allow ourselves to find consolation in statements such as Sir Kenneth Calman's partly because we want to–the alternative, after all, is rather unpleasant to contemplate–and partly because they seem to be justified by the past. Great strides are being taken, and there is reason for optimism. Yet progress is not easy. What stands in the way is not only the recalcitrance of the natural world, but organizational failings too. To provide ourselves with the vaccines we need, and quickly, we need to do things better, more effectively. But how? The answer to this question depends upon the way in which vaccine development is seen as taking place, and in this respect–I shall now argue–a change has taken place that parallels the structural changes discussed above. We can think of it as the replacement of one metaphor (one representation of how the vaccine innovation system works) by another.

By the 1970s vaccines were widely viewed as an effective tool of preventive health. Earlier scepticism, shown by the hesitant responses of some national public health authorities to the availability of vaccines,[40] had abated. And science was making gigantic strides forward, as the new viral vaccines showed. Nevertheless, vaccine development in the 1970s was not only risky and uncertain, it was scientifically and technically difficult, requiring, in Maurice Hilleman's words:

> the cooperative team play of a wide variety of disciplines, including, at the very least, the fields of virology, cell biology, biochemistry, biophysics, pathology, clinical medicine, epidemiology and applied biology. The effort is doomed from the outset unless the cooperating scientists of these diverse disciplines can be brought to focus on the multifaceted problems which are involved and for whose solution the guidelines may be hazy or nonexistent.[41]

Reflecting on such issues, a few years later Jonas Salk suggested a kind of discursive integration. He proposed the concept of "vaccinology" to refer to "the study and application of the basic requirements for effective immunization."[42] Salk elaborated his concept a few years later:

> "Vaccinology" might be defined as the study and application of the requirements for effective immunization. This body of knowledge would include an understanding of the fundamental properties of the immune system and of specific immunogens.... Applied vaccinology would involve the application of basic knowledge and practical solutions to the development of effective vaccination programs suitable for particular population groups.[43]

Anne-Marie Moulin has explained further what Salk intended with his neologism. "For the study of vaccines," she writes, "Salk called upon all disciplines, including the human sciences. Indeed, vaccinology brings together the research laboratory, the pharmaceutical industry, the governments, international agencies, epidemic cycles and the suffering flesh, body and psyche."[44] Vaccinology was thus conceived as a single body of knowledge: a field of science in which not only the biomedical, but also the social and cultural considerations underlying development, provision, and acceptance of vaccines have their place.

The concept of vaccinology not only pointed to a shared endeavor, it also helped constitute a shared past. By providing a rhetorical integration of two powerful and reassuring images, it permitted the construction of a common history and a common culture. The concept of vaccinology could draw on two well-established images: that of the successful fight against disease and the promise of science. It then became possible to state that "Of all the branches of modern medicine, vaccinology can claim to be the one that has contributed most to the relief of human misery and the spectacular increase in life expectancy in the last two centuries."[45]

What vaccine history there was, a decade ago, fitted rather well with the success story as well as with Salk's metaphorical integration.[46] The successes of vaccinology give rise to historical accounts that are not only reasonable and inspirational. Thanks to their constant reiteration they are also familiar, they are authoritative, and they are welcome. Faced with what can seem to be a fearful reservoir of pathogens laying in wait in the animal kingdom, they give us grounds for confidence. Even when current problems have to be acknowledged, new science always gives grounds for hope.[47] On the whole, we are happy to accept such histories of vaccinology. As they imply, the development, production, and use of vaccines against infectious diseases *can be* conceived as a single and remarkably successful medical discipline.

Within a few years of Salk's suggestion, concerns were shifting in such a way that a new integrative metaphor would be needed. Convinced that development and effective deployment of new vaccines was hampered by cognitive and social gaps between the contributing disciplines, Jonas Salk had conceived of an integrative *discipline*–vaccinology–as the means to overcome fragmentation. *Institutional* relationships, on the other hand, had been easy and unproblematic, as Cohen pointed out. For example, announcing the licence of the new rubella vaccine in 1969, *Science* noted simply and without comment that its development "resulted from the combined efforts of government, university, and industry scientists over an 8-year period."[48] This was now changing. Past successes have to be re-attributed, as Salk's integrative metaphor of a scientific discipline fades, to be replaced by a very different metaphor. Twenty years after Salk, the U.S. National Vaccine Advisory Committee wrote:

> The United States has been extraordinarily successful in vaccine research and development, contributing more than two thirds of all new vaccines approved worldwide in the last 20 years. This success is the product of a fragile network of interdependent industrial, governmental, and academic partners engaged in vaccine research and development in the United States. This highly effective, yet fragile, network was not designed, but evolved, in response to scientific, public health, and economic forces during the past 50 years.[49]

History is being rewritten. Past vaccine achievements are no longer the result of untiring efforts in the scientific field of vaccinology, but are now the result of an "unplanned" and "fragile" network of collaborations between heterogeneous institutions. And the problem, by the late 1990s, is no longer located in the laboratory, but in institutional relationships and in the marketplace.

In the mid-1980s, reports from the Institute of Medicine in the United States had detailed, separately, the vaccines needed domestically, and those needed in the developing world, and for which the basic knowledge was said to be available. Their list of vaccines needed in the developing world included those against rotavirus and *Shigella, Plasmodium* (responsible for malaria), hepatitis B, and the *Streptococci.* Some of these vaccines have since been developed, of course, but what–in the 1980s–were seen as the obstacles to their development? Laboratory research was not being translated into effective vaccines, despite unquestioned health care needs, in part because of the lack of market incentives. Pharmaceutical companies were devoting little or no effort to the search for a malaria vaccine (or indeed vaccines against any human parasitic diseases), because parasitic diseases were a problem of poor countries that would not be able to afford expensive new vaccines. Somehow or other, the incentive structure had to be changed. Perhaps the solution had to be found in new forms of collaboration between the public and private sectors, and in new mechanisms by which this collaboration could be orchestrated. The term that came to capture the new forms that would be needed was "public private partnerships." The editor of the *British Medical Journal* expressed the emerging consensus: one from which few would have dissented, the public and private sectors will need to work together in new ways to make vaccines and drugs available to the world's poor. The public sector alone cannot solve the problem because almost all new vaccines and drugs come from private companies. Yet private companies cannot solve the problem alone because their obligations to their shareholders mean seeking the highest returns—which tend to come from developing products for the rich world. [50]

Buse and Walt explain emergence of a range of Global Public Private Partnerships in terms of an ideological shift in the 1990s from "freeing" to "modifying" the market, of emerging notions of corporate responsibility, and as a response to changing notions of global governance.[51] A longer historical view suggests something else. We see how relationships that had been taken-for-granted, unworthy of comment, in the 1970s have now become the crux of the issue, providing us with a new metaphor: "Public-private partnerships exist at the nexus of several diverse organizations necessary to achieve equitable, improved treatment. Like a successful venture capital firm, partnerships must effectively orchestrate the resources within and across these organizations…"[52]

In the 1980s, the U.S. National Vaccine Program had been a response to the lack of leadership and coordination in the field. But the issue remained: a 1994 *Science* survey of leading vaccine scientists, business executives, and policy makers found many concerned at "lack of strong leadership and funding."[53] But at what level was this leadership required? What exactly was to be led? There is a second crucial aspect of the rhetorical construction that was emerging by the early 1990s. This is the emphasis on the "international" and, gradually, "the global."

The eradication of smallpox, certified by international declaration at the end of 1979, was one of the most magnificent and impressive successes of vaccination. The history of this success, as subsequently recounted by the health officials who masterminded it,[54] provided a powerful symbol of what was possible. For one thing, it showed that disease eradication was feasible. This was important because, at the time, conventional wisdom increasingly held that human pathogens were ecologically so well adapted that the concept of eradication was untenable.

No less important, the smallpox eradication program created a cadre of professionals whose ideas and enthusiasms continued to dominate the international immunization effort,[55] and it

> demonstrated the potential of WHO as an organisation within which all countries, whatever their beliefs and politics, could cooperate successfully in the pursuit of a common global objective. It encourages the hope that other challenges might likewise be addressed...an important impetus was provided for new initiatives in, for example, immunization, diarrhoeal disease control and the prevention of blindness.[56]

Inspired by these experiences, the World Health Organization launched the Expanded Program on Immunization (EPI) with the objective of taking vaccines of demonstrated value in the industrialized world and facilitating their use in developing countries. Despite the minimal starting point (less than 5 percent vaccine coverage overall) and lack of infrastructure in much of the world, the EPI rapidly succeeded in immunizing most children, even in the poorest regions, with its six chosen vaccines. A succession of international (or global) goals and initiatives followed: aimed in part at mobilizing financial and political support for immunization in the developing world.[57]

William Muraskin has provided a detailed study of one of the first and most influential global initiatives taken in the early 1990s, the Children's Vaccine Initiative (or CVI). In its beginnings, the CVI was a humanitarian endeavor, with as its initial goal "the creation of a single 'magic bullet' vaccine that could be given orally–at or near birth–for more than a dozen different diseases." [58] The CVI's founders hoped to establish a mechanism whereby the public sector could influence the way in which industry was deploying the new possibilities of biotechnology, and so get new and better vaccines to children in the Third World. Gradually, however, the goal diversified, to become nothing less than "rationalizing the entire system."[59] The CVI established a Task Force on Situation Analysis, and this it was that drove the transformation in the CVI's objectives. The Task Force began to address the whole range of issues: vaccine demand, procurement, production, relations with donors, global vaccine strategies...[60] However, the CVI found itself confronting insuperable difficulties in the international arena (turf battles between international organizations, differences in ideology between European and American donors, its own lack of resources) that led to its being closed down in 1999, in an atmosphere of bitter recrimination. Lessons had been learned, however, and the institutions that followed, though recognizably related, were to be differently structured.

Like the CVI, today, too, the public-private partnerships that have to do the orchestrating are not national or international, but global in scope. For example, in considering how barriers to the development and delivery of a vaccine against HIV/AIDS can best be overcome, a group of experts drawn from the Gates Foundation, the WHO, the NIH, and many other organizations plead for "a well-coordinated global enterprise."[61]

A metaphor such as this is but one small element in the discursive framework that serves to underpin the transformed vaccine innovation system. Many more elements can be identified. Here is one. Basing his account on the SARS outbreak a few years ago, and its containment, David Fidler argues that the era of national approaches to public health problems (which he refers to as "Westphalian public health") is now over.[62] Collaboration between nation states is no longer adequate. If this is assumed, then the need for global initiatives in the field of vaccine development is justified in a way they never could have been previously. Another element is the changed language used to characterize public sector vaccine institutes and their roles in the system. Under resourced, badly managed, ineffectively regulated, at the mercy of political whim, these institutions are said to be ill-equipped to compete in a world in which vaccine economics have changed dramatically. Their contribution can but be a strictly limited one.

Perhaps most intriguing and significant of all is the global logic that has been crafted over the past decade: a representational structure in which the proper place of each country and each organization, as well as the relationships between them, can be rationally characterized. In the early 1990s, whilst working at the WHO, Amie Batson and Peter Evans developed a graphic representation, a Grid, on which countries were plotted according to their income and population size. This Grid played an important role in the work of the CVI Task Force on Situation Analysis (on the staff of which Batson and Evans served), and, most important of all, it provided a guide to the optimal use of resources that donor organizations could use. Rich countries with large populations can be assumed to have the resources needed to produce vaccines for their own use, and populations large enough to make production viable. In other words, a large population implies a large enough market and so provides an economic justification for local production facilities. Where the population is large but the country is poor, though the potential for local production exists, technical assistance from outside is required if it is to be realized. Such countries, for example, Indonesia, should be helped to attain vaccine self-sufficiency. In poor small countries the assumption is that local production cannot be justified, so that donor support should be directed towards subsidizing procurement.[63]

The emergence of this discursive framework, and its associated global logic, has itself been critically deconstructed. Nicholas B. King has suggested that its roots lie in the perception of *emergent diseases* as a major threat to the national security of the United States.[64] Viewing disease emergence as the result of the interplay of various factors, dislocations and crises, a 1992 study by the National Academy of Sciences proposed that steps be taken in the areas of surveillance, training and basic research, vaccine development and coordination between local, national and international public health institutions.[65] This report, media coverage, popular books such as Laurie Garrett's 1994 bestseller[66] and a later (1997) report from the Institute of Medicine[67] were turning the threat of emerging diseases into a crucial new challenge to United States security and economic interests. King notes that the 1997 report laid great stress on the notion of global interconnectedness, and the importance of cooperative actions and solutions. New, according to King, is a "set of anxieties and solutions, envisioning a world in which the security of territorial borders has faded, to be replaced by one in which vast networks are not only conduits of infection but also prophylactic tools."[68]

The United States, according to the view that King teases out of a number of reports from the CDC and other central institutions, can best protect itself against this envisaged threat, by "the use of American technoscience in the establishment of global networks of information and exchange. 'International' projects, conducted through treaties between and cooperation among sovereign states, would be replaced by 'global' projects, conducted by coalitions of public, private and non-governmental organisations"[69] Drawing in particular on the 1997 Institute of Medicine report, King argues that in the course of the 1990s, the dominant view in the United States was becoming one in which the nation's interest in protecting the health and security of its citizens was best served by a global system that ensured the efficient production, distribution and consumption of vaccines and other products of the pharmaceutical industry in all corners of the globe.

The metaphorical shift implied in moving from a disciplinary integration to the concept of a network of institutions, a "global enterprise," or something "like a venture capital firm," represents acknowledgment and acceptance of two transformations in the vaccines world no less fundamental than the science and technology deployed. Focusing on the science suggests a trajectory of constant progress, stretching back to Pasteur and endlessly forwards. A focus on the ways in which the metaphors of global business are now used to represent vaccine development offers far less comfort. So too does an analysis of the changing locus of innovation, and the difficulty–today–of innovating in the health interests of a territorially defined population.

Charting the History of the Vaccine Innovation System

The starting point of this paper was the claim that perceptions of vaccine history are dominated by notions of progress, reaching back to Jenner and Pasteur and forwards to the conquest of HIV/AIDS, malaria, and tuberculosis. The vaccine literature is replete with expressions of what Daniel Sarewitz calls the "myth of infinite progress."[70] A myth it may be, but it is a powerful and a consoling one. Professional historians, in so far as they have interested themselves in vaccines, have tended to tell rather different stories, relating (for example) vaccination policies to national cultures or politics, public health aspects of colonial relations, or the association between vaccination and compulsion or the use of force.[71] Where and how vaccines are developed, produced and supplied (and to whom) has tended to receive little attention. Even James Colgrove's recent history of vaccine politics in the United States has little to say about debates regarding the role of the government in developing and producing vaccines.[72] One of few major contributions to the "history of the vaccine innovation system" is Galambos's study of Merck, Sharp & Dohm, and valuable though this is, I have tried to suggest that what is needed is more complex and more heterogeneous. The history that remains to be written is one that will acknowledge and explore the differential impact of the changes that have occurred: changes that have impacted on (national) institutions and their interrelations, on the roles of states, and on the articulation of vaccine innovation with responsibilities and priorities in the field of public health.

This paper has suggested that the scope for state action, for vaccine innovation driven by assessment of national public health needs, has declined. That is the principal conclusion of my analysis of Dutch public sector vaccine development. In discussing the social organization of vaccine development, I concluded that it seems to be increasingly difficult to make choices, or pursue a line of development work, on the basis of the public health needs of a defined population. As in the Netherlands, in Britain too there has recently been heated discussion of the desirability of switching from the whole cell pertussis vaccine to the new acellular vaccine. When Elliman and Bradford write, in the *British Medical Journal*, "The voice in the wilderness is not always wrong, and we should resist the temptation to change our policy just to conform,"[73] they put their finger on a critical feature of current vaccine politics. The "temptation" is becoming an irresistible pressure. It seems that today, whatever the scientific and technical competences available, it is difficult–if not impossible–for choices to be made on the basis of what is believed to be the public health interest of a territorially defined population. Similarly, an Indian scholar has suggested that "vaccine policy in India, rather than being determined by disease burdens and demand-pull, is increasingly driven by supply push, generated by the industry and mediated by international organisations."[74] Focusing specifically on the controversial introduction of hepatitis B vaccination in India, she argues that decisionmaking took place in the absence of adequate epidemiological data and equivocal results from the cost-efficacy studies that were conducted. Far more important, according to Yennapu Madhavi, were pressures from industry (both multinational and local manufacturers) and from international organizations.

I have suggested that social organization of vaccine development and production and its metaphorical representation are related, and that both are key elements of a history of the vaccine innovation system. Thirty years ago, vaccine history helped legitimate faith in future progress. The infectious diseases that threatened us would be conquered with new vaccines in the future, just as they had been in the past. Today, as threats have become globalized, so—it is taken for granted—must responses be too. The metaphorical representation of vaccine development and vaccine history, constantly reiterated and constantly enacted, is slowly being adjusted to changes in the social organization of the vaccine field. With threats of global epidemics, or pandemics, constantly held before us, the need for a global approach to public health seems self-evident: far removed from debates on economic globalization. Yet, as we consider what it might mean to write the history of the emerging global vaccine system, we should bear in mind the question preoccupying political scientists. Have states, asks Suzanne Berger in reviewing the political science literature on globalization, "lost the ability to sustain…distinctive configurations of market and non-market institutions that reflect societal preferences and national traditions?"[75]

Notes

The author would like to thank the Wellcome Trust Programme in the History of Medicine for support of much of the research on which this paper is based, and Ulrike Lindner for comments on an earlier draft.

1. A. R. Hinman, W. A. Orenstein, J. M. Santoli, L. E. Rodewald and S. L. Cochi, "Vaccine Shortages: History, Impact, and Prospects for the Future," *Annual Reviews of Public Health*, 2006, *27*: 235-59.
2. Sir Kenneth Calman, "Foreword" to *Immunisation Against Infectious Diseases*, ed. D. M. Salisbury and N. T. Begg (London: HMSO, 1996), (no page number).
3. See, for example, C. Abel "External Philanthropy and Domestic Change in Colombian Health Care: The Role of the Rockefeller Foundation, c. 1920-1950,"*Hispanic American Historical Review*, 1995, *75*: 339-76; Ilana Löwy "Epidemiology, Immunology and Yellow Fever: The Rockefeller Foundation in Brazil, 1923-1939" *Journal of the History of Biology*, 1997, *30*: 397-417; A. Soloranzo "Sowing the Seeds of Neo-imperialism: The Rockefeller Foundation Yellow Fever Campaign in Mexico," *International Journal of Health Services*, 1992, *22*: 529-54.

4. Ilana Löwy "Yellow Fever in Rio de Janeiro and the Pasteur Institute Mission (1901-1905): The Transfer of Science to the Periphery," *Medical History*, 1990, *34*: 144-63; Kimberly Pelis, "Prophet for Profit in French North Africa: Charles Nicolle and the Pasteur Institute of Tunis, 1903-1936," *Bulletin of the History of Medicine*, 1997, *71*: 583-622.

5. For a personal account of this work, see Frederick C. Robbins "Reminiscences of a Virologist," in *Polio 1997,* ed. T. M. Daniel and F. C. Robbins (Rochester, New York: University of Rochester Press, 1997), pp. 121-34.

6. Maurice R. Hilleman, "Six Decades of Vaccine Development–A Personal History," *Nature Medicine, Vaccine Supplement*, 1998, *4*: 507-14.

7. Louis Galambos, with Jane Eliot Sewell, *Networks of Innovation: Vaccine Development at Merck, Sharp & Dohme, and Mulford, 1895-1995* (Cambridge: Cambridge University Press 1995), pp. 79-99.

8. In February 1976 an influenza virus, believed to be identical to the one that had caused the flu pandemic of 1918 (to which twenty million people succumbed), was isolated from the body of an American army recruit. The decision was made to vaccinate the whole United States population with this virus. A series of disasters followed: including delays in producing the vaccine; unwillingness of manufacturers to assume responsibility for any damage caused by the vaccine; poor sero-conversion rates; and then vaccine damage on a large scale. The Director of what was then known as the Center for Disease Control (CDC) was fired. Much has been written about this episode. For contemporary studies, providing very different interpretations, see Richard E. Neustadt and Harvey V. Fineberg, *The Swine Flu Affair: Decision-Making on a Slippery Disease* (Washington, D.C.: U.S. Department of Health, Education, and Welfare, 1978), and Arthur M. Silverstein, *Pure Politics and Impure Science: The Swine Flu Affair* (Baltimore, Maryland: Johns Hopkins University Press, 1981). For a recent interpretation by two participants in events, see D. J. Sencer and J. D. Millar, "Reflections on the 1976 Swine Flu Vaccination Program," *Emerging Infectious Diseases*, 2006, *2*: 29-33.

9. Office of Technology Assessment (OTA), *Review of Federal Vaccine and Immunization Policies* (Washington, D.C.: U.S. Government Printing Office, 1979).

10. OTA, *Review*, p. 27.

11. Cited by OTA, *Review*, p. 35.

12. Institute of Medicine, *Vaccine Supply and Innovation* (Washington, D.C.: National Academies Press, 1985); David C. Mowery and Violaine Mitchell, "Improving the Reliability of the U.S. Vaccine Supply: An Evaluation of Alternatives," *Journal of Health Policy Politics and Law*, 1995, *20*: 973-1000.

13. William Jordan, "History and Commentary," in *The Jordan Report 20th Anniversary: Accelerated Development of Vaccines, 2002*, ed. Carole Heilman, Pamela McInnes, and Sarah Landry (Bethesda, Maryland: National Institutes of Health, 2002), p. 7. At http://www.niaid.nih.gov/dmid/vaccines/jordan20/.

14. Rachel Nowak, "U.S. National Program is Going Nowhere Fast," *Science*, 1994, *265*: 1376.
15. Barry R. Bloom, "The United States Needs a National Vaccine Authority," *Science*, 1994, *265*: 1378-80.
16. Henry G. Grabowski and John M. Vernon, *The Search for New Vaccines: The Effects of the Vaccines for Children Program* (Washington, D.C.: American Enterprise Institute, 1997).
17. Seung-il Shin, "The Global Vaccine Enterprise: A Developing World Perspective," *Nature Medicine, Vaccine Supplement*, 1998, *4*: 503-4.
18. Galambos and Sewell, *Networks of Innovation.*
19. Galambos and Sewell, *Networks of Innovation*, p. 244.
20. Mowery and Mitchell, "Improving the Reliability of the U.S. Vaccine Supply," p. 978.
21. I am grateful to Diana Obregón for this information.
22. The Scandinavian countries, Denmark, Finland, Norway and Sweden, had comparable public sector institutes at that time–as did a number of countries in Asia and Latin America.
23. What follows is based on Stuart Blume, "Lock in the State and Vaccine Development: Lessons from the History of the Polio Vaccines," *Research Policy*, 2005, *34*: 159-73.
24. Interview with P. Stœckel , cited in Blume, "Lock in," p. 170.
25. Stanley A. Plotkin "The Ten Most Important Discoveries in Vaccinology During the Last Two Decades," *The Jordan Report*, pp. 19-22.
26. E. J. Gangarosa, A. M. Galazka, C. R. Wolfe, L. M. Phillips, R. E. Gangarosa, E. Miller and R. T. Chen, "Impact of Anti-Vaccine Movements on Pertussis Control: The Untold Story," *Lancet*, 1998, *351*: 356-61.
27. The account that follows is based on Stuart Blume and Mariska Zanders, "Vaccine Independence, Local Competences, and Globalization: Lessons from the History of Pertussis Vaccines" *Social Science and Medicine*, 2006, *63*: 1825-35.
28. Grabowski and Vernon, *Search for New Vaccines*, p. 2.
29. Stanley A. Plotkin and Michel Cadoz, "The Acellular Pertussis Vaccine Trials: An Interpretation," *Pediatric Infectious Disease Journal*, 1997, *16*: 508-17.
30. Plotkin and Cadoz, "Acellular Pertussis Vaccine Trials," p. 515.
31. In 2003, the RIVM's responsibilities for vaccine supply were transferred to a new entity called the Netherlands Vaccine Institute. The two organizations are located side-by-side in Bilthoven.
32. Interview with physician-microbiologist at the NVI. Quoted in Blume and Zanders, "Vaccine Independence," p.1834.
33. Paul DiMaggio and Walter Powell, "The Iron Cage Revisited: Institutional Isomorphism and Collective Rationality in Organizational Fields," *American Sociological Review*, 1983, *48*: 147-60.
34. Quoted in Stuart Blume and Ingrid Geesink, "Vaccinology: An Industrial Science?" *Science as Culture*, 2000, *9*: 61.

35. Interview with Hans Cohen, quoted by Blume and Geesink, "Vaccinology," pp. 60-61.
36. Mowery and Mitchell, "Improving the Reliability," p. 976.
37. Phyllis Freeman and Anthony Robbins, "The Elusive Promise of Vaccines," *The American Prospect*, Winter 1991, pp. 80-90.
38. Hinman et al., "Vaccine Shortages," p. 240.
39. Wolf Lepenies and Peter Weingart, "Introduction," in *Functions and Uses of Disciplinary Histories*, ed. Loren Graham, Wolf Lepenies and Peter Weingart (Dordrecht: Reidel, 1983), p.xvi.
40. On American and British scepticism regarding BCG, see Linda Bryder, "'We shall not find salvation in inoculation': BCG Vaccination in Scandinavia, Britain and the U.S.A., 1921-1960," *Social Science and Medicine*, 1999, *49*: 1157-67; on skepticism in Germany that delayed introduction of polio vaccine, see Ulrike Lindner and Stuart Blume, "Vaccine Innovation and Adoption: Polio Vaccines in the U.K., the Netherlands and (West) Germany, 1955-65" *Medical History*, 2006, *50*: 425-46.
41. Hilleman, "Six Decades," p. 513.
42. Jonas Salk and Darrell Salk, "Control of Influenza and Poliomyelitis with Killed Virus Vaccines," *Science*, 1997, *195*: 834-46.
43. Darrell Salk and Jonas Salk, "Vaccinology of Poliomyelitis," *Vaccine*, 1984, *2*: 59-74.
44. Anne-Marie Moulin, "Philosophy of Vaccinology," in *Vaccinia, Vaccination and Vaccinology: Jenner, Pasteur and their Successors*, ed. Stanley Plotkin and Bernadino Fantini (Paris: Elsevier, 1996), p. 17.
45. F. E. André, "Vaccinology: Past Achievements, Present Roadblocks and Future Promises," *Vaccine*, 2003, *21*: 593-95.
46. An important exception was Allan M. Brandt, "Polio, Politics, Publicity and Duplicity: Ethical Aspects in the Development of the Salk Vaccine," *International Journal of Health Services*, 1978, *8*: 257-70. Particularly concerned by the laissez-faire attitude of government, Brandt explains the ethical inadequacies of the vaccine's introduction in terms also of exaggerated publicity and the National Foundation for Infantile Paralysis (March of Dimes) that had funded Salk's work and the field trials being unable to manage its conflicting responsibilities in fundraising, research, testing, and overseeing production and distribution.
47. Thus Hilleman writes, "Pioneering new vaccine development, in the period since 1985, has been remarkably sterile and filled with 'gonna's and promises' but few successes." Nevertheless, "The platforms of knowledge developed during the 20th century are ripe for exploitation and for anticipated successes early in the 21st century. It is not unreasonable to be optimistic…" Maurice Hilleman, "Vaccines in Historic Evolution and Perspective: A Narrative of Vaccine Discoveries," *Vaccine*, 2000, *18*: 1436-47, at p. 1445.
48. M. Mueller, "Rubella Vaccine is Licensed," *Science*, 1968, *165*: 48.

49. National Vaccine Advisory Committee, "United States Vaccine Research: A Delicate Fabric of Public and Private Collaboration," *Pediatrics*, 1997, *100*: 1015.

50. R. Smith, "Vaccines and Medicines for the World's Poorest," *British Medical Journal*, 2000, *320*: 952-53.

51. K. Buse and G. Walt, "Global Public-Private Partnerships: Part 1–A New Development in Health?" *Bulletin of the World Health Organization*, 2000, *78*: 549-61.

52. Craig Wheeler and Seth Berkeley, "Initial Lessons from Public-Private Partnerships in Drug and Vaccine Development," *Bulletin of the World Health Organization*, 2001, *79*: 728-34.

53. Jon Cohen, "Bumps on the Vaccine Road," *Science*, 1994, *265*: 1371-73.

54. Frank Fenner, D. A. Henderson, I. Arita, Z. Jezek, and I. D. Ladniyi, *Smallpox and Its Eradication* (Geneva: WHO, 1988).

55. Peter F. Wright, "Global Immunization–A Medical Perspective," *Social Science & Medicine*, 1995, *41*: 609-16.

56. Fenner et al., *Smallpox*, p. 1366.

57. Anita Hardon and Stuart Blume, "Shifts in Global Immunisation Goals (1984-2004): Unfinished Agendas and Mixed Results," *Social Science & Medicine*, 2005, *60*: 345-56.

58. William Muraskin, *The Politics of International Health: The Children's Vaccine Initiative and the Struggle to Develop Vaccines for the Third World* (Albany, New York: SUNY Press, 1998), p. viii.

59. Muraskin, *Politics of International Health*, p. viii.

60. Muraskin, *Politics of International Health*, pp. 101-2.

61. R. D. Klausner, A. S. Fauci, et al., "The Need for a Global HIV Vaccine Enterprise," *Science*, 2003, *300*. 2036 39.

62. David P. Fidler, *SARS, Governance and the Globalization of Disease* (London and New York: Palgrave Macmillan, 2004).

63. See Violaine S. Mitchell, Nalini M. Philipose and Jay P. Stanford, eds. *The Children's Vaccine Initiative: Achieving the Vision* (Washington, D.C.: National Academies Press, 1993), p. 70.

64. Nicholas B. King, "Security, Disease, Commerce: Ideologies of Postcolonial Global Health," *Social Studies of Science*, 2002, *32*: 763-89.

65. Joshua Lederberg, R. E. Shope, and S. C. Oaks, Jr., *Emerging Infections: Microbial Threats of Health in the United States* (Washington, D.C., National Academies Press, 1992).

66. Laurie Garrett, *The Coming Plague: Newly Emerging Diseases in a World Out of Balance* (New York: Farrar, Strauss & Giroux, 1994).

67. Institute of Medicine, *America's Vital Interest in Global Health: Protecting Our People, Enhancing Our Economy, and Advancing Our International Interests* (Washington, D.C.: National Academies Press, 1997).

68. King, "Security, Disease, Commerce," p. 773.

69. King, "Security, Disease, Commerce," p. 774.

70. Daniel Sarewitz, *Frontiers of Illusion: Science, Technology and the Politics of Progress* (Philadelphia: Temple University Press, 1996).

71. On the use of force, see in particular, Paul Greenough, "Intimidation, Coercion and Resistance in the Final Stage of the South Asian Smallpox Eradication Campaign, 1973-1975," *Social Science and Medicine*, 1995, *41*: 633-45.

72. James Colgrove, *States of Immunity. The Politics of Vaccination in Twentieth-Century America* (New York, Berkeley and London: University of California Press/Milbank Memorial Fund, 2006).

73. D. Elliman and H. Bradford, "Perhaps It Is Not Time to Switch from Whole Cell to Acellular Pertussis Vaccine," *British Medical Journal*, 2000, *321*: 451.

74. Yennapu Madhavi, "Manufacture of Consent? Hepatitis B Vaccination," *Economic and Political Weekly*, 14 June 2003, pp. 2417-24.

75. Suzanne Berger, "Globalization and Politics," *Annual Reviews of Political Science*, 2000, *3*: 43-62.

Molecularization and Infectious Disease Research: The Case of Synthetic Antimalarial Drugs in the Twentieth Century

Leo Slater

In fact, the effort is already being made to co-operate with biology; it is clear that a section of the forces of organic chemistry is being directed once more towards the goal from which it set out. The separation from biology was necessary during the past century while experimental methods and theories were being elaborated; now that our science is provided with a powerful armoury of analytical and synthetical weapons, chemists can once more renew the alliance both to its own honour and to the advantage of biology. Indeed, the prospect of obtaining a clearer insight into the wondrous series of processes which constitute animal and vegetable life may well lead the two sciences to work with definite purpose to a common end.[1]

Emil Fischer (1852-1919), 1907

How might historians characterize the trajectory of infectious disease in a biomedical context? In the nineteenth century, physicians and biologists created the germ theory, establishing and solidifying the microbial etiology of infectious disease; one hundred years ago, this was the growing consensus on infectious disease. Yet the intervening years have certainly seen infectious disease research and interventions still more dramatically transformed. So what can historians say to characterize the study of infectious disease in the twentieth century? This paper argues that fit and specificity, grounded on molecular–that is, chemical–understandings of living things and their environmental interactions, describe much that has become essential about today's understandings of infectious disease.[2] This was not momentary transformation, but was part of a project and a process that spanned the whole of the twentieth century. Furthermore, this process of molecularization has extended far beyond infectious disease research into every aspect of biomedicine.[3] Indeed, this logical pursuit argues that the molecule has become the explanatory tool for the study of the body, mind, environment, and many other areas of the "technoscientific" society of the twenty-first century.

Molecularization and a concomitant mechanistic rationalization have driven biomedicine. In the historiography of twentieth-century biomedicine, the impact of molecular thinking has been most clearly illustrated by molecular genetics and molecular biology. But this paper shows how a more specific and carefully drawn view of molecularization can allow historians to analyze productively many fields of biomedical endeavor: A focus on molecules in living systems was not limited to disciplines–such as molecular biology–branded as "molecular." The conceptualization of living things as profoundly chemical in their fundamental constituents allowed new modes of representation and intervention. This world view–superficially reductionist–actually revealed the profound connections between all living things and between them and their environments. Deploying even a narrow example from the field of malaria chemotherapy can reveal the power and reach of the molecular understanding in biological and disease systems.

For the chemotherapy of infectious disease, the molecular (rational) approach–often defined in opposition to a random approach or pure empiricism–meant seeking a molecular understanding of disease processes and interventions. Rationalization and molecularization enabled the search for drugs and vaccines. Several disciplines contributed tools to this project, not least organic chemistry, biochemistry, and immunology. These tools were both intellectual and physical, the former including chemical structure theories and concepts of chemical shape and affinity, and the latter involving the techniques of visualization from stains to immunofluorescence–and a growing number of electronic instruments which supplemented traditional microscopes. Basic immunological concepts, such as the determination of self versus non-self, were chemically defined. Instrumentation and visualization supported rationalization and molecularization. Across the whole of the twentieth century, the complexity of biological understanding grew. And for infectious disease, an increasing array of etiological organisms became the targets of investigations: bacteria, such as pneumococcus, staphylococcus, and streptococcus; larger parasites, such as the malaria-causing *Plasmodium*; the mycobacterium of tuberculosis; *Rickettsia*; and viruses such as smallpox, poliomyelitis, influenza, and HIV. This list, of course, goes on and on. To develop this theme, this paper draws on examples from malaria. Issues around rationalization and molecularization–much like the themes of instrumentation and visualization–easily pass beyond the boundaries of infectious disease, *per se*, but again these pages here are limited to a small example from malaria history: the development of synthetic antimalarials from the late nineteenth century through the middle decades of the twentieth century.

methylene blue

For synthetic chemicals employed against malaria, the story begins in Berlin, Germany, with methylene blue, a bright blue synthetic dye. In the mid-1880s, Paul Ehrlich (1854-1915) investigated the selective staining of nerve tissue by methylene blue.[4] Ehrlich was a physician and chemist of great insight and would go on to win the 1908 Nobel Prize in Physiology or Medicine.[5] He was fascinated by the specificity of dyes, the way in which they would stain some tissues and not others. Ehrlich was particularly interested in the way *living* tissues reacted to stains. From his methylene blue observations, he had two questions: "1. Why does methylene blue stain nerves?" and "2. Why are nerves stained by methylene blue?"[6] The answer to the first question was chemical in nature. Ehrlich observed that while methylene blue contained sulfur, another quite similar dye, Bindschedler's green, lacked this sulfur. Ehrlich concluded that the green dye could not stain living nerves because of its lack of sulfur. Chemical constitution controlled staining specificity.

methylene blue   **Bindschedler's green**

Methylene blue's specific constitution gave it the ability to bind to the nerve tissue. With regard to the second question, Ehrlich found that in higher animals not all nerve tissue was the same. "I have shown it probable that these differences between the individual nerve-endings are not due to different degrees of avidity for methylene blue, but rather to certain associated environmental conditions; for bluing of the nerves is intimately associated with the degree of oxygen saturation, inasmuch as it is precisely at those places which are best supplied with oxygen that staining of the nerve endings by methylene blue also occurs."[7] The chemical environment conditioned the behavior of the biological material. Ehrlich continued: "Further, one can easily ascertain that the nerve fibres that stain have also an alkaline reaction; and thus oxygen saturation and alkaline reaction provide the conditions which make possible the staining of nerve endings by methylene blue."[8] Notice that Ehrlich here described the biological functioning of the living tissue in chemical terms. Ehrlich was an influential prophet of the molecularization of living systems in general and of infectious disease in particular. His work on the chemotherapy of syphilis is well known, but he also pursued malaria.

For Ehrlich, methylene blue was not just useful as a stain for nerve tissue. It was also employed to stain malaria parasites in both fresh blood and fixed preparations. In 1891, while continuing his studies on the affinity of dyes for certain tissues, Ehrlich and his co-worker reported an antimalarial activity for methylene blue in the clinical cases of two malarial patients.[9] Methylene blue, which selectively stained parasites *in vitro*, acted against the disease, and Ehrlich's patients improved to some extent. But the dye was not as harmless as Ehrlich had initially believed. Ehrlich's findings with regard to methylene blue would not yield a useful tool in the fight against malaria, not directly anyway. In the 1920s, German chemists would revisit methylene blue and launch a more comprehensive and successful chemical attack on malaria.

But chemists in the late nineteenth century had another compound leading them on in the quest to create a synthetic antimalarial. This lead was quinine, the natural extract of cinchona tree bark that had been used against malaria for centuries. Starting from the simpler chemical constituents of quinine–the products of chemical degradations–they pursued quinine's antimalarial property in a synthetic form.[10] Notable among these attempts were those of the chemist Otto Fischer (1852-1932), cousin and collaborator of Emil Fischer, and of Ludwig Knorr (1859-1921), then working with Emil Fischer at the University of Erlangen in Germany.[11] Emil Fischer was a major proponent of the structure theory, a synthetic organic chemist of great ability and influence, and the author of an oft-cited analogy for biochemical specificity known as lock-and-key. Cousin Otto, pursuing quinine's active essence, eventually synthesized Kairine, one of the first planned syntheses of a drug.

N.B. Both drugs, Kairine and quinine, contain a quinoline-like structure.

Though Kairine showed modest fever-reducing activity, it was found to be toxic and ineffective against malaria. Knorr's efforts, however, resulted in the synthesis of Antipyrine, a less toxic anti-fever drug, in 1883.[12]

Antipyrine

Phenacetin

In 1888, the German dye firm of Meister, Lucius, and Brüning at Hoechst (Frankfurt) am Main, launched Antipyrine. Along with Bayer's Phenacetin (synthesized in 1887) it was one of the first mass produced synthetic pharmaceuticals. Bayer at Wuppertal-Elberfeld near Cologne was a major player in the German chemical industry and a producer of dyes with a growing interest in drugs. Commercial medications such as Antipyrine and Phenacetin–though not active against malaria– helped move dye firms into the pharmaceutical business and showed the promise of synthetic chemistry as a source of biologically active materials for medical interventions. In the coming decades, Ehrlich's anti-syphilis drugs would further pique interest in chemical interventions in infectious disease. Ehrlich died in 1915, but one further comment on his contributions to immunity and chemotherapy is merited here.

Ehrlich pioneered many aspects of the study of immunology and chemotherapy. Indeed, in 1907, it was he who coined the term chemotherapy. Ehrlich's notions of specificity with regard to immunology were not immediately translated to his chemotherapy work, but by the first decade of the twentieth century, the state of knowledge suggested connections between immunity and chemotherapy, as related modes in the body's fight against disease.[13] Ehrlich came to believe that natural immunity, the ability of the body to defeat or resist infection–the kind of immunity observed in vaccination, for example–operated by the same kind of chemical mechanism as drugs did. Historian Timothy Lenoir has written that the "suggestive analogy between pharmacological action and immunity was further strengthened by the researches of Röhl, Franke, and Browning in Ehrlich's institute."[14] In fact, it was one of these junior collaborators, Wilhelm Roehl (Röhl), who would move on with this suggestive analogy to a renewed interest in methylene blue. Born in Berlin, Roehl (1881-1929) was a German physician with training in physiological chemistry. This paper cannot dwell on Ehrlich's intellectual development, but emphasizes his fundamental characterization of biological systems in terms of fit and specificity, shape and affinity supported by chemical properties and interactions. In this, of course, he was not alone.

While the mode of action of antimalarial drugs was not well understood in the first half of the twentieth century, the chemical shapes and structures of these drugs, both natural and synthetic were knowable, as were their activities against parasites. Chemists' structural drawings, like those in this paper, were a shorthand way of showing the chemical, physical, and biological properties of chemical compounds.[15] The chemists and their collaborators could establish structure-activity relationships which allowed them to use chemical structures as models for biological activity: add a carbon atom here and toxicity goes down, add a nitrogen there and activity goes up. For example, Wilhelm Roehl–having moved on from Ehrlich's Frankfurt laboratory to Bayer's chemotherapy institute in Elberfeld–could map chemical composition and shape against the activity of potential drugs in birds and humans. Scientists at Bayer in Elberfeld were able to screen hundreds of compounds using a system of canaries infected with an avian malaria, *Plasmodium relictum*.[16] Roehl had developed this animal model based on his previous work with mice and other infectious diseases organisms such as trypanosomes. As Roehl commented: "Since 1911, a large series of preparations of the [quinine] and [quinoline] group, as well as basic substances of dye stuffs and other origin, have been submitted to me by the chemists of the 'Farbenfabriken;' these were usually tested on trypanosomes [on which Roehl had also worked when at Ehrlich's institute], they were tried in bird malaria, unfortunately always without success."[17]

Chemotherapy research at Bayer involved not just random screening but the development of a series of structure-activity relationships. Beginning with quinine, several workers sought to alter chemically the natural drug itself and to synthesize various related quinoline compounds. Quinine provided a starting point from which to explore chemical space; it was the first structural model for a possible synthetic drug. A "lead" compound, such as this, generally showed some desired properties and could lead chemists to compounds whose properties more and more closely matched those they sought. For Bayer, the desired property was antimalarial activity. Along the path to new compounds with this property might be compounds with other properties as well, such as low toxicity, ready availability from simple starting materials (low cost), or the ability to kill multiple life stages of the parasite. Bayer began with quinine, making "chemical attacks on the positions indicated by arrows," as in the diagram below.[18]

Quinoline nucleus and quinine structure with points of modification indicated by arrows.

As Werner Schulemann (1888-1975), a leader of the Bayer team, said, "It was generally assumed that an anti-malarial drug must contain a quinoline nucleus, with an aliphatic basic group bound by a carbon bond to the fourth position of quinoline. In spite of much excellent synthesis, however, the desired goal was not reached."[19] For Schulemann, quinine was the lead compound in a class of compounds having an attachment at the fourth position of the quinoline nucleus. Bayer's chemists modified the natural product as a first attempt on this structural class of compounds. Quinine was complex and proved a poor model. Investigations into it and closely related substances did not result in compounds with significant, or enhanced, antimalarial activity.[20] While Schulemann and his colleagues abandoned quinine, they would return to its quinoline nucleus.[21] Their concerns with chemical structure and shape were part of a broader shift toward a molecular understanding of medicine. Indeed, Bayer published many of their results in a series titled *Medicine in its Chemical Aspects*.[22]

Schulemann and his collaborators also pursued another structural line of inquiry employing Ehrlich's methylene blue and again using Roehl's malarial canaries as an assay. These, alongside methylene blue, were some of the compounds synthesized at Bayer to follow up on this lead:[23]

methylene blue

Compounds from the methylene blue series.

Compounds I and II, where the dimethyl sidechains of methylene blue had been slightly lengthened, were found slightly more effective than the parent compound. Structural changes in compounds I and II increased their antimalarial properties relative to methylene blue. However, their therapeutic index–the ratio of the effective dose to the tolerable dose–was still very low, around 1-to-1. Bayer's chemists found that they could improve this ratio by adding basic groups to the amino sidechains, as in compounds III and IV. The amino groups on the sidechains were those with the nitrogen (N) in them. They were "basic"–in the sense of a base as the opposite of an acid–because they formed salts when combined with acids. The chemists found another promising sidechain with this compound, V:

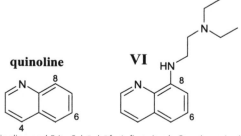

V   methylene blue

They extended to other classes of compounds this principle that effectiveness could be enhanced and toxicity reduced by the addition of basic alkyl attachments (nitrogen-containing sidechains). The other classes of compounds were primarily other dyes. Bayer was, after all, a synthetic dye firm. It was in a quinoline series, however, that success came first.

Having established in the methylene blue series the hypothesis that certain nitrogen-containing sidechains could increase the antimalarial activity and decrease the toxicity of a given chemical structure, Schulemann and the Bayer chemists began anew from a simpler starting point, the bare quinoline nucleus. To this they attached their active sidechains.[24] Using this quinoline nucleus as a starting point simplified the chemical exploration of antimalarial properties of the quinoline compounds by disposing of the structural and stereochemical complexity of the intact quinine molecule. Adding the promising sidechain not at the 4-position, as in quinine, but at the 8-position, Bayer chemist Fritz Schönhöfer (1892-1965) produced a series of quinoline compounds. He originally sought to add the amino group to the quinoline nucleus at the 6-position, but each attempt yielded only tarry goo. Then the chemists moved on to the 8-position. The 8-substituted compounds proved promising.[25] Even Schönhöfer's first simple 8-aminoquinoline, compound VI, proved active, showing several times the activity of quinine in the Roehl-canary test.

quinoline   VI

Quinoline and Fritz Schönhöfer's first simple 8-aminoquinoline.

Schulemann and his group pursued a range of shapes and structures in developing their several series of compounds. They varied the sidechains attached to their central structures, while keeping an eye on the lead compounds that showed the best activity, such as quinine and methylene blue. To illustrate the variety of compounds synthesized and tested, Schulemann constructed a sidechain diagram, giving a sample of the many chemical attachments that the chemists tried out.

Schulemann's Sidechain Diagram.[26]

The shape and chemical composition of each of these sidechains allowed Bayer further to refine the requirements of antimalarial compounds.

Schulemann pursued other modifications of the promising 8-amino series. He reasoned that they should add a methoxy-group ($-OCH_3$), which was essential for activity in quinine. Schönhöfer added this methoxy-group at the 6-position, producing a compound that Roehl termed A-prochin. Schönhöfer then proceeded through a whole series of compounds, A-prochin, Be-prochin, Ce-prochin, etc., each one a slight variation. It was Beprochin that excelled. Produced in 1924, Roehl found this compound well tolerated by his canaries and very active—more than 30-fold more—than other compounds in the series. Bayer marketed Beprochin under the name plasmochin.

quinoline   plasmochin

With a therapeutic index of 1:30, plasmochin was the first successful synthetic antimalarial.[27] The process that generated plasmochin was rational drug discovery, a set of practices that included the development of structure-activity relationships and, for some other drugs, an understanding of how the drug was taking the place of natural compound or substrate.[28] Nevertheless, Bayer often had to fall back on random screening to develop new lead compounds. What was lacking was a molecular understanding of how the drug worked, of its mode of action. With structure-activity relationships, chemists could only visualize one half of the lock-and-key that was the drug and its molecular target. If they knew the shape of the target–the lock–then they could grasp a more powerful approach to drug development: rational drug design. This would have to await more powerful tools for the visualization and analysis of molecules in the postwar period.

By the 1920s, modes of action for drugs and biologically active chemical compounds were still not well explored or well understood.[29] Wilhelm Roehl explored drugs–including plasmochin–as potential activators of the immune system or as possibly functioning like *in vitro* antiseptics. For Roehl: "The most insistent question is how the action of Plasmochin is produced. Does this involve an inhibition of parasite reproduction and a lethal action upon the parasites by the blood, or does the drug call into play dormant protective powers in the sense that immunity substances are newly formed or that the parasiticidal cells of the body develop greater capacity for inhibiting or destroying the micro-organisms of the disease?"[30] Roehl tested the capacity of his drug to switch on the immune system: "In any event, Plasmochin does *not* act by producing a general increase in the defensive powers of the body. For if mice inoculated with trypanosomes or with spirochetes of relapsing fever be treated with Plasmochin, the infections develop as when no therapy is employed."[31]

Nor did Roehl find his drug to trigger an immune response against malaria in his canaries. "But when canaries are given preliminary treatment with Plasmochin…and are inoculated two hours later with plasmodia, the infection takes its ordinary course as if no preliminary treatment had been given…. Hence, the assumption of an indirect action of Plasmochin is not confirmed by experiments."[32] The activity of plasmochin seemed not to be mediated by the immune system. Roehl also pursued the antiseptic analogy comparing the action of his new drug to that of the disinfectant mercuric chloride ("mercury bichlorid"): "Plasmochin inhibits the development of parasites, even in solutions of 1:1500 to 1:50,000, thus within very wide limits. Such a wide limit of inhibitory effect is known to us [through] the direct action of mercury bichlorid upon bacteria...."[33]

In subsequent decades, others, such as the University of Chicago's malaria group, continued to pursue the relationship between chemotherapy and immunity in malaria.[34] For example, they established that quinine's mechanism of action was not by increase in immune response.[35] The mode of action of antimalarial drugs remained an area of great interest and mystery. Nevertheless, chemists, pharmacologists, and others continued to view these drugs as chemical agents whose activity relied on shape and structure and specific molecular interactions with biological materials.

In the early 1930s, Bayer had a second synthetic success against malaria.[36] They screened more compounds from their dye programs, and another drug emerged: atabrine. The atabrine story paralleled the plasmochin story in key ways, though atabrine had unique problems and properties. Bayer's scientists continued to mold the conception of disease around chemical shapes and structures. The chemists developed structure-activity relationships for a new series of potential drug candidates. As with plasmochin, they characterized these compounds with a therapeutic index—the ratio of the effective dose to the tolerable dose—using canaries and *Plasmodium relictum*. Their new starting structure, borrowed from a series of dyes, was the acridine nucleus. The acridine nucleus replaced the quinoline nucleus that had yielded plasmochin. As in plasmochin's development, a large series of compounds were synthesized and tested. Two of Bayer's organic chemists, Hans Mauss (1901-1953) and Fritz Mietzsch (1896-1958) supplied many of these.[37] Atabrine emerged as the best of more than 300 acridine compounds screened against bird malaria in canaries.[38] It was far less toxic than plasmochin, but atabrine was still an acridine dye with a strong yellow color. In fact, the chemists' report on its preparation even included tassels of test fibers dyed bright yellow by the new drug.[39] (The sulfa drugs, too, were developed from dye stuffs, beginning with Prontosil in 1932. Bayer chemists Fritz Mietzsch and Josef Klarer synthesized Prontosil.[40])

acridine   **atabrine**

As the Bayer chemists explained, the fundamental structural difference between plasmochin and atabrine was that plasmochin was built around the quinoline nucleus while atabrine contained the acridine structure.[41]

quinoline   **acridine**

Bayer also screened the acridine compounds against streptococcal and staphylococcal bacteria, producing a number of antibacterial agents. Atabrine, like plasmochin, went first to Düsseldorf for testing in neuro-syphilis patients.[42] In the fall of 1930, it was tested against naturally occurring malaria in Romania.[43] For further trials against human malaria, atabrine traveled to the Hamburg Institute for Tropical Medicine and on to Latin America with two of the institute's researchers.[44] Following its successful tests, atabrine went on the market in 1932.[45]

With atabrine's international sales growing, Bayer's chemists and pharmacologists pursued new leads back in Germany. Mauss and Mietzsch had supplied Roehl's successor, Walter Kikuth (1896-1968), and his group with the acridine compounds from which they selected atabrine. Kikuth was a physician with a substantial background in tropical medicine research. Two other Bayer chemical scientists in Elberfeld, Fritz Schönhöfer and Hans Andersag (1902-1955), delivered a new series of aminoquinolines to Kikuth for screening.[46] In 1934, Andersag synthesized a colorless antimalarial, Resochin. What Bayer called Resochin would later be named chloroquine in the United States.

The loss of the right-hand ring (circled) of yellow atabrine transformed this compound into the white (colorless) chloroquine:

A change in structure altered the compound's properties: its color, its toxicity, and its antimalarial activity. Resochin (chloroquine), unlike atabrine, never made it past the Düsseldorf neurosyphilitics. This compound's antimalarial activity may have been overlooked by the Germans because of their reliance on the Roehl test for preliminary toxicity data or because it erroneously showed toxicity in the Düsseldorf tests. After the war, Schönhöfer and Kikuth suggested that the latter explanation was correct, saying that the "toxicity of this substance [was], however, so great in comparison to its effect, that it was treated no further."[47]

Nevertheless, this series of 4-aminoquinolines was promising. Bayer moved forward with another compound, sontochin, closely related to chloroquine. Sontochin was a methylated chloroquine.

Sontochin was chloroquine with an added methyl group, as indicated by the arrow.

After Kikuth had tested sontochin in animals, it, too, went to Düsseldorf for testing in neurosyphilitics in 1937. Believing sontochin to be less toxic and just as effective as Resochin, the Bayer workers dropped Resochin (chloroquine), having made less than a kilogram of this compound. By the end of 1938 and the beginning of 1939, the Hamburg Institute for Tropical Medicine had successfully tested the new methylated drug against naturally occurring malaria in sick sailors arriving in the German port city.[48] Neither of these chlorinated 4-aminoquinolines–sontochin or chloroquine–would be marketed in the United States before the outbreak of war in Europe. The antimalarial program at Bayer continued through World War II,[49] with sontochin seeing continued development. World War II also saw the United States and Britain each pursuing their own programs.[50] The British developed a successful and novel drug, Paludrine (also called proguanil or chlorguanide), while the United States wartime antimalarial project identified chloroquine as the postwar drug of choice. Though they missed chloroquine, the interwar German effort was the first sizable and systematic attempt to identify a synthetic substitute for quinine.

The United States antimalarial program was very large in comparison to these German interwar efforts and covered many aspects of malaria prevention and treatment, with particular emphasis on chemoprophylaxis. In brief, the United States antimalarial program screened some 14,000 compounds for antimalarial activity, clinically ratified atabrine as the drug of choice in 1943, and, by war's end, identified chloroquine as a superior compound. The program also delved into animal models of disease, pharmacology, toxicology, malaria biology, and malaria vaccine research. The National Research Council (NRC) coordinated most of this work, with funding and administration coming from the Office of Scientific Research and Development. The NRC and others drew on a set of intellectual and organizational resources and models extending back to the German pharmaceutical and dye industries and to such domestic institutions as the Rockefeller Institutes and Foundation. When sontochin tablets were captured by the Allies in North Africa in 1943, the program revisited the 4-aminoquinoline series and rapidly developed chloroquine for the treatment and prophylaxis of malaria in both military and civilian domains. The program also expanded the chemical space occupied by 8-aminoquinolines, plasmochin's chemical family:

The United States tested a number of variations of plasmochin's side-chain, which eventually yielded primaquine in the years following the war. The program was arguably the largest biomedical research program up to this time, a program that helped to safeguard millions of GIs and served as a model for future large-scale biomedical research projects.

By the 1940s, the relationship between the body's immune responses and the mechanisms of chemotherapy had been resolved into different modalities. René J. Dubos (1901-1982), a French-born microbiologist at the Rockefeller Institute for Medical Research in New York, wrote in 1941:

> It is usually considered that chemotherapeutic agents and immune antibodies exert their protective effect against bacterial infections by entirely different mechanisms. Paul Ehrlich, however, believed that the laws of chemotherapeutic action and immunity could be formulated in the same general terms. The living cell was assumed to possess a number of chemically reactive groups, called "receptors," with which dyes, bactericidal substances, and immune bodies reacted selectively. Ehrlich regarded these "receptors" as definite chemical entities, capable of entering into union

with dyes, antiseptics, and antibodies. Characteristic staining reactions, differential susceptibilities to toxic substances, and specific reactions with immune bodies could all be explained by postulating the existence of a sufficient number of "receptors" in the bacterial cell.[51]

Much had changed since Ehrlich's time, but much, too, remained. The modes of action of immune bodies and chemotherapeutic agents were teased apart, but the underlying explanatory models remained molecular in substance. Dubos described the fall and rise of immunochemistry: "Unfortunately, neither Ehrlich nor his immediate followers succeeded in identifying the chemical nature of these 'receptors,' or even in demonstrating their existence as well defined entities; the receptor theory therefore fell into disrepute and was often considered an attempt to mask ignorance under a covering of words. During the past two decades, however, immunochemistry has in several cases given reality and chemical definition to the 'receptors' postulated by Ehrlich."[52] The interactions of cells–living entities–with their environment were chemically mediated. It is interesting to note that Dubos' later career was intimately associated with rise of environmentalism.[53]

With the function of the immune system separated from the function of drugs, Dubos still saw much that needed explication with regard to drug action:

> There are of course many ways in which it is possible to interfere with the parasitic career of a virulent organism, and it would be futile to try to force the mechanism of action of the different therapeutic agents into one and the same pattern. But in any case it appears justified to claim that the rational development of antisepsis and chemotherapy has much to gain from a better knowledge of the chemical architecture of the bacterial cell for, in Paul Ehrlich's words, "only such substances can be anchored at any particular part of the organism which fit into the molecule of the recipient combination as a piece of a mosaic fits into a certain pattern."[54]

Ehrlich and those who followed him transformed the understanding of drugs and immunity and made all these interactions *chemical* in a profound and fundamental way.

Following World War II, other concepts of molecular shape led to new antimalarial drugs. Pyrimethamine was a clever modification of proguanil (Paludrine or chlorguanide), the drug developed by the British wartime antimalarial program. George Hitchings (1905-1998), a biologically engaged chemist at the Wellcome Research Laboratories in New York State, thought that proguanil was active in its cyclized form. Visualizing the active drug's shape as a second six-membered ring yielded a new class of drugs with two hexagonal structures. This class of cyclic compounds—based on the straight-tailed proguanil—led to pyrimethamine.[55] Shape and structure were the key to Hitchings' chemical insight.

Proguanil shown curled around on itself to highlight its structural similarity to pyrimethamine.

This drug was only one to come from the fruitful collaboration of Hitchings and Gertrude Elion (1919-1999), a research chemist. The concept of shape and fit—Emil Fischer's lock-and-key—led them to broad concepts of drug design, for which Hitchings and Elion later shared the 1988 Nobel Prize in Physiology or Medicine with James Black.

Work on the mode of action of antimalarial drugs in the second half of the twentieth century merits mention here. Chloroquine—the drug synthesized, tested, and abandoned by Bayer in Germany in the 1930s and then identified by the United States wartime program as the antimalarial of choice—was a wonder drug in the 1940s and on into the 1960s, when resistance by the parasites began to undercut its effectiveness.[56] In spite of its status and its use around the world as a cheap and effective remedy and prophylactic, little was known about how it actually worked. Only in the 1980s, did ingenuity and advances in analytical instrumentation allow a French group to suggest a plausible and supportable theory for chloroquine's mode of action.[57] It was nuclear magnetic resonance spectroscopy, a postwar instrumental technology, which visualized chloroquine in action.

Chloroquine did not activate the host's immune system, nor did it attack the malaria parasite directly. Chloroquine indirectly poisoned the parasite. Malaria parasites invaded red blood cells and devoured the proteins they found inside. Of course, much of the protein in a red blood cell was hemoglobin, the oxygen-carrying protein that allowed the cell to function. And hemoglobin, in turn, contained heme, a multi-cyclic iron-carrying structure. Heme was toxic, and, as the parasite consumed the cell's protein, it had to sequester the heme in a stable, insoluble crystal. It was here that the chloroquine intervened. Chloroquine got into the cell, settled on the growing crystal, and blocked its further growth. Heme then built up and poisoned the parasite. Chloroquine was shaped and constituted so that it could get to just the right place in the cell and interfere with this essential function in the parasite's biology. And chloroquine did not interfere with any essential processes in human biology. Knowledge of this mode of action of the drug opened up new possibilities for the rational design of new drugs, but it was not necessary for the rational discovery of chloroquine.[58] Chloroquine's shape and structure could be tailored and refined with knowledge only of chemical structure and biological activity. Pharmaceutical development continues to rely on these fundamental principles operating in the epistemic space which organic chemistry has opened in the realm of biology. This is one part of the history of molecularization.

I am, of course, one of many who have pushed for historical analysis of molecularization. Soraya de Chadarevian and Harmke Kamminga in their fine edited volume, *Molecularizing Biology and Medicine*, outline the major trends across much of the twentieth century.[59] They, along with the volume's other contributors, make a strong case for the transformative impact of molecularization on biomedicine from the 1910s through the 1990s. Though the editors trace a satisfying narrative in their introduction, the essays that comprise *Molecularizing Biology and Medicine* yield no coherent meaning for molecularization, leaving the impression only of a provocative label for a project whose overall image is just dimly discernible. In the end, the book is a fine beginning. But I would like to see the process of molecularization maintained at the center of inquiry, rather than left in the background as it has been in many historical accounts. Certainly, historians should examine the molecularization project beyond the narrow bounds of molecular genetics, where most historical efforts have been focused.[60] Looking at fit and specificity helps to keep the molecules and the fundamentally chemical nature of much biological knowledge and biomedical intervention at center stage. In fields such as molecular biology and molecular genetics, the molecular level of explanation is clear. Yet I would prefer not to surrender "molecularization" to those who would limit its scope to molecular biology and molecular genetics. I want to argue that this is part of a far broader trend impacting many areas of science, technology, and medicine beginning in the late nineteenth century and continuing today.

For this reason, I suggest that we look at a long twentieth century to find the big picture of the molecularization project. While it is possible to find precursors in the earlier mechanical philosophies or the iatrochemical traditions, the increasingly successful interventions of synthetic chemists and the development of chemical structure theory in the late nineteenth century began a continuous, congruous, and growing understanding of atoms and molecules as having well defined size and shape.[61] Structure theory and a tetrahedral carbon atom were essential elements that made possible a fit-and-specificity understanding of synthetic dyes acting in biological systems. The synthetic dye industry itself was a location for the growth of the molecular vision.[62]

The British chemist, William Henry Perkin's (1838-1907) mid-century attempt to synthesize the natural antimalarial drug quinine from simpler precursors was a major catalyst for the birth of the synthetic dye industry.[63] Perkin had based his synthesis on the number and type of atoms in his starting materials and his target without attention to structure and shape, indicating that he was operating in a conceptual space quite different than that of the chemists of the 1880s and 1890s. Their acceptance of structure theory and the tetrahedral carbon atom added shape and size to the basic concepts of mass and number. Nevertheless, Perkin had in hand sufficient tools to alter organic molecules in complex and reproducible ways, so when his attempt at quinine yielded instead an intensely colored substance, he exploited his finding to produce a commercial synthetic dye. Perkin got not quinine from his reaction but the novel synthetic dye, mauve. And, as others followed his lead, new chemical industries arose based on synthetic dyes, pharmaceuticals, and fine chemicals. Together, the concepts of molecular shape and the growing array of chemical reactions and molecular interventions propelled chemical science and industry further into biology and medicine. Paul Ehrlich's work in chemotherapy and immunology illuminate this early interpenetration. And the twentieth-century molecularization of science and technology extends beyond medicine and biology.

Chemical thinking and chemical instruments have shaped industry and science from the second industrial revolution in the late nineteenth century through to the molecularly based revolutions in nanotechnology, genomics, and microelectronics at the end of the twentieth century. This molecular view brought with it a host of physical, instrumental technologies. X-ray crystallography spans the twentieth century as a method of accessing the dimension of molecules and atoms. Similarly, in the post–World War II period, nuclear magnetic resonance spectroscopy became a tool first of chemical scientists and then of biomedical researchers. With increasing sensitivity and processing power, these technologies and many others were able to visualize not just small molecular structures but macromolecules.[64] Today, this molecularization can be found in pharmaceutical sciences, proteomics, biology, the manufacture of computer chips, even the purification of isotopes for nuclear power and weapons.

Since the time of Paul Ehrlich, the concepts of molecular shape and biological function have been linked. Here, in the first decade of the twenty-first century, chemistry has profoundly shaped our view of the world and our place in it. Who are we? We are the products of genes, genes made of molecules. What are mind and emotion? They are chemical states of the brain; if one is not "normal," pills can correct that. Plastics, drugs, DNA, food, vitamins, pollution, fuel: all chemical entities, all possible only through a molecular interpretation of the world. The molecular sciences and technologies also penetrated deeply into agricultural and the environment, from the Green Revolution and DDT to the replacement of natural products with synthetics.[65] The same was true of biomedicine. And within infectious disease, chemotherapy and immunology, especially vaccine development, stand out as sites of molecularization and rationalization. In chemotherapy and immunology, organic chemistry and biology can be clearly seen, in Emil Fischer's words, to have worked "with definite purpose to a common end."

Notes

1. Emil Fischer, "Faraday Lecture: Synthetical Chemistry in its Relation to Biology," *Journal of the Chemical Society*, 1907, *91*: 1749-65, quote on p. 1765. The lecture was delivered on 18 October 1907. Fischer (1852-1919), a German, was one of the preeminent organic chemists of his generation. He won the 1902 Nobel Prize in Chemistry.

2. In immunology, these concepts have been hotly contested. See, for example, Pauline M. H. Mazumdar, *Species and Specificity: An Interpretation of the History of Immunology* (New York: Cambridge University Press, 1995).

3. Ilana Löwy puts chemotherapy into the context of the molecularization of medicine, see, Löwy, "Biotherapies of Chronic Diseases in the Interwar Period: From Witte's Peptone to Penicillium Extract," *Studies in History and Philosophy of Science Part C: Studies in History and Philosophy of Biological and Biomedical Sciences*, 2005, *36*: 675-95, especially p. 691.

4. For more on Ehrlich, see Arthur M. Silverstein, *Paul Ehrlich's Receptor Immunology: The Magnificent Obsession* (San Diego, California: Academic Press, 2002); Mazumdar, *Species and Specificity*; Timothy Lenoir, "A Magic Bullet: Research for Profit and the Growth of Knowledge in Germany Around 1900," *Minerva*, 1988, *26*: 66-88; John Parascandola, "The Theoretical Basis of Paul Ehrlich's Chemotherapy," *Journal of the History of Medicine and Allied Sciences*, 1981, *36*: 19-43; John Parascandola and Ronald Jasensky, "Origins of the Receptor Theory of Drug Action," *Bulletin of the History of Medicine*, 1974, *48*: 199-220; and C. H. Browning, "Emil Behring and Paul Ehrlich: Their Contributions to Science," *Nature*, 1955, *175*: (parts 1& 2) 570-75 & 616-19.

5. Ehrlich held a number of posts in Berlin before becoming a public health officer in Frankfurt-am-Main. Then, in 1899, he became director of the new Royal Institute of Experimental Therapy in Frankfurt. He was also given directorship of the neighboring Georg Speyerhaus, established by Franziska Speyer.

6. Paul Ehrlich, "Address Delivered at the Dedication of the Georg-Speyer-Haus," in *The Collected Papers of Paul Ehrlich*, volume III, *Chemotherapy*, ed. F. Himmelweit (New York: Pergamon Press, 1960), pp. 53-63, delivered 6 September 1906, questions on p. 55.

7. Ehrlich, "Address," p. 55.

8. Ehrlich, "Address," p. 55.

9. P. Ehrlich and P. Guttmann, "Über die Wirkung des Methylenblau bei Malaria," *Berliner klinische Wochenschrift*, 1891, *28*: 953-56.

10. For a quick tour of some of this chemistry, see the Royal Society of Chemistry's website: http://pubs.rsc.org/Education/EiC/issues/2005July/painrelief.asp, viewed 21 May 2007.

11. Otto Fischer, full name Philipp Otto Fischer, succeeded his cousin as professor of chemistry at Erlangen in 1885.

12. German Patent 29123, 8 June 1883, Ludwig Knorr, *Berichte der Deutschen Chemischen Gesellschaft*, 1883, *17*: 546; Knorr, "Einwirkung von Acetessigester auf Phenylhydrazin," *Berichte der Deutschen Chemischen Gesellschaft*, 1883, *16*: 2597-99; and Knorr, "Ueber die Constitution der Chinizinderivate," *Berichte der Deutschen Chemischen Gesellschaft*, 1884, *17*: 2032-49. For more on the development of the antipyretics, see Jan R. McTavish, *Pain and Profits: The History of the Headache and Its Remedies in America* (New Brunswick, New Jersey: Rutgers University Press, 2004).

13. For more on this relationship, see Parascandola and Jasensky, "Origins of the Receptor Theory."

14. Lenoir, "Magic Bullet," pp. 81-82.

15. For an understanding of chemical structure determination in this period and a discussion of structures as chemical shorthand, see Leo B. Slater, "Woodward, Robinson, and Strychnine: Chemical Structure and Chemists' Challenge," *Ambix*, 2001, *48*: 161-89.

16. For more on the history of avian malaria, see Leo B. Slater, "Malarial Birds: Modeling Infectious Human Disease in Animals," *Bulletin of the History of Medicine*, 2005, *79*: 261-94.

17. Dr. Roehl's "Plasmochin" report, sent by Winthrop Chemical Company with their letter of 16 December 1926, folder 500, box 50, series 100, Record Group 1, Rockefeller Foundation Archives, Rockefeller Archive Center, Sleepy Hollow, New York, p. 4. This report is essentially a slightly annotated translation of Roehl's article, W. Roehl, "Die Wirkung des Plasmochins auf die Vogelmalaria," *Archiv für Schiffs- und Tropen-Hygiene, Pathologie und Therapie exotischer Krankheiten, Beihefte*, 1926, *30*: 311-18.

18. August Wingler, "Dyes and Methylene Blue in Medico-Chemical Research," in *Medicine in its Chemical Aspects*, vol. 2 (Leverkusen: I. G. Farbenindustrie A.G., 1934), pp. 223-28, especially p. 225.

19. Werner Schulemann, "Synthetic Anti-Malarial Preparations: A Discussion of the Various Steps which Led to the Synthesis and Discovery of 'Plasmoquine' and a Brief Account of Its Use in Tropical Medicine," *Proceedings of the Royal Society of Medicine*, 1932, *25*: 898.

20. Wingler, "Dyes and Methylene Blue," pp. 224-25.

21. Harold King and his co-workers pursued similar structure-activity investigations, on a smaller scale, in Great Britain. See A. Cohen and Harold King, "Antiplasmodial Action and Chemical Constitution: Part I. Cinchona Alkaloidal Derivatives and Allied Substances," *Proceedings of the Royal Society of London, Series B*, 1938, *125*: 49-60; and A. D. Ainley and Harold

King, "Antiplasmodial Action and Chemical Constitution: Part II. Some Simple Synthetic Analogues of Quinine and Cinchonine," *Proceedings of the Royal Society of London, Series B*, 1938, *125*: 60-92.

22. See, for example, Interessengemeinschaft Farbenindustrie Aktiengesellschaft, *Medicine in its Chemical Aspects*, vols. 1-3 (Leverkusen: I. G. Farbenindustrie A.G., 1933, 1934 & 1935).

23. For more detail on Bayer and this work, also see Schulemann, "Synthetic Anti-Malarial Preparations;" and Wingler, "Dyes and Methylene Blue," pp. 224-25.

24. Published accounts of Bayer's contributions to synthetic antimalarials can be found in *From Germanin to Acylureidopenicillin: Research that Made History, Documentation of Scientific Revolution*, ed. Rosemarie Alstaedter (Leverkusen: Bayer AG, 1980), pp. 18-24; Horst-Bernd Dünschede, "Tropenmedizinische Forschung bei Bayer," *Düsseldorfer Arbeiten zur Geschichte der Medizin, vol. 2* (Düsseldorf: Michael Triltsch Verlag, 1971), pp. 55-82; Fritz Mietzsch, "Beiträge zur Entwicklung der Chemotherapie aus den Laboratorien der Farbenfabriken Bayer" *Arzneimittel-Forschung*, September 1956, *6(4)*: 503-8; Fritz Mietzsch, "Entwicklungslinien der Chemotherapie (Vom chemischen Standpunkt gesehen)," *Klinische Wochenschrift*, 1951, *29*: 125-34; and Schulemann, "Synthetic Anti-Malarial Preparations."

25. Fritz Schönhöfer, "40 Jahre Plasmochin," *Arzneimittel-Forschung*, 1965, *15*: 1256-58.

26. After Schulemann, "Synthetic Anti-Malarial Preparations," p. 900.

27. Wingler, "Dyes and Methylene Blue," pp. 226-27.

28. For the rational approach to antibiotics through an understanding of bacterial metabolism, see, for example, Paul Fildes, "A Rational Approach to Chemotherapy," *Lancet*, 1940, *238*: 955-57. This rational approach through metabolism was, in part, a complement to vitamin-type research. Both entailed the determination of essential nutrients for an organism, but in the case of antibiotic research the essential nutrients were replaced with altered analogs that might block the proper uptake of similar and essential compounds.

29. For another view into the state of chemotherapy in this period, see Walter A. Jacobs, "The Chemotherapy of Protozoan and Bacterial Infections," *The Harvey Lectures*, 1923-1924, 67-95. Lecture delivered 8 December 1923.

30. Roehl's "Plasmochin" report, p. 7.

31. Roehl's "Plasmochin" report, p. 7.

32. Roehl's "Plasmochin" report, pp. 7-8.

33. Roehl's "Plasmochin" report, p. 8.

34. E. M. Lourie, "Studies on Chemotherapy in Bird Malaria: I.–Acquired Immunity in Relation to Quinine Treatment in *Plasmodium Cathemerium* Infections," *Annals of Tropical Medicine and Parasitology*, 1934, *28*: 151-69; Lourie "Studies on Chemotherapy in Bird Malaria: II.–Observations Bearing on the Mode of Action of Quinine," *Annals of Tropical Medicine*

and Parasitology, 1934, *28*: 255-77; Lourie, "Studies on Chemotherapy in Bird Malaria: III.–Difference in Response to Quinine Treatment between Strains of *Plasmodium Relictum* of Widely-Separated Geographical Origins," *Annals of Tropical Medicine and Parasitology*, 1934, *28*: 513-23; William H. Taliaferro and Lucy Graves Taliaferro, "Reduction in Immunity in Chicken Malaria Following Treatment with Nitrogen Mustard," *Journal of Infectious Diseases*, 1948, *82*: 5-30; William H. Taliaferro, "The Role of the Spleen and Lymphoid-Macrophage System in the Quinine Treatment of *Gallinaceum* Malaria: I. Acquired Immunity and Phagocytosis," *Journal of Infectious Diseases*, 1948, *83*: 164-80; William H. Taliaferro and F. E. Kelsey, "The Role of the Spleen and Lymphoid-Macrophage System in the Quinine Treatment of *Gallinaceum* Malaria: II. Quinine Blood Levels," *Journal of Infectious Diseases*, 1948, *83*: 181-99; William H. Taliaferro and Lucy Graves Taliaferro, "The Role of the Spleen and Lymphoid-Macrophage System in the Quinine Treatment of *Gallinaceum* Malaria: III. The Action of Quinine and of Immunity on the Parasite," *Journal of Infectious Diseases*, 1949, *84*: 187-220.

35. Lourie, "Studies on Chemotherapy in Bird Malaria: II."

36. By the early 1930s, Bayer employed several dozen chemical scientists at Elberfeld to support these developments.

37. Hans Mauss and Fritz Mietzsch, "Atebrin, ein neues Heilmittel gegen Malaria," *Klinische Wochenschrift*, 19 August 1933, *12(33)*: 1276-78; H. Mauss and F. Mietzsch, "Notiz zur Arbeit von O. J. Magidson und A. M. Grigorowski: Acridin-Verbindungen und ihre Antimalaria-Wirkung (I. Mitteil.)," *Berichte der Deutschen-Chemischen Gesellschaft*, 1936, *69*: 641; and H. Mauss, "Acridinverbindungen als Malariamittel," in *Medizin und Chemie*, vol. 4 (Berlin: Verlag Chemie, 1942), pp. 60-72.

38. For Kikuth's account of atabrine in the avian model systems, see Walter Kikuth, "Zur Weiterentwicklung synthetisch dargestellter Malariamittel: I. Über die chemotherapeutische Wirkung des Atebrin" *Deutsche medizinische Wochenschrift*, 1932, *58*: 530-31.

39. Hans Mauss and Fritz Mietzsch "Atebrin," 31 January 1933, 30 pages, Bayer Archives, Leverkusen (hereafter BAL) Pharm. wiss. Labor Elberfeld, Berichte, Mietzsch, 103/17.E.2.c.

40. The Prontosil story is nicely connected to the antimalarial story in David Greenwood, "The Quinine Connection," *Journal of Antimicrobial Chemotherapy*, 1992, *30*: 417-27.

41. "Der grundlegende chemische Unterschied zwischen Plasmochin und Atebrin...," 12 April 1934, p. 2, BAL Pharma Produkte A-Z, Atebrin 1932-1939, 166/8.

42. Franz Sioli, "Zur Weiterentwicklung synthetisch dargestellter Malariamittel: II. Über die Wirkung des Atebrin bei der Impfmalaria der Paralytiker," *Deutsche medizinische Wochenschrift*, 1932, *58*: 531-33.

43. F. M. Peter, "Zur Weiterentwicklung synthetisch dargestellter Malariamittel: III. Über die Wirkung des Atebrin gegen natürliche Malaria," *Deutsche medizinische Wochenschrift*, 1932, *58*: 533-35.

44. Peter Mühlens, "Die synthetischen Malariamittel Plasmochin und Atebrin," *Münchener Medizinische Wochenschrift*, 1932, *79*: 537-40; P. Mühlens and O. Fischer, "Über Malaria behandlung mit Atebrin," *Archiv für Schiffs- und Tropen-Hygiene Pathologie und Therapie exotischer Krankheiten*, 1932, *36*: 196-207.

45. Quinacrine was marketed in Germany as Atebrin, in Britain as mepacrine, and in the United States as Atabrine or Chinacrin. One may also find it referred to as acrichin or acrichine.

46. Some of this work was published during the war. See, for example, Fritz Schönhöfer, "Über die Bedeutung der chinoiden Bindung in Chinolinverbindungen für die Malariawirkung," *Hoppe-Seyler's Zeitschrift für physiologische Chemie*, 1942, *274*: 1-8.

47. Combined Intelligence Objectives Sub-Committee, "Clinical Testing of Antimalarials by I. G. Farben," CIOS XXIII-13, 20 May 1945, p. 11.

48. Walter Menk and Werner Mohr, "Sontochin (Nivaquine) in seiner Therapeutischen Wirkung bei Malaria," *Zeitschrift für Tropenmedizin und Parasitologie*, 1950, *2*: 351-61. See also, Combined Intelligence Objectives Sub-Committee, "Pharmaceuticals and Insecticides at I. G. Farben Plants Elberfeld and Leverkusen," CIOS XXIII-12, [1945], p. 30.

49. For more on German antimalarial efforts during World War II, see Richard L. Kenyon, Joseph A. Wiesner, and C. E. Kwartler, "Chloroquine Manufacture," *Industrial and Engineering Chemistry*, 1949, *41*: 654-62, p. 655; Combined Intelligence Objectives Sub-Committee, "Pharmaceuticals and Insecticides at I. G. Farben Plants Elberfeld and Leverkusen," CIOS XXIII-12, [1945]; "Clinical Testing of Antimalarials by I. G. Farben," CIOS XXIII-13, 20 May 1945; "Professor Doctor Werner Schulemann Malariologist," CIOS XXIII-17, [1945]; "Pharmaceutical Targets in Southern Germany," CIOS XXIV-16; "Insecticides, Insect Repellents, Rodenticides and Fungicides: I. G. Farbenindustrie A. G., Elberfeld and Leverkusen," CIOS XXVI-73, 19-30 May 1945, and "Tropical Medicines and Other Medical Subjects in Germany," CIOS XXIX-35; and British Intelligence Objectives Sub-Committee, "Pharmaceuticals: Research and Manufacturing at I. G. Farbenindustrie," BIOS Final Report No. 116, 7-23 August 1945.

50. For more on the British project, see David Greenwood, "Conflicts of Interest: The Genesis of Synthetic Antimalarial Agents in Peace and War," *Journal of Antimicrobial Chemotherapy*, 1995, *36(5)*: 857-72; F. H. K. Green and Sir Gordon Covell, eds., *Medical Research, History of the Second World War, United Kingdom Medical Series*, (London: H.M. Stationery Office, 1953), pp. 155-60; F. L. Rose, "A Chemotherapeutic Search in Retrospect," *Journal*

of the Chemical Society, 1951, 2770-88; and various authors in *Annals of Tropical Medicine and Parasitology*, 1945, *39(3 & 4)*, (Liverpool School of Tropical Medicine).

51. René J. Dubos, "The Significance of the Structure of the Bacterial Cell in the Problems of Antisepsis and Chemotherapy," in *Chemotherapy* (Philadelphia: University of Pennsylvania Press, 1941), pp. 29-42, quote on p. 29.

52. Dubos, "Significance," p. 29.

53. For more on Dubos, see Jill Elaine Cooper, "Of Microbes and Men: A Scientific Biography of René Jules Dubos" (Ph.D. dissertation, Rutgers University, 1998) and Carol L. Moberg, *René Dubos, Friend of the Good Earth: Microbiologist, Medical Scientist, Environmentalist* (Washington, D.C.: ASM Press, 2005).

54. Dubos, "Significance," p. 40. Dubos cites Paul Ehrlich, *Proceedings of the Royal Society*, London, 1900, *66*: 424-48, Ehrlich quote on p. 432.

55. George H. Hitchings, Gertrude B. Elion, Henry VanderWerff, and Elvira A. Falco, "Pyrimidine Derivatives as Antagonists of Pteroylglutamic Acid," *Journal of Biological Chemistry*, 1948, *174*: 765-66; E. A. Falco, G. H. Hitchings, P. B. Russell, and H. VanderWerff, "Antimalarials as Antagonists of Purines and Pteroylglutamic Acid," *Nature*, 1949, *164*: 107-8; and E. A. Falco, L. G. Goodwin, G. H. Hitchings, I. M. Rollo, P. B. Russell, "2:4-diaminopyrimidines—A New Series of Antimalarials," *British Journal of Pharmacology*, 1951, *6*: 185-200.

56. By the 1990s, molecular biology techniques allowed for new understandings of drug resistance in malaria parasites. For more on the genetic basis of chloroquine resistance, see Thomas E. Wellems, Lindsey J. Panton, Ilya Y. Gluzman, Virgilio E. do Rosario, Robert W. Gwadz, Annie Walker-Jonah, and Donald J. Krogstad, "Chloroquine Resistance not Linked to *mdr*-like Genes in a *Plasmodium falciparum* Cross," *Nature*, 1990, *345*: 253-55; and Xin-zhuan Su, Michael T. Ferdig, Yaming Huang, Chuong Q. Huynh, Anna Liu, Jingtao You, John C. Wootton, and Thomas E. Wellems, "A Genetic Map and Recombination Parameters of the Human Malaria Parasite *Plasmodium falciparum*," *Science*, 1999, *286*: 1351-53. More generally on the history of microbial resistance, see Angela N. H. Creager, "Adaptation or Selection? Old Issues and New Stakes in the Postwar Debates over Bacterial Drug Resistance," *Studies in History and Philosophy of Biological and Biomedical Sciences*, 2007, *38*: 159-90.

57. S. Moreau, B. Perly, and J. Biguet, "Interactions de la chloroquine avec la ferriprotoporphyrine IX. Étude par resonance magnétique nucléaire," *Biochimie*, 1982, *64*: 1015-25; Serge Moreau, Bruno Perly, Claude Chachaty, and Colette Deleuze, "A Nuclear Magnetic Resonance Study of the Interactions of Antimalarial Drugs with Porphyrins," *Biochimica et Biophysica Acta*, 1985, *840*: 107-16; and Andrew F. G. Slater, "Chloroquine: Mechanism of Drug Action and Resistance in *Plasmodium Falciparum*," *Pharmacology and Therapeutics*, 1993, *57*: 203-35.

58. For more on the mode of action of chloroquine, see A. C. Chou, and C. D. Fitch, "Ferriprotoporphyrin IX Fulfills the Criteria for Identification as the Chloroquine Receptor of Malaria Parasites," *Biochemistry*, 1980, *19*: 1543–49; and Arnulf Dorn, Sudha Rani Vippagunta, Hugues Matile, Catherine Jaquet, Jonathan L. Vennerstrom, and Robert G. Ridley, "An Assessment of Drug-Haematin Binding as a Mechanism for Inhibition of Haematin Polymerisation by Quinoline Antimalarials," *Biochemical Pharmacology*, 1998, *55*: 727–36.

59. Soraya de Chadarevian and Harmke Kamminga, eds., *Molecularizing Biology and Medicine: New Practices and Alliances, 1930s-1970s* (Amsterdam: Harwood Academic Publishers, 1998).

60. Joseph Fruton laments the loss of *chemical* and *chemistry* in describing biological science as *molecular*. This seems an accident of history that we might accept. See, for example, Joseph S. Fruton, *Proteins, Enzymes, Genes: The Interplay of Chemistry and Biology* (New Haven, Connecticut: Yale University Press, 1999), pp. 16-19. Likewise, those who argue for the *informational* over the *structural* school of molecular biology might wish to minimize the *molecular*. I would argue that the information they value is chemically encoded and that theory testing and intervention are only possible and intelligible at the level of molecules and atoms, in terms of shape and specificity.

61. One account that traces the origins of chemotherapy back to Paracelsus is Iago Galdston, *Behind the Sulfa Drugs: A Short History of Chemotherapy* (New York: D. Appleton-Century, 1943). Galdston also treats Ehrlich and others on his way to the sulfa drugs.

62. For an excellent account of the early synthetic dye industry and the role—or lack thereof—of chemical structure theory, see Anthony S. Travis, *The Rainbow Makers: The Origins of the Synthetic Dyestuffs Industry in Western Europe* (Bethlehem, Pennsylvania: Lehigh University Press, 1993).

63. For more on Perkin, see Simon Garfield, *Mauve: How One Man Invented a Color that Changed the World* (New York: W. W. Norton, 2002).

64. For approaches to instrumentation in chemical science, see Peter J. T. Morris, ed., *From Classical to Modern Chemistry: The Instrumental Revolution* (London: Royal Society of Chemistry, 2002).

65. DDT (dichloro-diphenyl-trichloroethane) as public-health insecticide is intimately linked to malaria control. It is also notorious for its impact on the environment when used as an agricultural insecticide and in this role points up the complex chemical connections between living things and their environment.

Scientific Discoveries: An Institutionalist and Path-Dependent Perspective

J. Rogers Hollingsworth

This paper is a part of a research program analyzing how institutional and organizational factors facilitate or hamper the making of major discoveries in basic biomedical science.[*1] Most of the paper focuses on research organizations and institutions in the United States during the twentieth century, though there are occasional soft comparisons with the institutional environments and organizations of other societies. The research program as a whole examines research organizations in Britain, France, Germany, and the United States throughout the twentieth century.

Critical to this paper is the definition of a major discovery. A major breakthrough or discovery is a finding or process, often preceded by numerous small advances, which leads to a new way of thinking about a problem. This new way of thinking is highly useful to numerous scientists in addressing problems in diverse fields of science. Historically, a major breakthrough in biomedical science was a radical or new idea, the development of a new methodology, or a new instrument or invention.[2] It usually did not occur all at once, but involved a process of investigation taking place over a substantial period of time and required a great deal of tacit and/or local knowledge, if not both.[3]

The analysis is multilevel in nature. Research in most research organizations takes place in laboratories located in departments or divisions that are part of an organization; in turn such research organizations are embedded in a larger institutional environment. Figure One is a simplified perspective of the way each of these levels influences the process of making major discoveries. One of the major challenges facing the scientific community is to understand how activities at one level of analysis are related to those at other levels.[4] As the social science community lacks a good understanding of the way processes at multi-levels of societies operate, this paper is intended to make a modest contribution toward explaining how interactions occurring at multiple levels influence major scientific discoveries. The paper's perspective is nonlinear and co-evolutionary. The heavy downward arrows in Figure 1 indicate the dominant type of influence which institutions and organizations exert on laboratories and researchers. The direction is not one way, for activities at the level of the laboratory influence the behavior of entire organizations as well as institutional environments, and these in turn feed back on the activities of individual laboratories. Collectively, all of these factors help to explain why there is variation across laboratories in departments, across departments in organizations, across organizations in a society, and across societies themselves when it comes to the making of major discoveries. While each of these four levels is constantly changing, it is the institutional environment which is most enduring and resistant to change. Actors at lower levels are greatly constrained by the norms, rules, and systems of rules that by definition constitute the institutional makeup of a society.[5]

Figure 1. Factors at multiple levels influencing major discoveries.

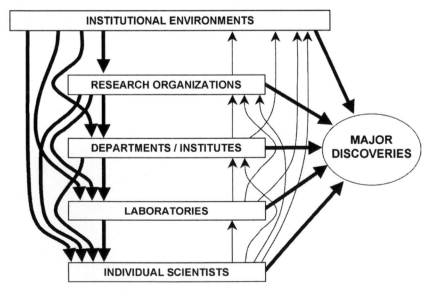

Institutional Environments and Research Organizations

The institutional environments of research organizations consist of a variety of variables, all of which are treated equally here. Institutional environments range from weak to strong.[6] Weak institutional environments exert only modest influence (1) over the appointment of scientific personnel of research organizations, (2) in determining whether a particular scientific discipline will exist in a research organization, (3) over the level of funding for research organizations, (4) in prescribing the level of training necessary for a scientific appointment (e.g., the habilitation), and (5) over scientific entrepreneurship (e.g., the existence of norms of individualism that socialize young people to undertake high-risk research projects).

Strong institutional environments are at the opposite end of the continuum on each of these characteristics. France is an example of a country that tended to have a strong institutional environment throughout the twentieth century, while research organizations in the United States have been embedded in a relatively weak institutional environment. However, the institutional environments of societies change over time, and the changes in the institutional environment may influence the capacity of a society to make major scientific discoveries. The data on the institutional environments of these four countries suggest that there is a high degree of complementarity among the five concepts constituting institutional environments: when one is weakly developed, the others tend to be weakly developed and vice versa. This perspective resonates with the concept of institutional complementarity, found in a variety of work within social science literature.[7]

The institutional environment in which research organizations are embedded has an impact on organizational behavior. The stronger the institutional environment is, the greater the organizational isomorphism—a factor that results in less diversity among the types and behavior of research organizations. When organizational isomorphism is high, there are strong pressures for organizations to converge in their behavior and culture. On the other hand, in weak institutional environments, diversity is greater with regard to types of research organizations and the structure and culture of the organizations. I have found that such a society possesses greater potential for multiple scientific breakthroughs.[8]

In societies in which external controls over organizations are highly institutionalized and strong, there has been less variation in the structure and behavior of research organizations. There, the connectedness[9] between research organizations and their institutional or external environments has generally been so strong that research organizations have had relatively little autonomy with which to pursue independent strategies and goals. Conversely, the weaker the institutional environment in which research organizations have been embedded, the greater the variation in the structure and behavior of research organizations. When the institutional environments have been more weakly developed, organizations generally have had greater autonomy and flexibility to develop new knowledge and to be highly innovative. Hence, in societies where institutional environments have been the most developed, rigid, and strong, there has been less organizational autonomy and flexibility, and fewer radical innovations have occurred in basic and applied science.[10]

Heterogeneity in the types of research organizations has tended to be greater in weak institutional environments than in strong ones. Hence, in the United States, with a relatively weak institutional environment, there have long been many more types of universities than in Germany, where universities that have been embedded in a strong institutional environment resemble one another much more.[11] In the United States, we find small, elite, private universities (Rockefeller University, California Institute of Technology, Rice University); medium-sized private universities (Johns Hopkins University, University of Chicago, Vanderbilt University, Princeton); and large private universities (Harvard, Stanford, MIT, NYU). In addition, there are the large public universities in California (Berkeley, UCLA, UCSB, UCSD) and the Midwest (Michigan, Indiana, Wisconsin, Illinois, Minnesota). Historically, each type of university featured a distinct type of population, somewhat differentiated from other types of research organizations, in part because their dominant competencies were not easily learned or transmitted across organizational populations.[12]

Of course, in both strong and weak institutional environments every organization is unique, meaning that heterogeneity always exists among organizations. But organizations of the same type, and in the same institutional environment, are likely to share many of the same attributes.[13] Even if weak institutional environments led to more heterogeneity among types of organizations, forces were nevertheless at work that led to increasing organizational isomorphism both across and within organizational types.

The society likely to have had numerous breakthroughs was one with a weak institutional environment that permitted a high degree of nonconformity and high-risk research. My in-depth, cross-national, and cross-temporal organizational study of 291 major discoveries in the twentieth century demonstrates that major discoveries tended to occur more frequently in organizational contexts that were relatively small and had high degrees of autonomy, flexibility, and the capacity to adapt rapidly to the fast pace of change in the global environment of science. As Table 1 illustrates, such organizations tended to have moderately high levels of scientific diversity and internal structures that facilitated the communication and integration of ideas across diverse scientific fields.[14] These organizations tended to have scientific leaders with a keen scientific vision of the direction in which new fields in science were heading and the capacity to develop a strategy for recruiting scientists capable of moving a research agenda in that direction.

Table 1. Characteristics of organizational contexts facilitating the making of major discoveries.*

- Moderately high scientific diversity
- Capacity to recruit scientists who internalize scientific diversity
- Communication and social integration of scientists from different fields through frequent and intense interaction
- Leaders who integrate scientific diversity, have the capacity to understand the direction in which scientific research is moving, provide rigorous criticism in a nurturing environment, have a strategic vision for integrating diverse areas, and have the ability to secure funding to achieve organizational goals
- Flexibility and autonomy associated with loose coupling with the institutional environment

* These characteristics were derived from intense, in-depth analysis of the organizational contexts in which major discoveries either occurred or did not occur through the twentieth century in Britain, France, Germany, and the United States (see J. Rogers Hollingsworth, Ellen Jane Hollingsworth, and Jerald Hage, eds., *The Search for Excellence: Organizations, Institutions, and Major Discoveries in Biomedical Science*, 2008).

Organizational contexts featuring such characteristics were Rockefeller University, the California Institute of Technology, the Salk Institute, and the Johns Hopkins University Medical School. Scientists at the relatively small Rockefeller University made more major discoveries in basic biomedical science than any other organization in the world during the twentieth century.[15]

Figure 2 portrays the kind of organizational context in which major discoveries are more likely to occur. These contexts possess a moderately high degree of scientific diversity and a high level of communication among scientists in diverse fields of science. Of course, as organizations acquire more and more diverse fields of science, they run up against limits to their ability to maintain communication across diverse fields.

Even in societies with relatively weak institutional environments, most organizational contexts hampered the making of major discoveries. Over time, most research organizations tended to become relatively large and more bureaucratic. They were divided into an increasing number of scientific disciplines, and communication diminished among scientists working in the various fields within the organization (see Table 2). Unlike Rockefeller University, most research universities were structured around

Table 2. Characteristics of organizational contexts constraining the making of major discoveries.*

- *Differentiation*: Organizations with sharp boundaries among subunits such as basic biomedical departments and other subunits, the delegation of recruitment exclusively to department or other subunit level, the delegation of responsibility for extramural funding to the department or other subunit level.

- *Hierarchical authority*: Organizations were very hierarchical when they experienced centralized (a) decisionmaking about research programs, (b) decisionmaking about number of personnel, (c) control over work conditions, (d) budgetary control.

- *Bureaucratic coordination*: Organizations with high levels of standardization for rules and procedures.

- *Hyperdiversity*: This was the presence of diversity to such a deleterious degree that there could not be effective communication among actors in different fields of science or even in similar fields.

* These characteristics were derived from intense, in-depth analysis of the organizational contexts in which major discoveries either occurred or did not occur through the twentieth century in Britain, France, Germany, and the United States (see J. Rogers Hollingsworth, Ellen Jane Hollingsworth, and Jerald Hage, eds., *The Search for Excellence: Organizations, Institutions, and Major Discoveries in Biomedical Science*, 2008).

departments and academic disciplines: for that reason they lacked organizational flexibility and acquired a great deal of organizational inertia—since academic departments have had a tendency to continue working in the same general problem areas.

Figure 2. The Impact of communication and cognitive distance on major discoveries.

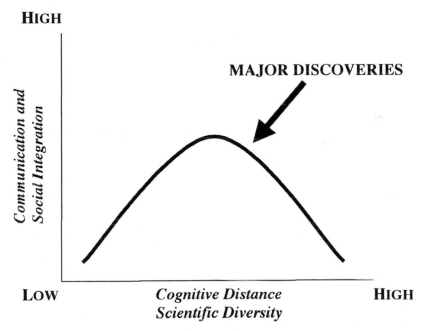

Institutional Environments and Isomorphism Within and Across Research Organizations

Societies vary in their capacity to produce major discoveries over time because they are influenced in various ways by several historical processes, notably organizational isomorphism and path dependency. Path dependency reminds us that the way things were previously organized influences the way they are organized today. Still, institutional environments, organizations, and individual actors are always changing. The stronger the institutional environment is, the greater the degree of organizational isomorphism and the greater the similarity of path-dependent processes among organizations. Even in societies with weak institutional environments, there are forces which lead over time to greater degrees of homogeneous behavior (i.e., organizational isomorphism) across and within organizations. Different populations of organizations in the same society develop a set of competencies and routines that become institutionalized but remain societally specific. As a result of these competencies, actors in both different and similar organizations engage in a great deal of common learning and socialization. Scientists, technicians, and administrators from different types of organizations in the same society acquire a great deal of common organizational know-how that is transmitted across time and organizations. Some years ago, DiMaggio and Powell[16] picked up on these ideas when they pointed out that organizations in the same society engage in many "mimetic processes." Later, Hodgson[17] developed the argument that routines are organizational metahabits which diffuse across populations of organizations within a particular institutional environment. To understand homogenizing forces across and within organizations in the same institutional environment, analysts have increasingly focused on control mechanisms of individuals in their socialization processes–although the control replicators are called many different things in the literature. Dawkins[18] used the term memes, Lumsden and Wilson[19] culturgens, Nelson and Winter[20] routines, and McKelvey[21] comps. Whatever the term, social scientists have been focusing for some time now on the way competition among organizational actors within an institutional environment is suppressed by norms, rules, habits, and conventions at the group and organizational levels.[22] Isomorphic pressures are especially strong when actors in highly saturated environments are competing for the same finite resources.[23]

Isomorphism, no matter how powerful a force, certainly does not sweep through history unimpeded. It occurs at a very moderate rate, constrained by many forces. One factor retarding organizational isomorphism is the existence of diverse types of research organizations in a society. Many years ago, Stinchcombe[24] made the astute observation that organizations founded at different points in time, even those of the same type, are influenced in their behavior for long periods of time by many of the cultural attributes of the social technologies current at the time of their foundation. When Stinchcombe made his observation, historians and social scientists had not explicitly developed the concepts of path dependency and organizational isomorphism, but his emphasis on how the history of organizations is permanently influenced by the moment of their creation is clearly suggestive of a path-dependency perspective. Stinchcombe was making the profound point that organizations do not necessarily closely track changes in their environment, but are somewhat inert, preserving certain nonadaptive qualities that often have deleterious effects on their capacity to be highly adaptive to their environments. Thus they resist isomorphic pressures; as a result, population heterogeneity persists despite forces leading to greater homogeneity.

There is a substantial body of literature suggesting that continuously high levels of radical innovation in modern societies require diversity in organizational forms and ideas, heterogeneity in organizational structures, and institutional environments with ample resources to nurture radical innovations.[25] Individual societies continuously confront contradictory pressures. On the one hand, they are subjected to processes that move organizational populations toward greater homogeneity and uniformity. On the other, homoeostatic forces within populations of specific types of organizations constrain evolutionary change and preserve nonadaptive forms, facilitating organizational inertia.[26] If a society is to be continuously creative and make radical innovations, it must have sustained variation and diversity in organizational forms and ideas, which are more likely to flourish in weak institutional environments.

However great the forces of isomorphism among populations of organizations are, new organizational forms may continue to emerge from time to time. Unfortunately, we lack sufficient theoretical tools to specify when and where radically new organizational types will emerge. For theoretical insights into this problem, some of our best sources are the biological literature on the processes of speciation. It is useful to think of the emergence of new organizational forms as an organizational mutant. Mutations occur all the time, among both biological and organizational species. However, most do not "take hold" as they are outnumbered in their population environments, crowded out, and "rapidly dissipate through the normal intermixing process."[27] Moreover, we know from numerous population-ecology studies that new organizations have low survival rates.[28]

Thought of as a mutation, a new organizational form is more likely to survive if it occurs in organizational environments that are sparsely populated, have ample resources to support such new development, and if it is not crowded out by the normal process of intermingling with other types of organizations. New surviving forms tend initially to be relatively autonomous from their environments. In such environments, organizational speciation may occur, and in the short term, a new form may be immune to the pressures of organizational isomorphism. Environments with resources exceeding demand offer a greater opportunity for a new organizational form to survive than do more competitively saturated environments.[29]

One example of the emergence of a new form of research organization is the establishment of several research institutions in the United States after 1960: the Salk Institute, the Scripps Research Institute (both in La Jolla, California), and the Fred Hutchinson Cancer Research Center (in Seattle, Washington). What was novel about these organizations compared with older ones (the Scripps Institute of Oceanography, the Rockefeller Institute, the various Carnegie Institutes, the Laboratory of Molecular Biology in the United Kingdom, the Institut Pasteur, the various Max Planck Institutes) was that this new form of research organization had no endowment, no permanent patron, and no assured source of financial support. These institutes, emerging in newly developing research environments in Southern California and Seattle, were managed by entrepreneurs skilled in raising money in the distinctive regional entrepreneurial landscape of the West Coast, where thousands of adventurous investors and philanthropists were in search of new, local investment niches. Traditional sources of capital–banks, the federal government, and more conservative philanthropists in the East who favored local organizations–tended to view these ventures with skepticism. Significantly, Silicon Valley emerged on the outskirts of Palo Alto, California, and the biotechnology industry also had much of its early success in the sparsely populated California landscape, not in the older centers of the United States where the industrial organizational density was quite high.

Since clusters of major discoveries tend to occur within relatively small organizations (see Table 1 and Figure 2), why is it that they may also occur within a large organization that is separated internally into various departments? Such rare occurrences tend to take place where the following two conditions exist:

- The organization must be extremely decentralized (permitting the actors making major discoveries to enjoy a high degree of autonomy and flexibility).
- The actors within the organization must have access to sufficiently diverse types of resources so that their scientific practices and administrative routines are not crowded out by those already institutionalized within the larger environment of the host organization.

The subunits of organizations where these clusters occur tend to have most of the characteristics listed in Table 1. According to evolutionary logic, those making major discoveries in a new scientific area of research tend to be in a better position to escape the institutionalized, homogenizing pressures of the existing research organizations and to possess the autonomy to intermix, interbreed, and reproduce their own intellectual progeny within their particular subunit of the larger organization.

The occurrence of a cluster of major discoveries in an organization, especially in a single department over thirty or forty years, is extraordinarily rare. Such a cluster of discoveries occurred in the Faculty of Arts and Sciences of Harvard University between the mid-1950s and the mid-1970s following the establishment of two new departments: the Department of Biochemistry and Molecular Biology, and the Department of Organismic and Evolutionary Biology. From each of these departments came a number of major discoveries. Significantly, these discoveries occurred in new departments, not in older ones encumbered by the inertia of the past.[30]

Over time, however, departments establish institutionalized routines, as do universities, and inertial processes set in, making it difficult for a highly creative subunit to continue being so innovative. At Harvard, as elsewhere, the level of innovativeness in a highly creative department eventually declined. Even organizations once highly decentralized, in which each subunit enjoyed a high degree of autonomy, tend to institutionalize a set of routines which diffuse across the organization, thereby establishing interlocking and conditional behaviors for all subunits of the organization. Eventually, a set of organizational routines becomes institutionalized throughout the organization, thus establishing shared collective capabilities, capacities, and behavior. In short, the organization emerges with a distinctive culture.[31]

Initially these two Harvard departments were headed by outstanding leadership with visionary agendas and staffed by scientists researching areas that were moderately high in diversity and very highly integrated scientifically—characteristics listed in Table 1 above. Even though each scientist within the department tended to pursue a separate body of research, the work was highly complementary to the research program of the entire department, which possessed a distinctive culture that glued it together.

Eventually, the distinctive scientific excellence of these departments declined. The scientific agenda of the new departments diffused to other organizations throughout the world, and many of the original members of the departments retired, died, or left. As scientific practices became routinized, no other leader emerged with a radically new agenda, capable of transforming the departments again into those on the cutting edge of science. The routines of the larger organization in which the departments were embedded slowly penetrated the departments. For all of these reasons, it is difficult for a research department to remain on the cutting edge of research for more than two or three decades. It is possible for a new department with a new scientific agenda to emerge, but seldom does such a department then proceed to produce clusters of pioneering discoveries in science. Rare indeed are the equivalents of within-organization mutations that are able to "take hold." Over the longer term, the distinctiveness of a "new departmental species" diminishes as it is constrained by the routines of the rest of the organization and other organizations in its institutional environment.

The Shift from a Weak to a Stronger Institutional Environment

Over time, the dynamics of the scientific enterprise embedded in a weak environment cause the institutional environment to become a much stronger one, and the institutional environment is transformed. In turn, the stronger institutional environment feeds back and alters the dynamics of the society's social system of science.

What is it about the scientific enterprise that leads to such change in the institutional environment of research organizations? For some time, the world has been experiencing an enormous expansion of new information and knowledge, which in turn begets ever more information and knowledge. For well over a century, the number of scientific papers and journals has been increasing exponentially, fueled by increases in the number of scientists and financial resources for science. For many years, developed economies also witnessed an exponential increase in the number of scientists and in the percentages of gross domestic product devoted to scientific research.[32] Of course, we have known since the time of Malthus that most forms of exponential growth must eventually come to a halt. No environment can continue to invest such extensive resources in scientific research: otherwise, at some point everyone would be a scientist and a society's entire gross national product (GNP) would be devoted to scientific research. Nevertheless, in all advanced industrial societies, the percentage of the population and of the GNP devoted to scientific research is continuing to increase, just not exponentially.[33]

Figure 3. Historical growth of investments in science.[34]

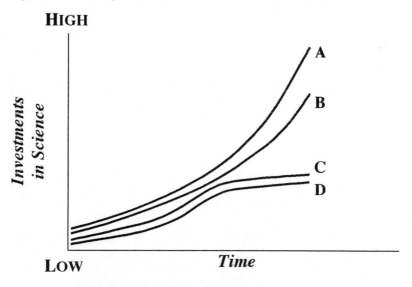

A Number of Scientific Papers
B Number of Scientific Journals
C Percent of Workforce in Research and Development
D Percent of Gross National Product for Research
   and Development

To understand these processes, we need to recall Max Planck's *Principle of Increasing Effort*: "with every advance in science, the difficulty of the task is increased; ever larger demands are made on the achievements of researchers, and the need for a suitable division of labor becomes more pressing."[35] With the expansion of knowledge comes increasing specialization, the development of new subspecialties, and the need for additional support staff. There are also increases in new instrumentation, leading to improved methods of measurement, which in turn lead to new fields of specialization and the need for even better instrumentation.

When new fields open up, the early investigators often make major breakthroughs: "the pickings are easier." As fields mature, the effort and resources required for significant advances increases continually. This constant "digging and searching" for significant findings as fields mature and broaden fuels an unending need for even more resources. As a result of this dynamic, the societal resources required to bring about a major discovery tend to increase exponentially. However, the number of major discoveries per annum increases very modestly–if at all. The idea that the number of important results stands as the square root of the total production of papers is frequently referred to as Rousseau's Law and is often attributed to Jean Jacques Rousseau.[36] Figure 4 illustrates the dramatic decline in the number of major discoveries relative to societal investments in science.

Figure 4. Number of major breakthroughs relative to scientific effort.[37]

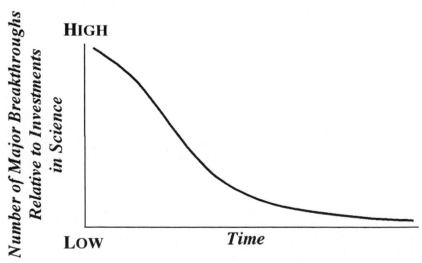

As the demand increased historically for more financial resources devoted to scientific research, central governments tended to become more involved in funding science and shoulder an increasing percentage of research expenditures, thus altering the institutional environment in which scientific research was embedded. This has had several consequences for the structure and culture of the social system of science. First, as central governments increased the proportion of their budgets spent on scientific research, politicians and government bureaucracies became more involved in making decisions about how funding should be allocated. Certain fields of science received an increasing proportion of investments while other areas were given only scant attention. Meanwhile, scientific communities have engaged in massive lobbying and public relations campaigns in an effort to influence the decisions of public officials. Second, as the amount of public sector money invested in science rose, governments increased their monitoring and auditing of research organizations in order to enhance research "efficiency and effectiveness" and to prevent fraud. Research organizations–like business firms–have increasingly become part of the "audit society."[38] Third, governments have acquired a taste for assessing the social benefits of scientific research, and have increasingly expressed little interest in funding the pursuit of knowledge for its own sake.[39] They increasingly support research that promises payoffs "here and now," in other words they prefer research with short-term societal benefits rather than high-risk research. Fourth, as central governments have become more involved in funding science and in making decisions about how the money should be used, research organizations have increasingly lost some of their autonomy. One consequence of these processes is an increasing convergence in the behavior of research organizations, a movement toward greater organizational isomorphism. Researchers have tended to gravitate toward scientific areas where there is funding. Since diversity in types of research organizations is associated with organizational autonomy and flexibility as well as scientific breakthroughs, an increase in the strength of the American institutional environment and the resulting greater organizational isomorphism has posed major problems for the capacity of American research organizations to continue making major breakthroughs.

Finally, the strengthening of the institutional environment of the American system of science has led to an increased commercialization of science. From a theoretical point of view, the strengthening of an institutional environment and an expanding role of the state in funding science has not necessarily led to the commercialization of science. This was quite contingent on a number of factors. In the United States case, the association between the strengthening of the institutional environment and the commercialization of science resulted primarily from the fact that the American scientific enterprise had historically been deeply embedded in a highly entrepreneurial culture.

To understand how this process has evolved in the American context, we must first recognize that social systems of science are somewhat bifurcated into public (i.e., communal) knowledge and private knowledge, and each of the two subsystems of knowledge had its own norms, incentives, and behavior.[40] Ironically, the increasing role of the government in funding science in the United States has led to a weakening in the development of public/communal knowledge/science. Historically, public knowledge has simply been knowledge owned by everyone in common. An example has been knowledge published in scientific journals to which everyone has had access: the reading of a scientific paper did not diminish its use for the next reader. This is very different from private knowledge, which is a private good, not available to all–in other words, if Jake eats his cake, no one else can eat it. If private knowledge has been patented or its use acquired by licensure, it is restricted to private use. These two systems of knowledge have had their own incentive structures. To most observers it has been relatively easy to understand the pecuniary motives of those who produce private knowledge for sale in the marketplace. But what have been the incentives that motivate those who produce knowledge owned in common by the community?

Merton[41] and others[42] observed that historically a major incentive to produce public knowledge was peer recognition. Societies bestowed rewards such as medals, prizes, and other forms of esteem on the discoverer. The scientist who was first in making a discovery received the credit, but unlike a sports tournament, there was little or no reward for being runner-up. Such an incentive system historically generated a great deal of competition among scientists and occasionally intense feuds as to who deserved recognition for priority. To facilitate the working of an effective incentive system and to assist in adjudicating priority disputes, the international scientific community has relied on scientific elites to determine which contributions to knowledge were important ones. Table 3 briefly describes the public science sector which has existed in the United States during the twentieth century.

While modern societies have had a scientific sector that produces public goods (i.e., public sector science), during the process of modernization, a for-profit sector has also produced science and technology at an accelerating rate. In the for-profit sector, the incentives for research have been primarily monetary in nature. During the past fifty years, the particular process of American industrialization has tended to diminish the proportion of individual scientists motivated to pursue communal obligations and the production of public knowledge and to increase the proportion of scientists engaged in the pursuit of pecuniary gain.[44] This process became one of the most important forces leading to a transformation in the American system of science. Table 4 summarizes the characteristics of the for-profit science sector in the United States.

Table 3. Public sector science in the United States.[45]

Property rights of scientific production: Science produced as a public good, belonging to the larger community.

Incentives to produce science: The reward was recognition of priority in discovery. Rewards came in the form of scientific awards, scientific citations, peer group esteem, salary increases.

Methods of funding: Sector funded by patrons, governments, grants, gifts, and contracts. If left to the market, the sector tended to be underfunded.

Locus of production: Heavy concentration in private non-profit and public sector organizations, although occasionally for-profit organizations produced public goods.

Vulnerability of sector: Sector tended to become bureaucratically funded over time. Funders tended to become less willing to finance high-risk projects. Research organizations became increasingly large and fragmented, hampering communication across diverse fields. As industrialization increased, an increasing proportion of scientists tended to seek monetary rewards rather than knowledge as an end in itself.

Long-term consequences of public sector science: Highly variable. Some knowledge had few or no effects on society; other knowledge often had great societal effects far in excess of the financial resources originally invested. Most major discoveries had significant payoffs only years later, though a few did have immediate benefits.

Table 4. For-profit sector science in the United States.[46]

Property rights of scientific production: Most of the science produced in this sector is proprietary in nature: Patents, copyrights, and licensing agreements are widely used for defining and protecting intellectual property rights.

Incentives to produce science: The rewards tended to be primarily monetary in nature.

Methods of funding: Sector predominantly funded by market forces in the private sector. Increasingly, universities and other non-profit organizations have been licensing discoveries made with federal funds and establishing science parks for private firms with strong affiliations to universities.

Locus of production: Historically heavily concentrated in for-profit organizations but in recent years, this sector has also had increasing activity in non-profit and public-sector research organizations.

Vulnerability of sector: The sector has been heavily dependent on decision makers with short-term horizons. As a result, the sector has tended to emphasize incremental research, designed to maximize profits in the short term.

Long-term consequences of heavy dependence on for-profit sector of science: If the society becomes excessively dependent on this sector for the production of knowledge, there is not likely to be enough new, basic knowledge necessary for high technological and economic growth over the long run.

While the for-profit sector of science has been expanding in the United States throughout the twentieth century, its rate of growth dramatically increased during the past twenty-five years. Ironically, the increasing role of the government in funding science in the United States has led to a weakening in the development of public, communal knowledge and science. The passage of the Bayh-Dole Act by Congress in 1980 did much to accelerate the expansion of the for-profit sector of science. This act stipulated that intellectual property resulting from federally (i.e., communally) funded research in universities could be patented, with universities and their researchers to be the beneficiaries of resulting royalties. The act stated that universities, as a condition for receiving federal research funds, had an obligation to make a good-faith effort to transfer resulting technological knowledge to the marketplace or to make it available in some other form for use by society. As a result, university linkages with industry increased dramatically. The number of patents issued to American universities tripled in a single decade (1984-1994). Numerous universities established intellectual property transfer offices, developed adjacent science parks, and dramatically increased their equity in firms located nearby and elsewhere. In 2000, American universities earned at least $1 billion by conservative estimates, primarily in royalties.[46]

Although an abundance of data is available on changes in patenting, the acquisition of patents by universities represents only the tip of the iceberg in the increasing commercialization of science in American research universities. My interviews with senior administrators and scientists in major research universities are consistent with other studies,[47] which indicate that patents amount to no more than 11 percent of the flow of knowledge with commercial value into the contemporary marketplace. The more important links between American universities and firms have been joint ventures between firms and individual university scientists, activities by university scientists in creating their own firms, efforts by universities and their affiliated foundations to act as venture capitalists and to become sole or part owners of new business ventures. Of course, a two-way interaction does take place between universities and firms, as firms in a number of sectors have substantially increased their investments in research conducted at universities. In recent years, major American universities have been at the forefront in developing new technologies that have spawned a transformation in the technology underlying a number of economic sectors: biotechnology, information technology, software, and computational biology. Because the knowledge created by American universities is so closely linked to these relatively new sectors, it is not surprising that the universities have been so intricately involved in their commercial development.[48]

In a twenty-five-year period following the passage of the Bayh-Dole Act, the historical relationship between public sector science and for-profit sector science has been significantly altered, bringing about a transformation in the culture and behavior of American universities. Historically, universities were sites which were primarily concerned with producing science as a public good, while for-profit firms were primarily engaged in producing science and technology as private goods, although the practices distinguishing these two types of organizations were never very clear cut. While the two types of organizations had somewhat different goals and reward structures, some universities and their faculties had long engaged in producing both public and private knowledge, as were also some for-profit organizations.[49] For example, the laboratories of AT&T and IBM had very enviable records for producing important basic scientific discoveries in the form of public science.[50] Nevertheless, in the aggregate the historical practices of American scientists in universities and in for-profit firms tended to be quite differentiated. In the past twenty-five years, the differences in the behavior of the two types of organizations have considerably narrowed.[51]

There is some evidence that in the short term the increasing commercialization of the American university is contributing to more technological innovations and to higher levels of economic productivity and growth. Clearly, a robust for-profit science sector has been an important stimulus to the American economy. However, sustainable increases in knowledge and technology are necessary in both public sector science and for-profit sector science. No one knows how to define the proper balance between the two sectors, but we have a great deal of evidence suggesting that, in the long run, public sector science will be underfunded should its financing be left to the market. Findings also indicate that the increasing commercialization of science and the bureaucratization of American research universities are beginning to discourage young investigators from conducting high-risk research.[52]

It is extremely difficult–perhaps impossible–to predict what the economic payoff is likely to be from particular discoveries, even important ones. For many years there has been considerable debate about the way advances in technology influence the agenda for fundamental and basic science. Historically, a great deal of interaction and co-evolution has occurred in the development of both science and technology. Yet, for long-term economic growth, a sustainable abundance of underlying advances in fundamental or basic knowledge is necessary. Indeed, the consequences of many fundamental advances in basic knowledge were only realized in the marketplace after long periods of time.[53] Moreover, most of the consequences were unintended. William H. Bragg and his son Lawrence were awarded the Nobel Prize in Physics in 1915 for work in crystallography, a field of science which many decades later is now transforming the biotechnology and pharmaceutical industries. The discovery by Oswald Avery in 1944 about the importance of DNA and the later discovery of the structure of DNA by Francis Crick and James

Watson had no short-term economic impact, even though in the long run they are perceived as being two of the most revolutionary discoveries in twentieth-century biology. Decades later, these three discoveries are contributing to the development of genetic engineering and numerous other forms of biotechnology. The same argument can be made about many other basic scientific discoveries which had little economic payoff in the short term, but reaped considerable dividends decades later. No doubt our societies have yet to realize the economic rewards of many other past basic discoveries. Of course, the economic significance of a few major, basic biomedical science discoveries was quickly picked up by business firms and the discoveries soon thereafter began to yield returns in the marketplace (e.g., the 1980 Nobel Prize in Chemistry awarded to Frederick Sanger and Walter Gilbert for their work on the sequencing of DNA; the 1978 Nobel Prize in Physiology or Medicine awarded to Daniel Nathans and Hamilton Smith for their research on the role of restriction enzymes in cutting up DNA, and the 1993 Nobel Prize in Chemistry to Kary Mullis for his development of the polymerase chain reaction).

The realization of economic rewards from fundamental discoveries in the biomedical sciences is a very inefficient and unpredictable process. There is no way of knowing in advance which discoveries will make a significant contribution to the wellbeing of society or when the consequences might be realized. What is clear from the historical record is that high-risk research and fundamental basic research are necessary for the general good of a society in the long run. There is no empirical evidence to suggest that the future wellbeing of societies will be any less dependent on fundamental discoveries and high-risk research than has been the case in the past. As Wolfgang Streeck has often reminded us, institutional environments that provide strong incentives for underinvestment and overconsumption in the short term are likely to result in an undersupply of productive assets in the longer term.[54]

As we consider the future of American science, it is helpful to engage in some historical perspective. In the late eighteenth and early nineteenth centuries, France was at the center of the global system of science.[55] Yet, by the middle of the nineteenth century, the center had already begun to shift to Germany, which retained its supremacy until the late 1920s.[56]

The center then shifted to Britain, which retained its supremacy through World War II. Since then, the United States has been the major center of Western science. The distribution of major prizes and rankings on citation indices make it unmistakably clear that the United States has been the hegemon in world science for at least a half century.

When we reflect retrospectively on these various centers, it becomes obvious that their decline in performance relative to other countries had already started just as they were thought to be at the height of their superior performance. The elite in each of these countries were so engaged in celebrating the achievements of their system that they failed to understand that the dynamics, the structure, and the contradictions inherent in each of their systems were leading to its decline. Future analysts engaging in retrospective analysis of American science at the end of the twentieth century are likely to observe a system which by most indicators was performing extraordinarily well. Yet, in retrospect, they are likely to note that the increasing organizational isomorphism both within and across its research organizations, combined with the increasing commercialization of science, had begun to impose fundamental limits on the ability of the American system to sustain its level of excellence.

Appendix 1

Interviews with scientists who were recognized for making major discoveries in American research organizations or other research organizations discussed in this paper.*

David Baltimore, Professor of Biology, Massachusetts Institute of Technology and former President of Rockefeller University. Interview in his MIT office, 28 April 1995.

Derek H. E. Barton (Sir), Professor of Chemistry, Texas A and M University and Professor Emeritus, Imperial College, London. Interview at the Beckmann Center, Scripps Research Institute, La Jolla, California, 6 February 1998.

Alan Battersby (Sir), Emeritus Professor of Chemistry, University of Cambridge. Interview in his office, 20 March 2002.

Seymour Benzer, Professor of Biology, California Institute of Technology. Interview in his office, 30 March 1994; second interview at Cold Spring Harbor Laboratory, New York, 26 August 1995; third interview at Neurosciences Institute, San Diego, California, 17 March 1996; fourth interview in his office, 22 December 1999.

Paul Berg, Professor of Biochemistry, Stanford University School of Medicine. Interview in his office, 6 May 2003.

Michael Berridge, Senior Research Fellow, Trinity College, Cambridge and Head of Cell Signalling Programme, Babraham Institute (U.K.). Interviews at Trinity College, 9 June 1999, 24 January 2002. Interview at Babraham Institute, 29 March 2002.

J. Michael Bishop, Professor of Microbiology, Director of Hooper Research Laboratory, University of California, San Francisco. Interview in his office, 10 August 1994.

James Black, Professor, King's College London. Interview at McGill University, 23 September 2004.

Günter Blobel, Professor at Rockefeller University and HHMI investigator. Interview in his office, 12 April 1995. Subsequent interviews in his office, 16 March 2001, 18 March 2001, 21 December 2004, 12 and 14 March 2007.

Konrad Bloch, Higgins Professor Emeritus of Biochemistry, Harvard University. Interview in his office, 25 April 1995.

Bernard S. Blumberg, Professor, Fox Chase Cancer Center (Philadelphia). Interview at Rockefeller Foundation Study Center, Bellagio, Italy, 21 May 1984.

Sydney Brenner, Professor Salk Institute, and Former Director of Laboratory of Molecular Biology (Cambridge, U.K.). Interview in La Jolla, California, 7 April 2003.

Francis Crick, President Emeritus and Distinguished Professor, Salk Institute; former scientist at Cambridge University and at the Laboratory of Molecular Biology. Interviews in his office in San Diego, 6 March 1996 and 11 March 1998. Interview at UCSD, 6 June 2002.

Renato Dulbecco, Emeritus President and Distinguished Professor, Salk Institute; Former Professor California Institute of Technology. Interview in his office in San Diego, 23 February 1996. Second interview in his office, 22 May 2000.

Gerald Edelman, Research Director, The Neurosciences Institute, San Diego, California, and former Professor and Dean, Rockefeller University. Interviews in Klosters, Switzerland, 17 January 1995, and at Neurosciences Institute, San Diego, 13 January, 16 January, 19 January, 30 January, 14 February, 20 February, 22 February, 5 March, 16 March, 17 March 1996; 12 February 1998; 4 April, 11 April, 18 November 2000. Telephone interview, 3 April 2001.

Manfred Eigen, Professor, Max-Planck Institut fur Biophysikalishe Chemie, Göttingen, Germany. Interview in Klosters, Switzerland, 16 January 1995.

Gertrude Elion, Scientist Emeritus, Wellcome Research Laboratories, Research Triangle Park, North Carolina. Interview in her office, 17 March 1995.

Martin Evans, Professor and Director of School of Biosciences, University of Cardiff. Telephone interview, 22 April 2002.

Daniel Carleton Gajdusek, Chief of the Laboratory for Slow Latent and Temperate Virus Infections and Chief of the Laboratory for Central Nervous System Studies at the National Institute for Neurological Disorders and Stroke. Interview at Neurosciences Institute, San Diego, California, 11 March 1996.

Robert Gallo, Chief of the Laboratory of Tumor Cell Biology, National Institutes of Health, Bethesda, Maryland. Interview at University of Wisconsin Union, 13 March 1994. Interview in Bethesda, Maryland, 29 June 1994. Interviews in his office, 31 August 1994, 4 September 1994, 4 March 1995, 17 November 1995.

Walter Gilbert, Carl M. Loeb University Professor at Harvard University. Interview in Chicago, 14 October 1993. Interview in his office at Harvard University, 26 April 1995.

Joseph Goldstein, Professor, Department of Molecular Genetics, University of Texas Southwestern Medical Center. Interview at Rockefeller University, 13 March 2007.

Paul Greengard, Professor at Rockefeller University. Interview in his office, 16 May 2001.

Roger Guillemin, Professor, Salk Institute. Interview in his office, May 8, 2000.

Stephen C. Harrison, Higgins Professor of Biochemistry and Molecular Biology and HHMI Investigator, Harvard University. Interview in his office, 18 December 2002.

Leroy Hood, Professor and Chairman, Department of Molecular Biotechnology, University of Washington (Seattle) and former Professor and Chair, Division of Biology at California Institute of Technology. Interview at his Seattle home, 29 July 1995. Telephone interview, 28 August 1996.

David Hubel, Professor, Harvard Medical School. Interview in San Diego, California, 13 March 1998.

Andrew Huxley (Sir), Emeritus Professor of Physiology, University of Cambridge, Former Master of Trinity College, University of Cambridge, and former President of the Royal Society. Interview in his room in Trinity College, 11 July 2000. Interviews 20 January and 4 March 2002.

François Jacob, Senior Scientist, Institut Pasteur. Interview at Cold Spring Harbor Laboratory, New York, 24 August 1995.

Eric R. Kandel, Director of Center for Neurophysiology and HHMI Investigator, Columbia University School of Physicians and Surgeons, member of Board of Trustees, Rockefeller University. Interview at Columbia University, 19 April 2001.

Aaron Klug, former Director, Laboratory of Molecular Biology (LMB), Cambridge, England, President of the Royal Society, Honorary Fellow of Trinity College. Telephone interview, 24 May 1999. Interview in his office at LMB, 11 July 2000. Interview at Trinity College, Cambridge, 3 April 2002.

Arthur Kornberg, Emeritus Professor of Biochemistry, Stanford University School of Medicine (Nobel laureate in Physiology or Medicine, 1959). Interview in his office, 5 May 2003.

Edwin Krebs, Professor of Biochemistry and HHMI Investigator, University of Washington School of Medicine, Seattle. Interview in his office, 2 August 1995.

Paul C. Lauterbur, Professor of Chemistry, University of Illinois. Interview in his office, 24 October 2005.

Joshua Lederberg, President Emeritus, Rockefeller University, former Chair, Medical Genetics, Stanford University School of Medicine, and former Professor of Genetics, University of Wisconsin (Madison). Interviews at Rockefeller University, 16 September 1993, 13 April 1995; telephone interview, 27 August 1999; interviews in his office 25 January 2001, 4 April 2001.

Rita Levi-Montalcini, Professor Emeritus of Biology, Washington University (St. Louis). Interview at her home in Rome, Italy, 15 June 1995.

Arnold Levine, President, Rockefeller University. Interview in his office, 14 May 2001.

Edward B. Lewis, Professor of Biology, California Institute of Technology. Interviews at Athenaeum and in his office, 25 March 1994, 21 December 1994.

William N. Lipscomb, Jr., Professor Emeritus of Chemistry, Harvard University. Interview in his office, 16 December 2002.

Roderick MacKinnon, Professor, Rockefeller University, and HHMI Investigator. Interview in his office, 1 March 2001.

Bruce Merrifield, John D. Rockefeller, Jr., Emeritus Professor, Rockefeller University. Interview in his office, 11 February 2000.

Vernon Mountcastle, Professor of Medicine, Johns Hopkins University. Interview, 7 March 1995. Second interview, 11 August 2000.

Daniel Nathans, Professor, Department of Molecular Biology and Genetics, Johns Hopkins University, Baltimore. Interview in his office, 21 July 1997.

Erwin Neher, Director of Department of Membrane Biophysics, Max Planck Institute for Biophysical Chemistry. Interview in his office, 15 April 2004.

Paul Nurse, President, Rockefeller University. Interviews in his office, 24 December 2004, 13 March 2007.

George Palade, Dean Medical School University of California, San Diego. Also former Professor at Yale University and Rockefeller University. Interviews in his office in San Diego, 7 March 1996, 13 March 1998.

Max Perutz, former Director, Laboratory of Molecular Biology, Cambridge, England. Interview at Peterhouse College, 15 March 1997; interview at Laboratory of Molecular Biology, 11 June 1999.

John Polanyi, Professor, University of Toronto. Interview at the Center for Advanced Cultural Studies, Essen, Germany, 5 September 2001.

Mark Ptashne, Professor Memorial Sloan-Kettering Cancer Center and former Professor and Chair, Department of Biochemistry and Molecular Biology, Harvard University. Interview in his New York City apartment, 24 May 2001.

Robert Roeder, Professor at Rockefeller University. Interviews at Rockefeller University, 24 April 2001, 8 May 2001.

Harry Rubin, Professor of Molecular and Cell Biology, University of California, Berkeley. Interview in his office, 4 January 1995.

William Rutter, Professor Emeritus of Biochemistry and Biophysics, University of California, San Francisco. Telephone interview, 11 August 1994.

Fred Sanger, Emeritus Staff, Laboratory for Molecular Biology, Cambridge, United Kingdom. Interview at Emmanuel College, University of Cambridge, 7 June 1999.

Philip Sharp, Chair and Professor of Biology, and former Director of Center for Cancer Research, Massachusetts Institute of Technology. Interview in his office, 3 May 1995.

Hamilton O. Smith, Professor, Department of Molecular Biology and Genetics, Johns Hopkins University, Baltimore. Interview in his office, 21 July 1997.

Michael Smith, former Director of Biotechnology Laboratory and Professor, University of British Columbia (Vancouver). Interview in his office, 5 February 1998.

Oliver Smithies, Professor of Molecular Genetics and Pathology, University of North Carolina (Chapel Hill), former President of Genetics Society of America. Interview in his office in Chapel Hill, 30 March 1996.

Solomon Snyder, Professor and Director of Neuroscience, Johns Hopkins University, Baltimore. Interview in his office, 18 July 1997.

Jack Strominger, Professor of Biochemistry, Department of Molecular and Cellular Biology, Harvard University. Interview in his office, 16 December 2002.

John Sulston (Sir). Former Director Sanger Institute (Hixton, U.K.), and former senior scientist, Laboratory of Molecular Biology (Cambridge, U.K.). Interview at St. John's College, Cambridge, 7 April 2006.

Howard Temin, Professor in McArdle Cancer Laboratory, University of Wisconsin (Madison). Interview at McArdle Cancer Laboratory, 26 November 1993.

Harold Varmus, Director of the National Institutes of Health and former Professor at University of California, San Francisco. Interview in his office, Bethesda, Maryland, 6 March 1995.

Bert Vogelstein, Professor of Oncology and HHMI investigator, Johns Hopkins University, Baltimore. Interview in his office, 18 July 1997.

James D. Watson, Director, Cold Spring Harbor Laboratory, New York. Interview at Cold Spring Harbor, 24 August 1995, and at Neurosciences Institute, San Diego, 20 February 1996.

Torsten Wiesel, President, Rockefeller University. Interviews in his office, 14 April 1995, 14 July 1997, 7 February 2001, 4 May 2001, 25 May 2001.

Don C. Wiley, John L. Loeb Professor of Biochemistry and Biophysics, Harvard University. Telephone interview, 4 November 1999.

Edward O. Wilson, Pellegrino University Professor and Curator of Entomology, Museum of Comparative Zoology, Harvard University. Interviews in his office, 4 May 1995, 17 December 2002.

Carl R. Woese, Professor of Microbiology, University of Illinois. Interview in his office, 26 October 2005.

K. Wuthrich, Professor of Bio-physics, Swiss Federal Institute of Technology (ETH) (Switzerland). Interview in his office, 12 December 1994.

* Titles are listed as of the time of the interview.

HHMI = Howard Hughes Medical Institute.

Ellen Jane Hollingsworth participated in many of these interviews on both sides of the Atlantic.

Appendix 2

Oral histories and public interviews (only of individuals recognized as having made a major discovery).

Paul Berg, Professor of Biochemistry, Stanford University. Interview available through Online Archive of California, UC Berkeley Regional Oral History Office. http://ark.cdlib.org/ark:/13030;kt1c6001df.

Konrad Bloch, Professor of Biochemistry (Emeritus), Harvard University. Interview with James J. Bohning, 22 March 1993. Transcript on deposit at Beckman Center for the History of Chemistry, Philadelphia, Pennsylvania. Copy in possession of J. Rogers Hollingsworth.

Herbert W. Boyer, former Professor, Department of Biochemistry, University of California San Francisco. Interview available through Online Archive of California, UC Berkeley Regional Oral History Office. http://ark.cdlib.org/ark:/13030/kt5d5nb0zs.

British Broadcasting Corporation (BBC) audiovisual interview with Lawrence Bragg, Francis Crick, John Kendrew, Max Perutz, James Watson, and Maurice Wilkins. First broadcast 11 December 1962. Tape located in Wellcome Trust Library, London.

Carl Cori, Professor of Biochemistry, Washington University Medical School. Interview with Harriet Zuckerman, 10 December 1963(CUL). Second interview with Paul G. Anderson, 18 October 1982 (WUA).

André Cournand, Professor in the College of Physicians and Surgeons at Columbia University. Interview with Harriet Zuckerman, 27 September 1963 (CUL).

E. E. Doisy, Professor of Biochemistry, University of St. Louis Medical School. Interview with Harriet Zuckerman, 12 December 1963 (CUL).

Vincent Du Vigneaud, Professor of Chemistry, Cornell University Medical College. Interview with Harriet Zuckerman, 2 October 1963 (CUL).

Joseph Erlanger, Professor of Physiology, Washington University Medical School. Interview with Harriet Zuckerman, 10 April 1964 (CUL).

Martin Evans, Professor, University of Cardiff. Interview with Virginia Papaionnou, 2001. http://www.laskerfoundation.org/awards/library/2001. Accessed 03/10/02.

Walter Gilbert, University Professor, Harvard University. "Autobiography." http://www.nobel.se/laureates/chemistry-1980-2-autobio.html.

Steve Harrison, Professor, Department of Molecular and Cellular Biology, Harvard University. Oral History (two parts). Recorded and edited by Sondra Schlesinger, March 30, April 1, 1999. http://medicine.wustl.edu/~virology/harrison.html.

Bertil Hille, Professor, University of Washington. Interview with Professor Eric Kandel, Columbia University, 1999 (HHMI).

Leroy Edward Hood, founder and Chairman of the Department of Molecular Biotechnology, University of Washington and co-founder of the Institute for Systems Biology in Seattle, Washington. "My Life and Adventures Integrating Biology and Technology: A Commemorative Lecture for the 2002 Kyoto Prize in Advanced Technologies," http://www.law.washington.edu/Casrip/classes/O'Connor/MyLifeandAdventures-KyotoP1%20(Hood).doc. Accessed 8/18/2003.

Gobind Khorana, Professor of Biology and Chemistry, Massachusetts Institute of Technology. Interview with H. S. Jones, July 1985 (BS).

Aaron Klug, former director, Laboratory of Molecular Biology, UK. and former President of the Royal Society. Autobiography and Nobel Lecture from Nobel Museum website. www.nobel.se/chemistry/laureates/1982.

Arthur Kornberg, Emeritus Professor, Department of Biochemistry, Stanford University "Biochemistry at Stanford, Biotechnology at DNAX." Oral interviews conducted by Sally Smith Hughes, Program in the History of the Biosciences and Biotechnology, Regional Oral History Office, Bancroft Library, University of California Berkeley.

Roderick MacKinnon, Professor, Rockefeller University. Interview by Professor Christopher Miller of Brandeis University, 1999 (HHMI).

Herman J. Muller, Professor of Genetics, Indiana University. Interview with Harriet Zuckerman, 12 December 1993 (CUL).

Paul Nurse, Director Imperial Cancer Research Fund. Broadcast on BBC Radio, 10 February 2002.

Paul Nurse, President Rockefeller University. Public Television interview with Charlie Rose, In New York City, December 2004 (Interview available through Office of Public Affairs, Rockefeller University).

Linus Pauling, Professor of Chemistry, California Institute of Technology. Interview with Harriet Zuckerman, 26 March 1964 (CUL).

Norman Pirie, Emeritus Professor, Rothamsted Experimental Research Station. Interview with W. S. Pierpoint. 27 June 1988 (BS).

Mark Ptashne, Professor, Sloan-Kettering Cancer Center. Interview by James Watson, 1999 http://www.laskerfoundation.org/library/ptashne/citation.html.

William Rutter, Former Professor of Biochemistry and Biophysics, University of California San Francisco. "The Department of Biochemistry and the Molecular Approach to Biomedicine at the University of California, San Francisco." 1998 interview. Online Archive of California, Regional Oral History Office, University of California, Berkeley.

Frederick Sanger, Emeritus Professor Laboratory for Molecular Biology (Cambridge, England). Interview with Horace Judson, 13 November 1987 (BS).

Frederick Sanger, Emeritus Professor Laboratory for Molecular Biology (Cambridge, England). Interview with Professor George G. Brownlee, 20 October 1992 (BS).

Edward Tatum, Professor of Biochemistry, Yale University. Interview with Harriet Zuckerman, 23 September 1963 (CUL).

Howard Temin, Professor, McArdle Laboratory for Cancer Research, University of Wisconsin. Interview with Barry Teicher and Margaret Andreasen, 26 July 1993 (OHAUW).

Alexander Todd, Emeritus Professor of Chemistry, University of Cambridge. Interview with Sir Hans Kornberg, 26 June 1990 (BS).

Harold Urey, Professor of Chemistry, University of California, San Diego. Interview with Harriet Zuckerman, 26 August 1963 (CUL).

Don C. Wiley, Professor, Department of Molecular and Cellular Biology, Harvard University. Oral History recorded and edited by Sondra Schlesinger, 1 and 5 April 1999 http://medicine.wustl.edu/~virology/wiley.htm.

BS = Biochemical Society (London) Archive

CUL = Columbia University Library

CITA = California Institute of Technology Archive

OHAUW = Oral History Archive, University of Wisconsin

WUA = Washington University Archive

HHMI = Website of Howard Hughes Medical Institute. www.hhmi.org/science/neurosci

Notes

* Acknowledgments: I am very grateful to Wolfgang Streeck, from whom I learned much about how institutional environments influence the performance of organizations. From Gerald Edelman, Ralph Greenspan and others at the Neurosciences Institute (La Jolla), I have gained enormously in my understanding of how the structure and culture of research organizations influence major scientific discoveries. Over many years, the person who has taught me most about innovations in organizations has been Jerald Hage, who has also been my co-investigator in the study of radical scientific innovations. For many years, my colleague David Gear has been of inestimable assistance in all my research. My good friend and colleague Karl Müller has contributed many valuable philosophical, sociological, historical, and comparative insights to my research agenda on major discoveries. But my greatest debt is to Ellen Jane Hollingsworth who has been my collaborator for many years, as we have studied how institutions and organizations either facilitate or hamper the making of major scientific discoveries over time and across organizations. Without her intellectual input, this paper would not have been possible. Finally I am very indebted to a variety of funding organizations for supporting my research on scientific discoveries: the Humboldt Stiftung, the National Science Foundation, the Andrew W. Mellon Foundation, the Rockefeller Archive Center, the Alfred P. Sloan Foundation, the Graduate School of the University of Wisconsin (Madison), the Swedish Council for Research on Higher Education.

1. To address these issues, I draw on the data from my study with Ellen Jane Hollingsworth and Jerald Hage of 291 major discoveries which occurred from 1901 through 1995 in four countries: Britain, France, Germany, and the United States. See J. Rogers Hollingsworth, Ellen Jane Hollingsworth, and Jerald Hage, eds., *The Search for Excellence: Organizations, Institutions, and Major Discoveries in Biomedical Science* (New York: Cambridge University Press, 2008, forthcoming).

2. This way of thinking is very different from the rare paradigm shifts analyzed by Thomas S. Kuhn in *The Structure of Scientific Revolutions* (Chicago: University of Chicago Press, 1962). Major breakthroughs about problems in basic biomedical science, as defined here, occur within the paradigms about which Kuhn wrote.

3. Depending on the scientific community to operationalize this definition, I consider major discoveries to be research that received one of the following forms of recognition: (1) the Copley Medal, awarded since 1901 by the Royal Society of London, insofar as the award was for basic biomedical research; (2) the Nobel Prize in Physiology or Medicine since the first award in 1901; (3) the Nobel Prize in Chemistry since the first award in 1901, insofar as the research had great relevance to biomedical science; (4) ten nominations in any three years prior to 1940 for a Nobel Prize

in Physiology or Medicine; (5) ten nominations in any three years prior to 1940 for a Nobel Prize in Chemistry if the research had great relevance to biomedical science; (6) prizeworthy designation for the Nobel Prize in Physiology or Medicine by the Karolinska Institute committee, which prepared a short list of possible prizewinners and recommended the winner(s); (7) prizeworthy designation for the Nobel Prize in Chemistry by the Royal Swedish Academy of Sciences committee, which prepared a short list of possible prizewinners and recommended the winner(s) (if the research had great relevance to biomedical science); (8) discoveries resulting in the Arthur and Mary Lasker Prize for basic biomedical science; (9) the Louisa Gross Horwitz Prize in basic biomedical science; (10) discoveries in biomedical science resulting in the Crafoord Prize, awarded by the Royal Swedish Academy of Sciences, if the discovery had high relevance to the biological sciences. I have had access to the Nobel Archives for the Physiology or Medicine Prize at the Karolinska Institute and to the Archives at the Royal Swedish Academy of Sciences in Stockholm for the period from 1901 to 1940. The archives are closed for the past fifty years for reasons of confidentiality, but I have used other prizes (Lasker, Horwitz, Crafoord) to identify major discoveries during the latter part of the twentieth century. I use prizes and other forms of recognition to identify major discoveries. My concern is not whether proper credit was assigned to individual scientists for major breakthroughs. Rather, I seek to understand the structure and culture of the organizational context where research did or did not result in a major discovery as described above. I have studied organizations, departments/institutes and laboratories, as well as the interactions among individuals. I am indebted to Professor Ragnar Björk of the University of Södertörn for conducting most of the research in the archives of the Royal Swedish Academy and the Karolinska Institute in Stockholm.

The research on major discoveries summarized here is based on a great deal of archival research, many interviews, and wide reading in many scientific fields. Archives have been used in the United States (e.g., Rockefeller Archive Center, American Philosophical Society, University of Wisconsin, Caltech, University of California Berkeley, University of California San Francisco, University of California San Diego, Harvard Medical School) and in Great Britain and Europe. I have conducted in-depth interviews with more than 500 scientists, administrators, and officers of major funding agencies on both sides of the Atlantic. Appendix 1 lists interviews that I conducted with scientists who were recognized for making major discoveries in American research organizations or other research organizations discussed in this paper. I also used as sources the oral histories and public interviews with individuals recognized as having made a major discovery listed in Appendix 2, as well as many others.

4. J. Rogers Hollingsworth and Robert Boyer, eds., *Contemporary Capitalism: The Embeddedness of Institutions* (Cambridge and New York: Cambridge University Press, 1997); J. Rogers Hollingsworth and Ellen Jane Hollingsworth, "Major Discoveries and Biomedical Research Organizations: Perspectives on Interdisciplinarity, Nurturing Leadership, and Integrated Structure and Cultures," in *Practicing Interdisciplinarity*, ed. Peter Weingart and Nico Stehr (Toronto: University of Toronto Press, 2000), pp. 215-44.

5. J. Rogers Hollingsworth, Karl Müller, and Ellen Jane Hollingsworth, eds., *Advancing Socio-Economics: An Institutionalist Perspective* (Lanham, Maryland: Rowman and Littlefield Publishers, 2002).

6. In writing this paper, I am especially indebted to a number of papers by Wolfgang Streeck who over the years has emphasized the important role of institutional environments in shaping the performance of organizations. For example, see the essays in Wolfgang Streeck, ed., *Social Institutions and Economic Performance: Studies of Industrial Relations in Advanced Capitalist Economies* (London and Beverly Hills, California: Sage Publications, 1992). Also see Richard Whitley, "Competition and Pluralism in the Public Sciences: The Impact of Institutional Frameworks on the Organisation of Academic Systems," *Research Policy*, 2003, *32*: 1015-29.

7. On the concept of institutional complementarity, see Bruno Amable, "Institutional Complementarity and Diversity of Social Systems of Innovation and Production," *Review of International Political Economy*, 2000, *7(4)*: 645-87; Peter A. Hall and David Soskice, *Varieties of Capitalism: The Institutional Foundations of Comparative Advantage* (Oxford: Oxford University Press, 2001); Martin Höpner, "What Connects Industrial Relations and Corporate Governance? Explaining Institutional Complementarity," *Socio-Economic Review*, 2005, *3(2)*: 331-58; Colin Crouch, Wolfgang Streeck, Robert Boyer, Bruno Amable, Peter A. Hall and Gregory Jackson, "Dialogue on 'Institutional Complementarity and Political Economy,'" *Socio-Economic Review*, 2005, *3(2)*: 359-82.

8. Jerald Hage and J. Rogers Hollingsworth, "Idea Innovation Networks: A Strategy for Integrating Organizational and Institutional Analysis," *Organization Studies*, 2000, *21*: 971-1004; J. Rogers Hollingsworth, "Institutionalizing Excellence in Biomedical Research: The Case of the Rockefeller University," in *Creating a Tradition of Biomedical Research: Contributions to the History of the Rockefeller University*, ed. Darwin H. Stapleton (New York: Rockefeller University Press, 2004), pp. 17-63; Hollingsworth, Hollingsworth, and Hage, eds., *Search for Excellence.*

9. On the concept of organizational and institutional connectedness, see Hage and Hollingsworth, "Idea Innovation Networks."

10. Hollingsworth, "Institutionalizing Excellence in Biomedical Research;" Hage and Hollingsworth, "Idea Innovation Networks;" Whitley, "Competition and Pluralism in the Public Sciences."

11. Abraham Flexner, *Universities: American, English, German* (New York: Oxford University Press, 1930); Joseph Ben-David, *The Scientist's Role in Society: A Comparative Study* (Englewood Cliffs, New Jersey: Prentice-Hall, 1971); Joseph Ben-David, *Centers of Learning: Britain, France, Germany, United States* (New York: McGraw Hill, 1977); Lothar Burchardt, *Wissenschaftspolitik im Wilhelminischen Deutschland* (Göttingen, Germany: Vandenhoeck and Ruprecht, 1975); Charles E. McClelland, *State, Society, and University in Germany, 1700-1914* (New York: Cambridge University Press, 1980); Charles E. McClelland, "Professionalization and Higher Education in Germany," in *The Transformation of Higher Learning, 1860-1930,* ed. Konrad H. Jarausch (Chicago: University of Chicago Press, 1983), pp. 306-320; Jonathan Harwood, *Styles of Scientific Thought: The German Genetics Community, 1900-1933* (Chicago: University of Chicago Press, 1993); Peter Lundgreen, ed., *Reformuniversität Bielefeld, 1969-1994: Zwischen Defensive und Innovation* (Bielefeld, Germany: Verlag für Regionalgeschichte, 1994); Lynn K. Nyhart, *Biology Takes Form: Animal Morphology and the German Universities* (Chicago: University of Chicago Press, 1995); Mitchell G. Ash, ed., *German Universities Past and Future* (Providence, Rhode Island: Berghahn, 1997).

12. Bill McKelvey, *Organizational Systematics: Taxonomy, Evolution, Classification* (Berkeley: University of California Press, 1982), p. 192; Howard Aldrich, Bill McKelvey and Dave Ulrich, "Design Strategy from the Population Perspective," *Journal of Management*, 1984, *10*: 69.

13. J. Rogers Hollingsworth, Philippe Schmitter, and Wolfgang Streeck, eds., *Governing Capitalist Economies: Performance and Control of Economic Sectors* (New York: Oxford University Press, 1994).

14. The results reported in Tables 1 and 2 were derived from an analysis of major research universities across the twentieth century. In the United States, there were only about 15 such universities in 1920, and approximately 100 by 2000.

15. Hollingsworth, "Institutionalizing Excellence in Biomedical Research;" Hollingsworth and Hollingsworth, "Major Discoveries and Biomedical Research Organizations."

16. Paul DiMaggio and Walter W. Powell, "The Iron Cage Revisited: Institutional Isomorphism and Collective Rationality in Organizational Fields," *American Sociological Review*, 1983, *48*: 147-60.

17. Geoffrey Hodgson, "The Mystery of Routine: The Darwinian Destiny of an Evolutionary Theory of Economic Change," *Revue Economique*, 2003, *34*: 355-84.

18. Richard Dawkins, *The Selfish Gene* (New York: Basic Books, 1976).

19. Charles J. Lumsden and Edward O. Wilson, *Genes, Mind, and Culture: The Coevolutionary Process* (Cambridge, Massachusetts: Harvard University Press, 1981).

20. Richard R. Nelson and Sidney G. Winter, *An Evolutionary Theory of Economic Change* (Cambridge, Massachusetts: Harvard University Press, 1982).

21. McKelvey, *Organizational Systematics*.

22. Douglass Cecil North, *Institutions, Institutional Change, and Economic Performance* (Cambridge: Cambridge University Press, 1990); Donald T. Campbell, "A Naturalistic Theory of Archaic Moral Orders," *Zygon*, 1991, *26*: 91-114; Joel A. C. Baum, "Whole-Part Coevolutionary Competition in Organizations," in *Variations in Organization Science*, ed. Joel A. C. Baum and Bill McKelvey (Thousand Oaks, California, and London: Sage Publications, 1999), pp. 113-35; Peter J. Richerson and Robert Boyd, *Not by Genes Alone: How Culture Transformed Human Evolution* (Chicago: University of Chicago Press, 2005).

23. Amos Hawley, *A Theory of Community Structure* (New York: Ronald Press, 1950); McKelvey, *Organizational Systematics*.

24. Arthur Stinchcombe, "Social Structure and Organizations," in *Handbook of Organizations*, ed. James March (Chicago: Rand McNally, 1965), pp. 153-93.

25. Bart Nooteboom, "Innovation, Learning and Industrial Organization," *Cambridge Journal of Economics*, 1999, *23*: 127-50; Salvatore Rizzello, *The Economics of the Mind* (Cheltenham: Edward Elgar, 1999); Raghu Garud and Peter Karnøe, eds., *Path Dependence and Creation* (Rahway, New Jersey: Lawrence Erlbaum Associates, 2001); Salvatore Rizzello and Margherita Turvani, "Subjective Diversity and Social Learning: A Cognitive Perspective for Understanding Institutional Behavior," *Constitutional Political Economy*, 2002, *13*: 210-14; Hage and Hollingsworth, "Idea Innovation Networks."

26. Stephen Jay Gould, "Is a New and General Theory of Evolution Emerging," *Paleobiology*, 1980, *6*: 119-30; W. Graham Astley, "The Two Ecologies: Population and Community Perspectives on Organizational Evolution," *Administrative Science Quarterly*, 1985, *30*: 224-41; Joel A. C. Baum and Bill McKelvey, eds., *Variations in Organization Science: In Honor of Donald T. Campbell* (Thousand Oaks, California: Sage Publications, 1999); Ernst Mayr, *What Evolution Is* (New York: Basic Books, 2001).

27. Ernst Mayr, *Animal Species and Evolution* (Cambridge, Massachusetts: Harvard University Press, 1963); Mayr, *What Evolution Is*; Astley, "Two Ecologies," p. 232. For a discussion of the influence of the natural sciences on the social sciences, see Renate Mayntz, "The Influence of Natural Science Theories on Contemporary Social Science," in *European Social Science in Transition,* ed. Meinolf Dierkes and Bernd Biervert (Frankfurt/Main: Campus, 1992), pp. 27-79.

28. Michael Hannan and John Freeman, "Structural Inertia and Organizational Change," *American Sociological Review*, 1984, *29*: 149-64; Michael Hannan and John Freeman, eds., *Organizational Ecology* (Cambridge, Massachusetts: Harvard University Press, 1989).

29. McKelvey, *Organizational Systematics*.

30. The brief generalizations about these two Harvard departments are based on numerous interviews with scientists and administrators, as well as on archival materials at Harvard. These materials are reported in much more detail in the forthcoming study, Hollingsworth, Hollingsworth, and Hage, *Search for Excellence*.

31. Nelson and Winter, *Evolutionary Theory of Economic Change*.

32. National Science Board, *Science and Engineering Indicators 2004* (Arlington, Virginia: National Science Foundation, 2004.) *Indicators* is published every other year under the same title.

33. National Research Council Canada, *Looking Forward: S &T for the 21st Century–Foresight Consolidation Report, NRC Renewal Project* (August 2005). http://www.nrc-cnrc.gc.ca/docs/NRC-Foresight_Consolidation_Report_e.pdf.

34. Derived from National Science Board, *Science and Engineering Indicators* (various years); Nicolas Rescher, *Scientific Progress* (Pittsburgh, Pennsylvania: University of Pittsburgh Press, 1978); Derek J. de Solla Price, *Little Science, Big Science* (New York: Columbia University Press, 1963).

35. Max Planck, *Vorträge und Erinnerungen*, 5th ed. (Stuttgart: S. Hirzel, 1949); Rescher, *Scientific Progress*.

36. Rescher, *Scientific Progress*, p. 97. For a discussion of the historical literature on Rousseau's Law, see Rescher, *Scientific Progress*, pp. 96-98; and George K. Zipf, *Human Behavior and the Principle of Least Effort: An Introduction to Human Ecology* (Cambridge, Massachusetts: Addison-Wesley, 1949).

37. Derived from National Science Board, *Science and Engineering Indicators* (various years); Rescher, *Scientific Progress*; Price, *Little Science, Big Science*.

38. Michael Power, *The Audit Society: Rituals of Verification* (Oxford: Clarendon Press, 1997).

39. Uwe Opolka, ed., *Science between Evaluation and Innovation. A Conference on Peer Review, Max Planck Forum 6* (Munich: Max-Planck-Gesellschaft, 2003).

40. Partha Dasgupta and Paul A. David, "Toward a New Economics of Science," *Research Policy*, 1994, *23*: 487-521; Rebecca S. Eisenberg and Richard R. Nelson, "Public vs. Proprietary Science: A Fruitful Tension?" *Daedalus*, 2002, *131*: 89-101.

41. Robert K. Merton, *The Sociology of Science: Theoretical and Empirical Investigations* (Chicago: University of Chicago Press, 1973).

42. Dasgupta and David, "Toward a New Economics of Science;" Richard Whitley, *The Intellectual and Social Organization of the Sciences,* 2nd ed. (Oxford: Oxford University Press, 2000); Whitley, "Competition and Pluralism in the Public Sciences."

43. David F. Noble, *America by Design: Science, Technology, and the Rise of Corporate Capitalism* (New York: Knopf, 1977); David F. Noble, *Forces of Production: A Social History of Industrial Automation* (New York: Knopf, 1984); Henry Etzkowitz, *MIT and the Rise of Entrepreneurial Science* (London and New York: Routledge, 2002).

44. For discussion of the literature on public knowledge, consult Merton, *Sociology of Science*; Dasgupta and David, "Toward a New Economics of Science;" Eisenberg and Nelson, "Public vs. Proprietary Science."

45. For discussion of the literature on the for-profit science sector, see Dasgupta and David, "Toward a New Economics of Science;" Eisenberg, "Proprietary Rights and the Norms of Science in Biotechnology Research;" Eisenberg and Nelson, "Public vs. Proprietary Science;" Rebecca S. Eisenberg and Michael A. Heller, "Can Patents Deter Innovation? The Anticommons in Biomedical Research," *Science*, 1998, *280*: 698-701; Burton Weisbrod, ed., *To Profit or Not to Profit: The Commercial Transformation of the Nonprofit Sector* (New York and Cambridge: Cambridge University Press, 1998).

46. Etzkowitz, *MIT and the Rise of Entrepreneurial Science*, chap. 10; National Science Board, *Science and Engineering Indicators 2004*.

47. Wesley Cohen, Richard Florida, Louis Randazzese, John Walsh, "Industry and the Academy: Uneasy Partners in the Cause of Technological Advance," in *Challenges to the Research University*, ed. R. Noll (Washington, D.C.: Brookings Institution, 1998); Ajay Agrawal and Rebecca Henderson, "Putting Patents in Context: Exploring Knowledge Transfer from MIT," *Management Science*, 2002, *48*: 44-60.

48. Manuel Trajtenberg, Rebecca Henderson, and Adam Jaffe, "University Versus Corporate Patents: A Window on the Basicness of Invention," *Economics of Innovation and New Technology*, 1997, *5*: 19-50; Rebecca Henderson, Adam B. Jaffe, and Manuel Trajtenberg, "Universities as a Source of Commercial Technology: A Detailed Analysis of University Patenting, 1965-1988," *Review of Economics and Statistics*, 1998, *80*: 119-27; Samuel Kortum and Josh Lerner, "What Is Behind the Recent Surge in Patenting?" *Research Policy*, 1999, *28*: 1-22; Jinyoung Kim and Gerald Marschke, "Accounting for the Recent Surge in U.S. Patenting: Changes in R&D Expenditures, Patent Yields, and the High Tech Sector," *Economics of Innovation and New Technology*, 2004, *13*: 543-58.

49. Rima Apple, "Patenting University Research: Henry Steenbock and the Wisconsin Alumni Research Foundation," *Isis*, 1989, *30*: 375-94; Rebecca S. Eisenberg, "Proprietary Rights and the Norms of Science in Biotechnology Research," *Yale Law Journal*, 1987, *97(21)*: 177-231; Rebecca S. Eisenberg, "Patents and the Progress of Science: Exclusive Rights and Experimental Use," *University of Chicago Law Review*, 1989, *56*: 1017-86.

50. Nathan Rosenberg, "Why Do Companies Do Basic Research with Their Own Money?" *Research Policy*, 1990, *19(2)*: 165-74.

51. Sheila Slaughter and Larry Leslie, *Academic Capitalism: Politics, Policies and the Entrepreneurial University* (Baltimore: Johns Hopkins University Press, 1997); Walter W. Powell and Jason Owen-Smith, "Universities as Creators and Retailers of Intellectual Property: Life Sciences Research and Commercial Development," in Weisbrod, ed., *To Profit or Not to Profit*, pp. 169-93; Weisbrod, ed., *To Profit or Not to Profit*.

52. These observations became quite obvious as a result of the many interviews that I conducted.
53. Illinois Institute of Technology Research Institute, *Technology in Retrospect and Critical Events in Science, TRACES* (Washington, D.C.: National Science Foundation, 1968); Paul A. David, David C. Mowery, and W. Edward Steinmueller, "Analyzing the Economic Payoffs from Basic Research," *Economics of Innovation and New Technology*, 1991, *2*: 73-90.
54. Streeck, ed., *Social Institutions and Economic Performance*.
55. Ben-David, *Centers of Learning*; Martin. J. S. Rudwick, *Bursting the Limits of Time* (Chicago: University of Chicago Press, 2005).
56. Ben-David, *Scientist's Role in Society*; Burchardt, *Wissenschaftspolitik im Wilhelminischen Deutschland*.

Notes on Contributors

Stuart Blume was educated at the University of Oxford and has been Professor of Science Dynamics at the University of Amsterdam since 1982. Prior to moving to the Netherlands, Blume worked at the University of Sussex, the London School of Economics, and at various British government departments. From 1977 to 1980, he was Research Secretary of the Committee on Social Inequalities in Health (commonly known as the Black Committee). His main research interest, thereafter, has been in the development, assessment, and deployment of new medical technologies: most recently focused on vaccines against infectious diseases.

David Cantor works as a historian for the National Library of Medicine and the National Cancer Institute in Bethesda, Maryland. His scholarly work focuses on twentieth-century history of medicine, most recently the history of cancer. He is the editor of *Reinventing Hippocrates* (Ashgate, 2002), the guest editor of "Cancer in the Twentieth Century" a special issue of the *Bulletin of the History of Medicine* (Spring 2007), and series editor (edited collections) of *Studies in the Social History of Medicine* published by Routledge for the Society for the Social History of Medicine.

Angela N. H. Creager is Professor of History at Princeton University, where she specializes in the history of modern biomedical research. Author of *The Life of a Virus: Tobacco Mosaic Virus as an Experimental Model, 1930-1965* (2002), she is currently working on the legacy of the bomb project for postwar biology and medicine through a study of the Atomic Energy Commission's radioisotope program.

Gerald N. Grob is the Henry E. Sigerist Professor of the History of Medicine Emeritus at the Institute of Health, Health Care Policy, and Aging Research at Rutgers University in New Brunswick, New Jersey. He is the author of many articles and books dealing both with mental health policy and changing patterns of morbidity and mortality in the United States. Currently he is working on a book dealing with changing explanations and therapies in modern American medicine.

Caroline Hannaway is a Historical Consultant for the Office of NIH History. She has research interests in both eighteenth- and nineteenth-century French medicine and twentieth-century American medicine. At the NIH, she has edited, with Victoria A. Harden and John Parascandola, *AIDS and the Public Debate: Historical and Contemporary Perspectives*, and with Ingrid G. Farreras and Victoria A. Harden, *Mind, Brain, Body, and Behavior: Foundations of Neuroscience and Behavioral Research at the National Institutes of Health*. She is Associate Editor of the *Journal of the History of Medicine and Allied Sciences*.

J. Rogers Hollingsworth is Professor of Sociology and History and former Chairperson of the Program in Comparative History at the University of Wisconsin, Madison. At present, he is Director of the Institute for Biomedical Research. In recent years, he has also been a visiting scholar in the Institute for Nonlinear Science in the Department of Physics at the University of California, San Diego, as well as in the Neurosciences Institute in La Jolla, California. He earned his Ph.D. at the University of Chicago. He is the author or editor of eighteen books and dozens of scholarly papers, and he is a frequent consultant to research organizations on both sides of the Atlantic–primarily concerning how the structure and processes of medical systems influence their performance and how the structure and processes of research or research organizations hamper or facilitate the making of major discoveries in basic biomedical science.

Daniel J. Kevles is the Stanley Woodward Professor of History and Chair of the Program in History of Science and Medicine at Yale University. Educated at Princeton, he taught at the California Institute of Technology before joining the Yale faculty, in 2001. His works include *The Physicists, In the Name of Eugenics, The Baltimore Case*, and co-edited with Leroy Hood, *The Code of Codes: Scientific and Social Issues in the Human Genome Project*. He is currently at work on a history of innovation and ownership in living matter, a book about plant and animal breeding and intellectual property protection since the eighteenth century.

Susan E. Lederer is Associate Professor of History of Medicine, History, and African American Studies at Yale University. She is the author of *Subjected to Science: Human Experimentation in America Before the Second World War* (1995) and *Frankenstein: Penetrating the Secrets of Nature* (2002). Her most recent book is *Flesh and Blood: Transfusion and Transplantation in Twentieth-Century America* (2008).

Richard C. Lewontin is an evolutionary and population geneticist. He is Alexander Agassiz Research Professor at Harvard University. He spent many years as an NIH panel member on the Genetics Study Section and is the author of the American Academy of Arts and Sciences report on the funding of research in universities.

Buhm Soon Park, teaches science policy and history of science as Associate Professor of the Korea Institute of Science and Technology in Daejeon, Korea. He has been a member of the Office of NIH History for several years, first as a DeWitt Stetten, Jr., Memorial Fellow in the History of Biomedical Sciences and Technology from 1999 to 2004 and then as an Associate Historian. His research interests are in the history of the physical and biomedical sciences in the twentieth century. He has published several articles on the history of quantum chemistry, and is currently writing a book titled, *Biomedicine and Government: A History of Research Policies and Activities at the NIH*.

Leo B. Slater is Historian of the Naval Research Laboratory in Washington, D.C. A former pharmaceutical research chemist, he earned a Ph.D. in History from Princeton in 1997, and has held a number of positions and fellowships including the DeWitt Stetten, Jr., Memorial Fellowship in the History of Biomedical Sciences and Technology, Office of NIH History. He is just completing a history of antimalarial drug development in the twentieth century.

Darwin H. Stapleton is Executive Director of the Rockefeller Archive Center in Sleepy Hollow, New York. He holds an undergraduate degree from Swarthmore College and an M.A. and a Ph.D. from the University of Delaware. He has been an educator, administrator, consultant, and author. He has published widely on the transfer and diffusion of technology, the science-technology interface, public health and medicine, and Rockefeller philanthropy.

Carsten Timmermann is a Wellcome Research Fellow at the University of Manchester's Centre for the History of Science, Technology and Medicine. He has published on constitutional therapy and German medicine in the interwar period and, more recently, on medical research in postwar Germany and Britain, especially on high blood pressure and cardiovascular disease. He edited (with Julie Anderson) *Devices and Designs: Medical Technologies in Historical Perspective* (2006). Currently he is working on a book on the history of lung cancer.

Index

A

Acker, Caroline, 5
Action for Mental Health, 1961, 72-73
Ad Hoc Committee on Planning for
  Mental Health Facilities, 75
agricultural education, 11-12
agricultural research, 11-12, 15, 24
  funding of, 12, 15
Adams, James A., 180
AIDS,
  NIH contributions to research
    on, 4
AIDS and the Historian, 4
*AIDS and the Public Debate: Historical
  and Contemporary Perspectives*, 4
Allen, Ernest, 186
American Association for the
  History of Medicine
    AIDS History Group of, 4
American Association of University
  Professors, 24
American Board of Radiology, 114
American Cancer Society (ACS),
  172, 177, 178, 179, 180, 181,
  182, 183, 184, 188, 189, 190
American Civil Liberties Union
  and organ transplantation, 160
American College of Chest Physicians
  Committee on Heart
  Transplantation of, 165

American College of Medical
  Genetics, 212
American College of Surgeons,
  103, 112
  cancer clinics approved by,
    103, 112
American College of Surgeons-
  National Institutes of Health
  registry of heart transplants, 166
American Foundation
  report of, 173, 181, 183
American Heart Association, 165
American Lung Association, 173
American Medical Association
  (AMA), 72, 80, 83, 108
American Psychiatric Association
  (APA), 66, 70, 72, 85
American Psychological
  Association, 73
American Radium Society (ARS),
  102, 108
American Society for the Control
  of Cancer (ASCC), 99, 103, 105,
  173, 174, 179
Anderson, Hans, 300-1
Anfinsen, Christian B., 41
antimalarial drugs
  British work on, 302-3, 305
  German work on, 293-302
  synthetic, 287-315

testing in neurosyphilis patients,
300, 301
United States work on, 302-3, 305
World War II and, 40, 176, 302
antipyrine, 291-92
Appel, Kenneth E., 72
AT&T
laboratories of, 336
Atabrine, 299-300
Atomic Bomb Project, 14
as model for post-World War II
research, 16
Atomic Energy Commission (AEC),
17-18, 183, 189, 206
National Laboratories of, 17-18
Atwell, Robert, 75
Austoker, Joan, 233
Avery, Oswald T., 222-26
and DNA, 222-26, 336
and "transforming principle,"
223-26
avian flu
vaccine for, 271

B

bacteriophage
cooperation in research on, 206
Bailey, Charles, 149
Bailey, Pearce, 42, 43, 44-45
Baltimore City Hospitals, 41
gerontology clinic at, 39
Barnard, Christiaan, 147, 153, 154,
155-56, 158, 159, 164, 166
Barnard, Louwtjie, 158
Batson, Amie, 277-78
Bauer, Johannes, 223

Bayer Company, 292, 293, 294,
299, 305
chemists' research at, 293-98,
299-302
Bayh-Dole Act (Public Law 96-517),
1980, 334, 335
Beadle, George, 180
Beams, J. W., 223
Beit Memorial Fellowships, 237,
241, 243
Benison, Saul, 188
Beprochin, see plasmochin
Berger, Suzanne, 281
Bergström, Sune, 221
Berliner, Robert, 41
Bigelow, Newton, 73-74
Bignall, J. R., 246
Bindschedler's green, 289-90
Biochemistry of Cancer, 32
Biogen, 262
Biologics Control
Laboratory of, 36, 38
Biologics Standards
Division of, 38
biotechnology companies, 203, 204,
208, 210-11, 260, 262, 326, 337
Black, Edith, 55, 156
Black, James, 305
Blaiberg, Philip, 59
Blume, Stuart, 255-86, 355
Bone, Homer, 105-6
Boone, Bert R., 41
Bowers, R. V., 65
Bowman, Robert, 41
Bradford, H., 280
Bragg, Lawrence, 336
Bragg, William H., 336

Braunwald, Eugene, 41

Brenner, Sidney, 225-26

British Empire Cancer Campaign, 235, 244
  Scientific Advisory Committee at, 235

British Medical Journal, 274, 280

Brodie, Bernard B. (Steve), 41

Brompton Hospital for Diseases of the Chest, London, 246

Bronk, Detlev, 220

Brown, Bertram, 82

Brown, Clarence Robert, 165

Brownlee, John, 238, 239

Bryder, Linda, 233

Buse, K., 275

Bush, George W., 59

Bush, Vannevar, 14-15, 17, 171, 258
  and *Science—The Endless Frontier*, 14-15, 176

Butler University, Indianapolis, 24

C

California Institute of Technology, 320, 322

Calman, Kenneth, Sir, 256, 271

Cambridge University physiology and MRC, 233, 234, 238, 241

cancer
  and quackery, 99, 100, 105
  clinics, 103, 105, 112, 121-24, 244
  NCI radium loan program for treatment of, 109-16, 119-20
  research on, Britain, 235, 244-47
  research on, United States, 95, 96, 105, 106-7, 109

state health departments and, 103, 105, 112-13, 114
  therapies for, 97-100, 102, 190, 245-46
  war on, 12, 190

Cantor, David, 5, 95-146, 235, 355

Cape Town miracle, 147

cardiac research
  programs in the United States, 147, 149, 150, 151, 157

Carnegie Institutions, 326

Carrel, Alexis, 149, 218-19

Celebrezze, Anthony, 75, 78, 79

Celera, 207-8

Centers for Disease Control (CDC), originally Center for Disease Control, 259, 278

Centre d'études du polymorphisme humain, 208, 209

de Chadarevian, Soraya, 306

Chargaff, Erwin, 180

Chestnut Lodge, Maryland, 44

Children's Vaccine Initiative, 276-77
  Task Force on Situation Analysis at, 271, 277

chloroquine, 300, 301-2, 303, 305-6
  mode of action of, 306

Christie Hospital, Manchester, 244, 247

City-County Hospital, El Paso, Texas, 110

City-County Hospital, Los Angeles, California, 110

Civil War
  and federal government funding of research, 11

Clinical Center, NIH, 33, 35, 43, 44, 46

Clinical research
  definition of, 232
  in postwar Britain, 231-254
Clinical Research Board
  and MRC, 240
Cobb, W. Montague, 165-66
Cohen, Hans, 269-70, 273
Cohen, Henry, Sir
  report of, 240
Cohen, Robert A., 44
Cold War, 12, 16, 205, 206
Colgrove, James, 278-80
Colorado General Hospital,
  Denver, 110
Colorado Psychopathic Hospital,
  Denver, 62
Columbia Broadcasting System,
  147, 153
Columbia University, 35
Commonwealth Serum Laboratory,
  Australia, 262
Community Mental Health Centers
  (CMHCs), 77, 78, 79-80, 81-82,
  84-86, 87
  consequences of, 86-88
Compton, Karl, 179
Control Data Corporation
  computer of, 220
Cooley, Denton, 154, 161
Cooper, Theodore, 161, 162, 165
Cornell University Medical College,
  33, 219
Counter-current apparatus, 221
Craig, Lyman C., 221
Creager, Angela N. H., 171-201, 355
Crichton, Michael, 157
Crick, Francis, 336-37

D

Daft, Floyd S., 34, 35
Dale, Henry, 236, 238
  and NIMR, 238, 242
Darvall, Denise, 153, 156-57
Davis, Dorland J., 38-39
Davis, James, 102
Davis, Jefferson, 150
Davy, Humphrey, 204
Dawkins, Richard, 324
Dean, H. Trendley, 46-47
DeBakey, Michael, 151, 154, 157
DeCode, 208
Defense Advanced Research Projects
  Agency (DARPA), 17
Demerec, Milislav, 180
Department of Health, Education,
  and Welfare (DHEW), 63, 75,
  81, 84
DiMaggio, Paul, 324
Division of Infectious Diseases,
  NIH, 28, 36, 39
Division of Industrial Hygiene,
  NIH, 28
Division of Physiology, NIH, 28, 39
Division of Public Health Methods,
  NIH, 28
DNA, 203, 207, 208-9, 211, 222,
  224, 225, 226
Doll, Richard, 244-45
Double Helix, The,
  see Watson, James D.
Drosophila
  cooperation in research on, 206
Dubos, René J., 225, 303-5

Dupree, A. Hunter, 176
Dutch Institute of Public Health
    (RIV), 262, 263, 269
        and polio vaccination in the
            Netherlands, 263-65, 266
Dutch Vaccine Institute (NVI),
    266-68
Dyer, Rolla E., 40, 45-46

E

Eagle, Harold, 31-32
Earle, Wilton, 32
Ebaugh, Franklin G., 62
Ebony, 160
Edson, Lee, 161
Eighth Day of Creation, The,
    see Judson, Horace
Ehrlich, Paul, 303, 304, 305, 308
    and chemotherapy, 292, 308
    and immunology, 292-93, 308
    and methylene blue, 281-91, 294
    and receptor theory, 303-4
Eli Lilly, 259
Elion, Gertrude, 305
Elliman, D., 280
Elliott, Thomas Renton, 234, 237,
    238, 243
emergent diseases
    as global phenomena, 278
    NAS report on, 1992, 278
    report on, 278, 279
    threat to U.S. security, 278-279
Emerson, Sterling, 180
Emory University, 2
Enders, John, 257
Endicott, Kenneth, 120, 186

Erlanger, Joseph, 219
Experimental Biology and Medicine
    Institute (EBMI), 34, 46, 182
Evans, Peter, 277-78
Ewing, James, 98, 107, 108
    cancer center proposal of,
        107, 108, 109

F

Fales, Henry, 6
Fatteh, Abdullah, 164
Federal Security Agency
    (predecessor of DHEW), 63
Feldman, Myer, 75
Felix, Robert H., 42, 43, 44, 62, 63,
    64, 65-66, 67, 70, 71, 74, 75, 76,
    79, 81, 82, 83, 88
Fidler, David, 277
Fischer, Emil, 287, 291, 305, 309
Fischer, Otto, 291
Fisher, Donald, 234
Fletcher, Walter Morley, Sir, 233-34
Flexner, Abraham, 72
Fogarty, John E., 63, 77
Food and Drug Administration, 259
Foster, Michael, 237
    school of physiology of, 238
Foundation for Advanced Education
    in the Sciences, Inc. (FAES), 5
Fox, E. Brooke, 6
Fred Hutchinson Cancer Research
    Center, 326
Fredrickson, Donald, 147, 148,
    153-54, 157, 161, 166
Freis, Edward, 243

G

Galambos, Louis, 261, 262, 280
Galileo Galilei, 205
Galton, Francis, 241
Ganguly, Arupa, 211
Garrett, Laurie, 278
Gasser, Herbert, 219-20
Gates Foundation, 277
GenBank, central genomic
    database in U.S., 209
gene sequencing, 207-8
genes, human
        and breast cancer, 210-11
        patents for, 209-212
Genentech, 203
genomic databases
        status of, 207-9
Georgia Department of Public
    Health, 113, 114
germ theory of disease, 287
Gey, George, 32, 125
Gibbon, John H., 149
Gilbert, Walter
        and sequencing of DNA, 337
Gillick, Muriel, 151
Goldwater Memorial Hospital,
    New York, 31, 40-41, 180
Gorman, Mike, 71, 77
Gottesman, Michael, 5
Great Depression, 13, 61, 62, 69,
    96, 102
Green, Jerome C., 154
Greenstein, Jesse P., 32
Greenwood, Major, 236, 239
Griffith, Frederick, 222
Grob, Gerald N., 59-74, 356

Groote Schuur Hospital, Cape Town,
    154, 155, 156, 159
Groves, Leslie, 17
Gunn, Selskar M., 181-82

H

Haas, Victor H., 37-38
Hahnemann Hospital, Philadelphia,
    149
Hamburg Institute for Tropical
    Medicine, 300, 302
Hampstead Military Hospital, 237
Hannaway, Caroline, 1-7, 356
Harden, Victoria A., 1, 2-3, 4-5,
    6, 7
        and AIDS research at NIH, 4-5
        and *Inventing the NIH: Federal
        Biomedical Research Policy,
        1887-1931*, 2, 28
Hardy, James, 150
Harris, Oren, 79, 83
Hart, Philip d'Arcy, 247
Hartline, Haldan Keffer, 220-21
Harvard University, 35, 41, 105,
    114, 207, 242, 257, 320, 327-28
Hatch Act, 1887, 12
Haupt, Clive, heart donor, 159, 160
Heart Disease Epidemiology Study,
    Framingham, Massachusetts, 39
heart transplantation, 1, 147-170
        African Americans and, 163-66
        first, 153
        news media and, 149-50, 151-52,
        153, 159
        numbers performed, 148, 160-62

racial politics and, 155, 156, 159-60,161,163-66
surgery for, 147, 148, 149
Heller, John R., 32, 120
Henderson, Donald A., 259
Hill-Burton Act, 1946, 61, 81, 84
Hill, Archibald V., 219
Hill, Austin Bradford, 236, 239, 244-45, 246
Hill, Leonard, 238
Hill, Lister, 63, 79, 80
Hilleman, Maurice R., 258, 272
 virus vaccine research initiative of, 258
Himsworth, Harold, 237, 239
Hitchings, George, 305
HIV/AIDS, 210, 271, 277, 279; see also AIDS
Hodgson, Geoffrey, 324
Hoffenberg, Raymond, 158-59
Hogan, Michael F., 59
Hollander, Alexander, 17
Hollingsworth, J. Rogers, 218, 317-53, 356
Holly, Ellen, 160
Hooke, Robert, 205
Hopf, Otto, 218
Horning, Evan C., 41,
Hudson, Claude, 34
Human Genome Project, 203, 209
Hume, David, 154, 155, 158, 164
Hygienic Laboratory, Staten Island
 divisions of, 27-28
 forerunner of NIH, 1, 27-28, 33
hypertension
 British research on, 240-44
 drugs and control of, 242-44

I

IBM
 laboratories of, 336
Imperial Cancer Research Fund (ICRF), 234, 244
infectious disease, 36, 287-88
Institut Mérieux, later Fondation Mérieux, 265
Institut Pasteur, 257, 326
Institute of Medicine, United States, 278
 report on vaccines needed in developing world, 274, 278, 279
International Vaccine Institute (IVI), South Korea, 260
Iowa State University, 221

J

Jackson Laboratory, Bar Harbor, Maine, 96
Jefferson Medical College, Philadelphia, 149
Jenner, Edward, 256, 271, 279
Jewett, Frank, 179, 180
Johns Hopkins University, 31, 32, 41, 65, 107, 220, 221, 236, 320, 322
Johnson, Lady Bird, 158
Johnson, Lyndon B., 83, 153, 158
 Great Society programs of, 83
Joint Commission on Mental Illness and Health (JCMIH), 72, 74, 75, 76, 78
 reports of, 72, 73, 74
Jones, Boisfeuillet, 79
Jones, Cyril, 166
Jordan, William, 259

Journal of the American Medical Association (*JAMA*), 151, 174
Journal of the National Cancer Institute, 30
Journal of the National Medical Association, 165
Judson, Horace, 225

K

Kairine, 291
Kamen, Martin, 180
Kamminga, Harmke, 306
Kantrovitz, Adrian, 152-53, 157
    and heart transplantation, 152-53
Kasperak, Michael, 161
Kennedy, John F., 75, 77, 78, 80
    and JCMIH recommendations, 75
    and mental retardation, 75, 80
    Interagency Task Force of, 84
Kety, Seymour S., 43-44, 66
Kevles, Daniel J., 176-77, 188, 189, 203-15, 357
Kikuth, Walter, 300, 302
Kilgore, Harley, 177
King, Nicholas B., 278-79
Kirklin, John, 154
Klett, Joseph, 161, 163
Knorr, Ludwig, 291
Koch, Robert, 9
Kolb, Lawrence, 61, 62
Koop, C. Everett, 3
Korean War, 15, 16, 190
Kornberg, Arthur, 35
Kramer, Morton, 69, 70, 71
Kreshover, Seymour J., 48-49
de Kruif, Paul, 175

L

laboratory instruments
    at Rockefeller Institute for Medical Research, 217-30
Laboratory of Molecular Biology, U.K., 326
Langley, John, 237
Langsley, Donald G., 85
Lasker, Mary, 63, 69, 71, 179, 183
Lasker Award, 221
Lawrence, Christopher, 234-35
Leavitt, Sarah, 6
Lederer, Susan E., 147-80, 357
Lederle-Praxis Biologicals, 260
Leibniz, Gottfried, 205
Lemkau, Paul V., 65
Lenoir, Timothy, 292
Lewis, Thomas, 236, 237, 241
    research of, 236-37
Lewontin, Richard C., 9-25, 205, 357
Life, 151, 156
Lillehei, C. Walton, 154
Lincoln, Abraham, 11
Lindbergh, Charles, 149, 218-19
Lindbergh-Carrel perfusion pump, 218-19
Lindegren, Carl, 180
Little, Clarence Cook, 96, 108, 113, 116, 118, 119, 174
Lollobrigida, Gina, 153
London School of Hygiene and Tropical Medicine (LSHTM), 236, 238, 239, 241
Los Alamos National Laboratory, 17
Lower, Richard, 150, 154, 158, 161, 163, 164
Lumsden, Charles J., 324

lung cancer,
    and the MRC, 244-47
    as public health problem, 244-45
    cigarette smoking as cause, 245
    statement of MRC on cause
        (1957), 245
Luria, Salvador, 180
Lyons, Michele, 4

M

McCarty, Maclyn, 222, 223-24, 225
MacDonald, Jeanette, 151
McKelvey, Bill, 324
Mackenzie, James, 236
Macleod, Colin, 222, 223, 225
McMichael, John 237, 243
Madhavi, Yennapu, 280
Magnuson, Warren G., 105-6
Maimonides Medical Center,
    Brooklyn, 152, 153
Manhattan Project
    and federal government
        support of research, 14, 15
    and Los Alamos, 15
    and Oak Ridge, 15
malaria, 40, 271, 279
    avian form of, 293, 299
    chemotherapy for, 288, 299
    drugs for, 289, 291-92, 299
    history of, 289
Malthus, Thomas, 329
March of Dimes, 178, 179, 189,
    190, 191; see also NFIP
March, Michael, 79
Marine Hospital, Baltimore, 110,
    115, 121
Marks, Harry, 177

Massachusetts Institute of
    Technology (MIT), 179, 320
Mauss, Hans, 299, 300
Maverick, Maury, 105-6
Maxwell, Morris, 99
May and Baker, 243
Mayo Clinic, 34, 154
Max Planck Institutes, 326
Medicaid, 83, 86
Medical College of Virginia, 150,
    154, 161, 163, 164
medical education
    in Britain, 234-35
Medical Research Committee, U.K.,
    233, 235, 237; see also Medical
    Research Council
Medical Research Council, U.K.,
    1, 231-254
    Committee on the Evaluation
        of Different Methods of
        Cancer Therapy of, 245
    links with Cambridge of, 233,
        234, 237, 238, 241, 242
    National Institute of Medical
        Research of, see NIMR
    statement on the cause of
        lung cancer of, 245
    Statistical Unit of, 236, 238-39,
        245
    Tuberculosis Research Unit of, 24
Medicare, 83, 86
Medicine in its Chemical Aspects, 294
MedImmune, 262
Meister, Lucius, and Bruning, 292
Memorial Hospital, New York, 98
Mental Health Study Act, 1955, 72

mental illness,
  community clinics for, 65-66,
    68, 72-88
  drug treatment for, 70-72
  lobotomy for, 71
  shock therapy for, 71
Mental Retardation Facilities and
  Community Health Centers
  Construction Act, 1963, 59, 70,
  80-81, 86
Merck, Sharp and Dohme, 258,
  260, 261-62, 280
Merrifield, Bruce, 221
Merton, Robert K., 205, 332
Methodist Hospital, Houston, 151
methylene blue, 289-91, 294-95
Metzger, Henry, 5
Microbiological Institute, 30, 32,
  36-37, 182
Middlesex Hospital Medical
  School, 245
Mider, G. Burroughs, 30-31, 186
Mietzch, Fritz, 299, 300
Milbank Memorial Fund, 68
Mitchell, Violaine, 262
molecular biology, 172, 182, 207, 288
molecularization
  and infectious disease, 287-315
  history of, 287-89, 306-7, 308
Molecularizing Biology and Medicine:
  New Practices and Alliances,
  1930s-1970s, 306-7
Montreal Neurological Institute, 45
Moore, Stanfield, 226
Morrill Land Grant College Act,
  1861, 11
Morrow, Andrew G., 41-42
Moulin, Anne-Marie, 272

Mowery, David, 262
Moynihan, Daniel Patrick, 75, 85
Mullis, Kary, 337
Muraskin, William, 276-77
Myriad Genetics, 210-11

N

Napoleon, 204
Nathans, Daniel, 337
National Academy of Sciences,
  11, 179
National Advisory Allergy and
  Infectious Diseases Council, 38
National Advisory Cancer Council
  (NACC), 39, 95, 112, 115, 116-17,
  118-19, 125
National Advisory Dental Research
  Council, 46
National Advisory Heart Council, 40
National Advisory Mental Health
  Council, 64, 68
National Bureau of Standards,
  110, 116
National Cancer Act, 1936, 95, 109
National Cancer Act, 1971, 31, 95,
  97, 109, 174
National Cancer Control Program, 31
National Cancer Institute (NCI),
  2, 3, 28, 61, 66, 109, 110, 174,
  182, 183
  and radium loan program, 95-146
  and research of, 95, 107
  budget of, 95-96, 106-7, 116, 118
  intramural program of, 29-33
  structure of, 31
National Capitol Civil Liberties Union
  and organ donation, 165

National Center for Biological
Information, 209
National Childhood Vaccine Injury
Compensation Program, 1986,
260, 265
National Dental Research Act, 1948,
45
National Endowment for the
Humanities, 25
National Foundation for Infantile
Paralysis (NFIP), 172, 174-75,
178-79, 180, 182, 183, 185, 188,
189, 190
    Committee of Scientific
        Research of, 175
    Committee on Research for the
        Prevention and Treatment
        of After Effects of, 175
    Committee on Virus Research
        of, 175, 178
    funding of research by, 177-78
    March of Dimes fundraising
        campaigns of, 178, 179
National Health Act, 1948, U.K.,
239, 240
National Health Advisory Council
(of Surgeon General), 37, 181
National Health Service, U.K.,
231-32, 239, 244
National Heart Institute (NHI),
39, 147-48, 150, 152, 157, 182
    artificial heart program of, 150-51
    funding of research on heart
        transplantation, 147, 148,
        150, 153-54, 157-58, 166
    intramural programs of 39-42
    staff of, 41-42

National Heart, Lung, and Blood
Institute, 3
National Human Genome Research
institute, 207
National Institute for Medical
Research (NIMR)
    departments of, 237-38
    of MRC, 235, 237-39, 242
National Institute for Public Health
and the Environment (RIVM),
the Netherlands, 262, 266, 268
National Institute of Allergy and
Infectious Diseases (NIAID), 2,
3, 33, 107, 182, 259, 266
    appropriations for, 38
    origins, 36
    research programs of, 38
National Institute of Arthritis and
Metabolic Diseases (NIAMD),
32, 182-83
    creation of, 34
    intramural program of, 34-37
    structure of, 34
National Institute of Dental Research
(NIDR), 3, 45-49, 182
    fluoridation studies of, 47
    funding for, 47
    space problems of, 46-47
    staffing of, 47-48
    structure of, 46, 49
National Institute of Health, 28
    divisions of, 28
National Institute of Mental Health
(NIMH), 1, 3, 42-45, 59-88, 183
    joint program with NINDB,
        43-44

mental health policy of, 74-77,
81-83, 87-88
service orientation of, 76
structure of, 43-44
National Institute of Neurological
Disease and Blindness (NINDB),
42-45, 183
joint program with NIMH,
43-44
National Institute of Neurological
Disorders and Stroke, 3
National Institutes of Health (NIH),
15, 17, 42, 147, 183, 186, 189,
211, 212, 231, 259, 277
and Human Genome Project, 209
and patents, 203-4
categorical structure of, 28-29,
50, 182-83, 187
centennial of, 3-4, 27
extramural research programs
of, 18, 27, 177, 182
funding, 66, 67-68
internal organization of, 49-50
intramural research programs
of, 18-19, 27-58
Office of NIH History of, 1-7
research freedom of scientists
at, 19, 40, 43, 50, 185, 186
research funding of, 1, 7, 18,
27, 174, 177, 183
scientific directors of, 28-29,
32, 35-36, 40
National Mental Health Act, 1946,
64, 67, 81-82
National Microbiological Institute,
36, 37-38

National Museum of Health and
Medicine, 3
National Naval Medical Center, 44
National Neuropsychiatric
Institute, 61
National Psychiatric Institute, 63
National Radium Commission,
U.K., 115-16, 235
National Research Council (NRC),
11, 40, 71, 179, 203, 302
Committee on Growth of,
179-80, 181
National Science Foundation (NSF),
15, 17, 20, 25, 171, 177, 183,
185, 186
Special Committee on Medical
Research of, 187
National Tuberculosis Association
(NTA), 73
National Vaccine Program (NVP),
259-60, 262, 275
Neal, Paul A., 34-35
Nelson, Richard R., 324
New Deal
programs, 13, 74, 96, 116,
119, 174
for mice, 96, 108
New York Times, 156, 160
New York University, 40, 41, 48, 320
Newton, Isaac, 205
Nirenberg, Marshall, 4
Nobel Prize in Chemistry, 221, 336
Nobel Prize in Physics, 336
Nobel Prize in Physiology or
Medicine, 218, 220, 221, 225,
226, 257, 289, 305, 337

North Carolina State College of Agriculture and Engineering, 23
North Carolina State University, 23-24
North London Hospital for Consumption, 237

O

O'Connor, Basil, 175, 183, 188, 189
Oak Ridge National Laboratory, 17
Office for Scientific Research and Development (OSRD), 176, 186, 302
    Committee on Medical Research of, 176
Office of Naval Research, 17
Office of NIH History, 1-7
    advisory committee of, 3, 5, 6
    conferences of, 4, 6
    exhibits of, 3, 4, 5-6
    invention of, 1-7
    Pisano grants of, 6
    Stetten fellows program, 5-6
Office of Technology Assessment, U.S. Congress, 259
Olby, Robert, 225
Omnibus Medical Research Act, 1950, 34
Otago Medical School, Dunedin, New Zealand, 243
Oxford University, 242

P

Paludrine (proguanil), 302, 305
Park, Buhm Soon, 5, 27-58, 357
Parran, Thomas, 61, 62, 63, 105, 106, 108, 115

Pasteur, Louis, 10, 271, 279
Pasteur-Mérieux, 262, 269-70
patents, 334-35
    and science, 203-12
    for human genes, 210-12
    lack of for vaccines, 258, 270
    resistance to for life science products, 207
Path to the Double Helix, The, see Olby, Robert
Paton, William, 242-43
Patterson, James T., 105, 173, 191
Pearson, Karl, 239, 241
Pepper, Claude, 64
peptide synthesizer, 221
Perkin, William Henry, 307-8
Perlman, David, 151
pharmaceutical companies, 10, 40, 71, 257
    and antibiotics, 257
    and genomic databases, 208, 209
    and vaccines, 258-59, 260, 265, 268, 274
phenacetin, 292
Pickels, Edward, 223
Pickering, George White, 237, 241-42, 244
Pisano, John J., 6
Planck, Max
    Principle of Increasing Effort of, 330
plasmochin, 297, 298-99, 300, 303
Platt, Philip S., 182-83
Platt, Robert, 241
Plotkin, Stanley, 265
poliomyelitis,
    research on, 174-75, 185
    war against, 178, 189, 191

poliomyelitis vaccine trials, 175
Postgraduate Medical School,
    Hammersmith, 237, 243
Powell, Walter W., 324
President's Birthday Ball
    Commission, 175
President's New Freedom
    Commission on Mental
    Health, 2003, 59
Price, Derek de Solla, 217
Priest, J. Percy, 64
Princeton University, 320
Psychiatric Quarterly, 73
Public Health Service, see U.S.
    Public Health Service
Public Health Service Act, 1944,
    120, 177
pyrimethamine, 305

Q

Queen's Hospital, Hawaii, 110
Quigley, Daniel, 99-100
quinine, 291, 293, 294, 296
    synthetic forms of, 291-92, 307
quinoline, 293, 294, 296, 297,
    299, 300

R

Rader, Karen A., 96
radiotherapy
    trials of, 246-47
radium
    costs of, 100-102, 116
    distribution in Britain, 115-16,
        117, 235

hospitals receiving loans of,
    110-12,113, 119-20, 121-24
loans of, 31, 108, 116
purchase of by NCI, 95
sources of, 101
therapy, 97-100, 109, 115, 235,
    246-47
Radium Hsopital, Omaha,
    Nebraska, 100
radiumized paste, 99
randomized controlled trials, 245-48
Reagan, Ronald, 27
research organizations
    institutional environments of,
        318, 320-26, 328-38
    isomorphism of, 323-28
    scientific discoveries and
        322-23
Resochin, 300, 301, 302;
    see also chloroquine
Reward of Courage, 1921,
    ASCC movie, 99
Ribicoff, Abraham, 75
Rice University, 320
Richards, A. N., 181
Richmond Times-Dispatch, 165
Rivers, Thomas M., 175
Robbins, Frederick, 257
Roberts, John Alexander Fraser, 241
Rockefeller Foundation, 179, 182,
    188, 219, 223, 225, 236, 239,
    257, 302
    International Health Board of,
        173-74
    International Health Division
        of, 222-23, 225

Rockefeller Institute for Medical
Research, 2, 149, 302, 303, 326
and neurophysiology, 219-21
centrifuges at, 222-23
computers at, 220-21
instrumentation at, 217-226
Rockefeller University, 320, 321
Rocky Mountain Laboratory, 36
Rocky Mountain spotted fever,
2, 3, 30
Roehl, Wilhelm, 292-93, 296,
297, 298-99
canary test of, 293, 295, 296,
297, 298, 299
Rogers, Paul, 79
Roosevelt, Franklin D., 14, 174-75,
189-90
Ross, Donald, 160-61
Rothen, Alexandre
and ultracentrifuge, 223, 224, 225
Rousseau, Jean Jacques
Law of, 330
Royal College of Physicians, 234, 245
Royal Marsden Hospital, London, 244
Royal Society, 11, 233, 234
Russell, Louis B., 165
Rwamaro, Vincent, 159

S

Sabin, Albert B., 255, 263
polio vaccine of, 263-265, 268
Salk, Jonas, 255, 263, 265, 271, 272
and concept of "vaccinology,"
272
polio vaccine of, 263-265, 268
Salk Institute, La Jolla, California,
322, 326

Samuelson, Paul, 14
San Francisco Chronicle, 151
Sanger, Frederick
and sequencing of DNA, 337
Sapir, Philip, 74
Sarewitz, Daniel, 279
Sarnoff, Stanley J., 41
SARS, 271, 277
Scadding, J. G., 246
Schechter, Alan, 5
Scheele, Leonard A., 30, 31, 46
Schereschewsky, Joseph W., 105,
109, 114, 115, 118
Schönhöfer, Fritz, 296, 300-1
Schrire, Velva, 156
Schulemann, Werner, 294, 296-97
science,
and national security, 205-6
competition in, 205-6
cooperation in, 204-5, 206
priority disputes in, 205
Science, 184, 275
Science—The Endless Frontier,
see Bush, Vannevar
scientific directors,
at NIII, 5, 28-29, 32, 40, 43,
45, 48
scientific discoveries
an institutionalist and path-
dependent perspective on, 317-53
characteristics of organizations
constraining, 322
characteristics of organizations
facilitating, 321
definition of, 317
incentive for, 332-33

Scripps Institute of Oceanography, 326
Scripps Research Institute, 326
Sebrell, William Henry, Jr., 34, 49, 50
Sedgwick County Hospital, Wichita, Kansas, 110
Sewell, David, 164
Shannon, James A., 39, 40-42, 43, 44, 166
Sharples Company
    centrifuge of, 223-24, 225
Shell Oil Company
    sponsor of research, 185
Shin, Seung-il, 260-61, 262
Shock, Nathan, 41
Shriver, Eunice Kennedy, 75
Shryock, Richard Harrison, 176
Shumway, Norman, 148, 150, 152, 154, 155, 157, 158
    and heart transplants in dogs, 150, 151, 155, 156
    and human heart transplantation, 151-52
Shy, G. Milton, 45
Sigerist, Henry E., 107
Silicon Valley, 326
Skolnick, Mark, 211
Slater, Leo, 5, 287-315, 358
smallpox eradication program, 255, 259, 275-76, 289
Smirk, Frederick Horace, 237, 243-44
Smith, Hamilton, 337
SmithKline Beecham, 270
Smithsonian Institution, 2, 3
Snyder, Carl, 149
Society for History in the Federal Government, 4

sontochin, 301, 302
Spencer, Roscoe R., 30-31
Der Spiegel, 153
Squibb and Sons, 258
St. Elizabeths Hospital, 44
St. Louis University School of Medicine, 83
St. Luke's Hospital, Denver, 110
St. Mary's Hospital Medical School, 241, 242
Stadtman, Earl, 6
Stadtman, Thressa, 6
Stanford University, 149, 150, 151, 320
Stanley, Wendell, 175, 185
Stapleton, Darwin H., 217-30, 358
Starling, E. H., 236
Starr, Paul, 189
Starzl, Thomas, 154
State Agricultural Experiment Stations, 12
State Bacteriological Laboratories, Sweden, 262
State mental hospitals, 60-61, 65-66, 67, 70, 72, 73, 74, 76, 77, 78, 81, 82-83, 85, 86-88
Steenbock, Harry, 207
Stein, William H., 226
Stetten, DeWitt, Jr., 2-3, 5, 35-36, 50
Stetten, Jane, 3
Stinchcombe, Arthur, 324,
Stoeckel, Philippe, 265
Storck, John, 178
Streeck, Wolfgang, 337
Strickland, Stephen P., 177
Sulston, John, 208

Svedberg, Thè,
    inventor of ultracentrifuge,
        223, 225
Swedish Hospital, Seattle, 110
Switzer, Mary, 63
synthetic dyes, 289-91, 307-8

T

Tansey, E. M. (Tilly), 238
Temple University, 41
Terry, Luther L., 41
Thompson, Lewis R., 118-19
Time, 148, 149, 151, 153
Timmermann, Carsten, 231-54, 358
Tiselius, Arne, 225
Tobacco mosaic virus (TMV),
    175, 182
Topping, Norman, 40
Transforming Principle, The,
    see McCarty, Maclyn
tranquilizing drugs, 70, 71, 72
Truman, Harry S., 61, 64
Tucker, Bruce O.
    concern over removal of his heart
        for transplantation, 163-65
Tucker, Grover, 163
Tucker, William, 163-64

U

Udenfriend, Sidney, 41
U.S. Bureau of the Budget, 75, 79
U.S. Bureau of Mines, 101
U.S. Coast Guard Academy, 62
U.S. Congress, 12, 15, 30, 36, 46,
    50, 63, 64, 67, 68, 71, 72, 75, 77,
    78-79, 83, 95, 96-97, 102, 103,
    107, 108-9, 116, 118, 150, 259, 260

U.S. Department of Agriculture
    funding of research by, 174, 188
    tasks of, 11-12
U.S. Department of Commerce, 101
U.S. Department of Defense (DOD),
    24, 44, 189
U.S. Department of Energy (DOE),
    17, 24; see also Atomic Energy
    Commission
U.S. Department of Labor, 75
U.S. federal government
    and mental health policy, 59,
        62, 63-64
    consequences of research
        spending by, 19-25
    research spending by, 9, 11-13,
        14-16, 17, 19-25
U.S. National Vaccine Advisory
    Committee, 273-74
U.S. National Vaccine Program,
    259-260, 275
U.S. Patents and Trademarks Office
    (USPTO), 204, 207, 211-12
U.S. Public Health Service, 28, 30,
    31, 32, 34, 36, 37, 39, 42, 45, 61,
    63, 97, 105, 106, 108, 112, 113,
    119, 174, 177, 186
    Bureau of Medical Services
        of, 45
    Bureau of State Services of,
        37, 39, 45, 66, 81, 120
    Division of Mental Hygiene
        of, 61, 62
    Division of Research Grants
        of, 40, 177
    Division of Venereal Disease
        of, 32

University College, London, 219, 236
University College Hospital,
    London (UCH), 234, 235, 236,
    239, 241, 243
University of California,
    Berkeley, 320
    Los Angeles, 221, 320
    Santa Barbara, 320
    San Diego, 320
University of Chicago, 17, 20,
    299, 320
University of Colorado, 62
University of Indiana, 320
University of Illinois, 320
University of Michigan, 320
University of Minnesota, 150,
    154, 320
University of Mississippi, 150
University of Pennsylvania, 41,
    43, 48
University of Rochester, 32, 33
University of Southern California, 178
University of Toronto, 207
University of Virginia, 33, 223
University of Wisconsin, 207, 320

V

vaccination
    in U.S., 255-56, 292
vaccine
    acellular, 265-66, 270
    DTP, 255, 256
    hepatitis B, 270, 280
    Hib, 256
    influenza, 38, 270
    measles, 255, 256

    mumps, 256
    pertussis, 255, 260
    pneumonia, 257, 259, 270
    poliomyelitis, 255, 259, 263-65,
        268, 270
    rubella, 256
    smallpox, 255, 256
    tetanus, 255
    varicella, 270
vaccine development and production,
    272, 309
    privatization of, 270
vaccine history
    ideas of progress in, 255-56,
        271, 279-80
    writing on institutional changes
        in, 256-57, 279-81
vaccine research
    changes in field of, 269
    government, 259-60
    support of by U.S. federal
        government, 259-60
vaccines
    cost of, 270
    in the Netherlands, 266-67
    success of, 255
Vaccines for Children Act, 1993,
    260, 262
Valier, Helen, 239
Van Slyke, Cassius J., 39-40
Vanderbilt University, 320
Venter, J. Craig, 203, 207
Veterans Administration, 42, 154
Vitamin D, 207
Voegtlin, Carl, 29-30, 114
Vincent, George, 174

viruses
>funding of research on, 172,
>>179-80, 182
>studies of, 172, 182
voluntary health organizations,
>171-201; see also ACS, NFIP
>and NIH
>>fundraising activities of, 173,
>>>178-79
>>relationship with research,
>>>174-75, 177-78, 181-82,
>>>183, 190, 192

W

Walt, G., 275
Walter Reed Army Institute of
>Research, 258
Wangensteen, Owen, 154, 158
war
>and legitimating state
>>intervention, 10-11, 12
>and science research funding,
>>175-76
>and socialization of research,
>>10-11
>on cancer, 12, 190
>on disease, 12
>on drugs, 12
>on poliomyelitis, 189-90
>rhetoric of, 12, 177, 187
Warren State Hospital,
>Pennsylvania, 69
Washington Post, 101, 116, 117, 159
Washington University School of
>Medicine, St. Louis, 35, 219
Washkansky, Louis, 153, 156-57

Watson, James D., 245, 336-37
Weed, Lewis, 180
Wellcome Physiological
>Laboratories, 238
Weller, Thomas, 257
Western Electric, 219
Wilder, L. Douglas, 164
Wilder, Russell M., 34
Williams, Richard H., 74
Wilson, E. B., 181
Wilson, Edward O., 324
Wilson, Woodrow, 11
Windeyer, Brian W., 245
Windsor, Duke of, 151
Winter, Sidney, 324
World War I, 12, 14, 205, 237
World War II, 9, 13, 14, 15, 16, 21,
>22, 23, 28, 29, 36, 40, 59, 60, 61,
>69, 72, 171, 177, 188, 189, 190,
>205, 206, 231, 233, 239, 241,
>244, 257, 302, 308, 338
Worm Breeder's Gazette
>database on *c. elegans* gene, 208
Woolley, Wayne, 221
World Health Organization, 259,
>265, 268, 270, 276, 277
>Expanded Program on
>>Immunization of, 276
Wycoff, Ralph, 223
Wyngaarden, James B., 3

XYZ

Yale University, 48, 178
Yolles, Stanley, 75, 83
Young, James Harvey, 2